Your *Clinics* subscription just got better!

You can now access the FULL TEXT of this publication online at no additional cost! Activate your online subscription today and receive...

- Full text of all issues from 2002 to the present
- Photographs, tables, illustrations, and references
- Comprehensive search capabilities
- Links to MEDLINE and Elsevier journals

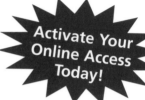

Activate Your Online Access Today!

Plus, you can also sign up for E-alerts of upcoming issues or articles that interest you, and take advantage of exclusive access to bonus features!

To activate your individual online subscription:

1. Visit our website at **www.TheClinics.com**.

2. Click on "Register" at the top of the page, and follow the instructions.

3. To activate your account, you will need your subscriber account number, which you can find on your mailing label (note: the number of digits in your subscriber account number varies from six to ten digits). See the sample below where the subscriber account number has been circled.

This is your subscriber account number

```
******************************************3-DIGIT 001
FEB00   J0167   C7   (123456-89)   10/00   Q: 1

J.H. DOE, MD
531 MAIN ST
CENTER CITY, NY  10001-001
```

4. That's it! Your online access to the most trusted source for clinical reviews is now available.

theclinics.com

ELSEVIER

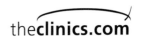

ANESTHESIOLOGY CLINICS OF NORTH AMERICA

Current Concepts in Postoperative Pain Management

GUEST EDITOR
Girish P. Joshi, MB, BS, MD, FFARCSI

CONSULTING EDITOR
Lee A. Fleisher, MD

March 2005 • Volume 23 • Number 1

SAUNDERS
An Imprint of Elsevier, Inc.
PHILADELPHIA   LONDON   TORONTO   MONTREAL   SYDNEY   TOKYO

W.B. SAUNDERS COMPANY
A Division of Elsevier Inc.

The Curtis Center • Independence Square West • Philadelphia, Pennsylvania 19106

http://www.theclinics.com

ANESTHESIOLOGY CLINICS OF NORTH AMERICA   Volume 23, Number 1
March 2005   ISSN 0889-8537
Editor: Robert G. Gardler   ISBN 1-4160-2806-4

The ideas and opinions expressed in *Anesthesiology Clinics of North America* do not necessarily reflect those of the Publisher. The Publisher does not assume any responsibility for any injury and/or damage to persons or property arising out of or related to any use of the material contained in this periodical. The reader is advised to check the appropriate medical literature and the product information currently provided by the manufacturer of each drug to be administered to verify the dosage, the method and duration of administration, or contraindications. It is the responsibility of the treating physician or other health care professional, relying on independent experience and knowledge of the patient, to determine drug dosages and the best treatment for the patient. Mention of any product in this issue should not be construed as endorsement by the contributors, editors, or the Publisher of the product or manufacturers' claims.

Anesthesiology Clinics of North America (ISSN 0889-8537) is published quarterly by the W.B. Saunders Company Corporate and editorial offices: The Curtis Center, Independence Square West, Philadelphia, PA 19106-3399. Accounting and circulation offices: 6277 Sea Harbor Drive, Orlando, FL 32887-4800. Periodicals postage paid at Orlando, FL 32862, and additional mailing offices. Subscription prices are $84.00 per year (US student/resident), $175.00 per year (US individuals), $210.00 per year (Canadian individuals), $270.00 per year (US institutions), $330.00 per year (Canadian institutions), $230.00 per year (foreign individuals), and $330.00 per year (foreign institutions). To receive student and resident rate, orders must be accompanied by name of affiliated institution, date of term, and the *signature* of program/residency coordinator on institutions letterhead. Orders will be billed at individual rate until proof of status is received. Foreign air speed delivery is included in all *Clinics'* subscription prices. All prices are subject to change without notice. POSTMASTER: Send address changes to *Anesthesiology Clinics of North America*, W.B. Saunders Company, Periodicals Fullfillment, Orlando, FL 32887-4800. Customer Service: 1-800-654-2452 (US). From outside of the US, call 1-407-345-4000. E-mail: hhspcs@harcourt.

Anesthesiology Clinics of North America is also published in Spanish by McGraw-Hill Interamericana Editores S. A., P.O. Box 5-237, 06500 Mexico D. F., Mexico.

Anesthesiology Clinics of North America is covered in *Index Medicus, Current Contents/Clinical Medicine, Excerpta Medica, ISI/BIOMED,* and *Chemical Abstracts.*

Printed in the United States of America.

CONSULTING EDITOR

LEE A. FLEISHER, MD, Robert D. Dripps Professor and Chair, Department of Anesthesia; and Professor, Department of Medicine, University of Pennsylvania School of Medicine, Philadelphia, Pennsylvania

GUEST EDITOR

GIRISH P. JOSHI, MB, BS, MD, FFARCSI, Professor of Anesthesiology and Pain Management; and Director of Perioperative Medicine and Ambulatory Anesthesia, University of Texas, Southwestern Medical Center, Dallas, Texas

CONTRIBUTORS

TIMOTHY J. BRENNAN, PhD, MD, Associate Professor, Departments of Anesthesiology and Pharmacology, University of Iowa College of Medicine, Iowa City, Iowa

JENNIFER J. DAVIS, MD, Assistant Professor, Department of Anesthesiology, University of Utah School of Health Sciences, Salt Lake City, Utah

MARCEL E. DURIEUX, MD, PhD, Professor, Department of Anesthesiology and Neurological Surgery, University of Virginia Health System, Charlottesville, Virginia

HOLLY EVANS, MD, FRCP(C), Associate, Department of Anesthesiology, Duke University Medical Center, Durham, North Carolina

NOOR M. GAJRAJ, MD, FRCA, DABPM, Baylor Center for Pain Management, Baylor University Medical Center, Frisco, Texas

TONG J. GAN, MB, FRCA, Professor of Anesthesiology, Duke University Medical Center, Durham, North Carolina

ASHRAF S. HABIB, MBBCh, MSc, FRCA, Assistant Professor of Anesthesiology, Duke University Medical Center, Durham, North Carolina

RAAFAT S. HANNALLAH, MD, Professor, Departments of Anesthesiology and Pediatrics, The George Washington University Medical Center; Chief, Division of Anesthesiology, Children's National Medical Center, Washington, District of Columbia

KEN B. JOHNSON, MD, Associate Professor, Department of Anesthesiology, University of Utah School of Health Sciences, Salt Lake City, Utah

GIRISH P. JOSHI, MB, BS, MD, FFARCSI, Professor of Anesthesiology and Pain Management; and Director of Perioperative Medicine and Ambulatory Anesthesia, University of Texas, Southwestern Medical Center, Dallas, Texas

HENRIK KEHLET, MD, PhD, Professor, Section for Surgical Pathophysiology, The Juliane Marie Centre Rigshospitalet, Copenhagen, Denmark

STEPHEN M. KLEIN, MD, Assistant Professor, Department of Anesthesiology, Duke University Medical Center, Durham, North Carolina

PAMELA E. MACINTYRE, BMedSc, MBBS, FANZCA, MHA, FFPMANZCA, Director, Acute Pain Service, Department of Anaesthesia, Hyperbaric and Pain Medicine, Royal Adelaide Hospital and University of Adelaide, North Terrance, Adelaide South Australia, Australia

KAREN C. NIELSEN, MD, Assistant Professor, Department of Anesthesiology, Duke University Medical Center, Durham, North Carolina

BABATUNDE O. OGUNNAIKE, MD, Assistant Professor, Department of Anesthesiology and Pain Management; and Director, Anesthesia Surgical Services at Parkland Health and Hospital System, University of Texas Southwestern Medical Center, Dallas, Texas

ESTHER M. POGATZKI-ZAHN, MD, PhD, Department of Anesthesia and Intensive Care Medicine, University of Muenster, Muenster, Germany

NARINDER RAWAL, MD, PhD, Professor, Department of Anesthesiology and Intensive Care, Örebro University Hospital, Örebro, Sweden

JEFFREY M. RICHMAN, MD, Assistant Professor, Department of Anesthesiology and Critical Care Medicine, The Johns Hopkins University, Baltimore; Department of Anesthesiology, The Johns Hopkins Hospital, Baltimore, Maryland

SUSAN M. STEELE, MD, Professor, Department of Anesthesiology, Duke University Medical Center, Durham, North Carolina

JEFFREY D. SWENSON, MD, Associate Professor, Department of Anesthesiology, University of Utah School of Health Sciences, Salt Lake City; and Director of Acute Pain Service, University of Utah School of Health Sciences, Salt Lake City, Utah

MARCY S. TUCKER, MD, PhD, Assistant Professor, Department of Anesthesiology, Duke University Medical Center, Durham, North Carolina

SUSAN T. VERGHESE, MD, Associate Professor, Department of Anesthesiology and Pediatrics, The George Washington University Medical Center; Division of Anesthesiology, Children's National Medical Center, Washington, District of Columbia

J. LEE WHITE, MD, Associate Professor, Department of Anesthesiology, University of Virginia Health System, Charlottesville, Virginia

CHRISTOPHER L. WU, MD, Associate Professor, Department of Anesthesiology and Critical Care Medicine, The Johns Hopkins University, Baltimore; Department of Anesthesiology, The Johns Hopkins Hospital, Baltimore, Maryland

PETER K. ZAHN, PhD, Department of Anesthesia and Intensive Care Medicine, University of Muenster, Muenster, Germany

CONTENTS

Foreword   xi
Lee A. Fleisher

Preface   xiii
Girish P. Joshi

Mechanisms of Incisional Pain   1
Timothy J. Brennan, Peter K. Zahn, and Esther M. Pogatzki-Zahn

> Postoperative, incisional pain is a unique but common form of acute pain. Because effective postoperative analgesia reduces morbidity following surgery, new treatments continue to be sought. It is through the development of investigational models and studies of the mechanisms that perioperative medicine can be advanced. This article reviews studies on a rat plantar hindpaw model for postoperative pain and proposes mechanisms for enhanced excitability of sensory neurons caused by incisions.

Consequences of Inadequate Postoperative Pain Relief and Chronic Persistent Postoperative Pain   21
Girish P. Joshi and Babatunde O. Ogunnaike

> Inadequately controlled pain has undesirable physiologic and psychologic consequences such as increased postoperative morbidity, delayed recovery, a delayed return to normal daily living, and reduced patient satisfaction. Importantly, the lack of adequate postoperative pain treatment may lead to persistent pain after surgery, which is often overlooked. Overall, inadequate pain management increases the use of health care resources and health care costs. This article reviews the physiologic and psychologic consequences of inadequately treated pain, with an emphasis on chronic persistent postoperative pain.

Postoperative Care of the Chronic Opioid-Consuming Patient   37
Jeffrey D. Swenson, Jennifer J. Davis, and Ken B. Johnson

Recently, there has been a significant increase in the use of opioid analgesics for chronic pain in the outpatient setting. As a result, anesthesiologists are commonly presented with the dilemma of treating acute postoperative pain in patients who do not receive adequate analgesia with conventional doses of opioid. This article presents a practical approach to treating postoperative pain in the chronic opioid-consuming patient. Specifically, a technique based on pharmacokinetic modeling is described that predicts safe and therapeutic opioid dosing in these patients.

Role of Cyclooxygenase-2 Inhibitors in Postoperative Pain Management   49
Noor M. Gajraj and Girish P. Joshi

Cyclooxygenase (COX)-2 inhibitors are as efficacious as nonselective nonsteroidal anti-inflammatory drugs for the treatment of postoperative pain but have the advantages of a better gastrointestinal side-effect profile as well as a lack of antiplatelet effects. There have been recent concerns regarding the cardiovascular side effects of COX-2 inhibitors. Nonetheless, they remain a valuable option for postoperative pain management. The pharmacology of these agents and available studies are reviewed.

Clinical Pharmacology of Local Anesthetics   73
J. Lee White and Marcel E. Durieux

Whereas currently available local anesthetics may be suitable for intraoperative and in-hospital postoperative use, long-acting analgesia after outpatient procedures will require new techniques and drugs. Catheter delivery systems are rapidly gaining clinical acceptance and allow for great flexibility in dosing. Encapsulated local anesthetics can provide the slow release of drugs. Novel, long-acting local anesthetics are being investigated but are not yet ready for clinical use. In addition to the effects on the sodium channel, other actions of these novel compounds need to be explored, because both beneficial and detrimental effects may be induced with these compounds.

Role of Analgesic Adjuncts in Postoperative Pain Management   85
Ashraf S. Habib and Tong J. Gan

Postoperative pain remains a major problem. A multi-modal analgesic approach is recommended to optimize pain management and reduce opiate-related adverse effects. Several analgesic adjuncts have been investigated, and many have proved to have a useful analgesic effect. This article reviews the literature regarding use of analgesic adjuncts in the perioperative period.

Intravenous Patient-Controlled Analgesia: One Size Does Not Fit All   **109**
Pamela E. Macintyre

> Patient-controlled analgesia was introduced as a technique that would allow greater flexibility in opioid delivery for the management of acute pain. However, so far, any benefit compared with conventional methods of pain relief appears to be small. This article reviews some of the factors that could limit the usefulness of intravenous patient-controlled analgesia in the clinical setting and what strategies might allow patient-controlled analgesia to become more effective.

Epidural Analgesia for Postoperative Pain   **125**
Jeffrey M. Richman and Christopher L. Wu

> Epidural analgesia provides superior analgesia compared with other postoperative analgesic techniques. Additionally, perioperative epidural analgesia confers physiologic benefits, which may potentially decrease perioperative complications and improve postoperative outcome. However, there are many variables (eg, choice of analgesics, catheter-incision congruency, and duration of analgesia) that may influence the efficacy of epidural analgesia. In addition, the use of epidural analgesia should be evaluated on an individual basis because there are risks associated with this technique.

Peripheral Nerve Blocks and Continuous Catheter Techniques   **141**
Holly Evans, Susan M. Steele, Karen C. Nielsen, Marcy S. Tucker, and Stephen M. Klein

> Peripheral nerve blocks provide intense, site-specific analgesia and are associated with a lower incidence of side effects when compared with many other modalities of postoperative analgesia. Continuous catheter techniques further prolong these benefits. These advantages can facilitate a prompt recovery and discharge and achieve significant perioperative cost savings. This is of tremendous value in a modern health care system that stresses cost-effective use of resources and a continued shift toward shorter hospital stay as well as outpatient surgery.

Postoperative Pain Management in Children   **163**
Susan T. Verghese and Raafat S. Hannallah

> There is increased awareness of the need for effective postoperative analgesia in infants and young children. A multi-modal approach to preventing and treating pain usually is used. Mild analgesics, local and regional analgesia, and opioids when indicated, frequently are combined to minimize adverse effects of individual drugs or techniques.

Multimodal Analgesia Techniques and Postoperative Rehabilitation 185

Girish P. Joshi

The concept of multimodal analgesia involves the use of different classes of analgesics and different sites of analgesic administration to provide superior dynamic pain relief with reduced analgesic-related side effects. Although multimodal analgesia techniques have assumed increasing importance in the management of perioperative pain, it has become increasingly apparent that postoperative outcome may not be improved. Nevertheless, the integration of multimodal analgesia techniques with a multimodal and multidisciplinary rehabilitation program may enhance recovery, reduce hospital stay, and facilitate early convalescence.

Procedure-Specific Postoperative Pain Management 203

Henrik Kehlet

Procedure-specific postoperative pain management guidelines arguably are more helpful to the clinician than general pain guidelines or guidelines based on the use of the Oxford League Tables. Two sources, the United States Veteran's Health Administration and the European Prospect Working Group, offer websites that include surgical procedure-specific postoperative pain management guidelines, which are available and currently updated.

Organization, Function, and Implementation of Acute Pain Service 211

Narinder Rawal

Undertreatment of postoperative pain continues to be a major problem internationally. The solution does not seem to be the development of new analgesic drugs or technologies but the development of an appropriate organization that utilizes existing expertise. Evidence suggests that the introduction of an Acute Pain Service (APS) reduces patients' pain intensity, but other outcome benefits are modest. Although the number of hospitals with an APS is increasing, the literature is unclear about the optimal structure, staffing, and function. There is a need for the development of well-defined APS criteria with which to assess performance and compare with national standards.

Index 227

FORTHCOMING ISSUES

June 2005
> **Issues in Transfusion Medicine**
> Terri G. Monk, MD, and
> Lawrence T. Goodnough, MD, *Guest Editors*

September 2005
> **Obesity and Sleep Apnea**
> Peter Rock, MD, FCCP, MBA, *Guest Editor*

December 2005
> **Pediatric Anesthesiology**
> Andrew T. Costarino, Jr, MD, and
> B. Randall Brenn, MD, *Guest Editors*

RECENT ISSUES

December 2004
> **Transplantation**
> Randolph H. Steadman, MD,
> Marie Csete, MD, PhD, and
> William T. Merritt, MD, MBA, *Guest Editors*

September 2004
> **Infectious Disease and Bioterrorism**
> Samuel C. Hughes, MD, and
> James D. Marks, MD, PhD, *Guest Editors*

June 2004
> **Vascular Anesthesia**
> Michael J. Murray, MD, PhD, *Guest Editor*

THE CLINICS ARE NOW AVAILABLE ONLINE!

For more information about Clinics:
http://www.theclinics.com

ELSEVIER
SAUNDERS

Anesthesiology Clin N Am
23 (2005) xi–xii

ANESTHESIOLOGY
CLINICS OF
NORTH AMERICA

Foreword

Current Concepts in Postoperative Pain Management

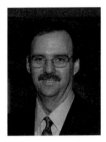

Lee A. Fleisher, MD
Consulting Editor

Pain has become the fifth vital sign and is now a critical focus of patient care. The relief of pain has always been part of the anesthesiologist's role in the most immediate postoperative period, and the development of acute postoperative pain services has extended this interest beyond the postanesthesia care unit. There is also increasing evidence that optimal pain management can impact outcome beyond the intraoperative period. Therefore, it is increasingly common for perioperative pain management to begin in the operating room using multimodal approaches, particularly in high-risk patients. This issue of the *Anesthesiology Clinics of North America* provides an update on the advances in perioperative pain management with an emphasis on multimodal approaches and special patient populations.

In choosing a Guest Editor for this issue, I enlisted the expertise of Girish Premji Joshi, who is currently Professor of Anesthesiology and Pain Management and Director of Perioperative Medicine and Ambulatory Anesthesia at the University of Texas Southwestern Medical Center at Dallas. Dr. Joshi has been an extremely active investigator in the area of pain relief after surgery for over a decade, with 39 original articles and numerous book chapters and case reports to his credit. He has also been active in numerous societies—most notably the

doi:10.1016/j.atc.2005.01.001
anesthesiology.theclinics.com

Society for Ambulatory Anesthesia, where he has served on numerous committees as well as the Board of Directors. He is therefore extremely well qualified to elicit contributions from an outstanding international group of authors. I believe this issue will help those anesthesiologists who participate in postoperative pain management through their intraoperative care (ie, all anesthesiologists) as well as those individuals who focus on postoperative pain management as a primary interest.

Lee A. Fleisher, MD
Departments of Anesthesia and Medicine
University of Pennsylvania School of Medicine
3400 Spruce Street, Dulles 690
Philadelphia, PA 19104, USA
E-mail address: fleishel@uphs.upenn.edu

ELSEVIER
SAUNDERS

Anesthesiology Clin N Am
23 (2005) xiii–xiv

ANESTHESIOLOGY
CLINICS OF
NORTH AMERICA

Preface

Current Concepts in Postoperative Pain Management

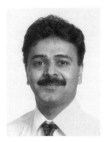

Girish P. Joshi, MB, BS, MD, FFARSCI
Guest Editor

It is estimated that the surgical workload will keep increasing and that the predominant increase will be in ambulatory procedures. With more extensive and potentially more painful surgical procedures being performed on an outpatient basis and with the acceptance of the concept of "fast-track" surgery, the need for effective and prolonged postoperative pain relief has become evident. Alleviation of pain may contribute to improved clinical outcomes, hasten recovery, and reduce the need for hospitalization, as well as expedite rehabilitation and return to daily living.

However, the provision of adequate analgesia continues to be a major challenge, and undertreatment of postoperative pain remains a problem. It is hoped that improvements in our understanding of the pathophysiology of acute pain may increase the analgesic armamentarium and allow mechanism-specific analgesic therapy. While we search for newer ways to prevent and treat postoperative pain, appropriate application of currently available analgesic therapies is a prerequisite to adequate pain relief.

Although numerous unanswered questions remain, it is clear that a multimodal approach is required to achieve optimal analgesia and balance the amount of pain relief with avoidance of undesirable side effects. Because opioid-related side effects delay recovery and rehabilitation, opioid-free analgesic techniques

doi:10.1016/j.atc.2004.12.001

are recommended. Regional analgesic techniques, particularly continuous peripheral nerve blocks and epidural analgesia, are the cornerstones of a multi-modal analgesia technique as they provide intense dynamic pain relief. We need to explore innovative delivery systems for currently available analgesics, which would allow greater flexibility in drug delivery. Although the benefits of regional analgesia are well demonstrated, additional research showing improved patient outcome is necessary. Other nonopioid analgesics (eg, acetaminophen and non-specific nonsteroidal anti-inflammatory drugs or COX-2–specific inhibitors) should be used whenever possible with the aim of reducing opioid requirements. However, many studies reporting reduced opioid requirements with nonopioid analgesics have not been able to show reduced opioid-related side effects. Fur-thermore, the efficacy of analgesic adjuncts such as ketamine and clonidine remains controversial, and additional well-designed studies are necessary before their routine use can be recommended. Of note, nonpharmacologic interventions should become a standard component of multimodal analgesia techniques.

Most importantly, the choice of analgesic techniques needs to be individu-alized for each patient and procedure. However, there are insufficient data re-garding the optimal patient-specific and procedure-specific multimodal analgesic technique. Nevertheless, organized acute pain services and quality improvement initiatives are critical components of pain management and need to be im-plemented in every institution. It is also mandatory to integrate multimodal analgesic therapy into surgical care as a continuum from the preoperative pe-riod through the convalescence period, which will require a close cooperation between the anesthesiologists and surgeons.

This issue of the *Anesthesiology Clinics of North America* reviews the current controversies in postoperative pain management. The contributors, all of whom are regarded as experts in their field, have provided us with current information on postoperative pain management. The management of postoperative pain in special patient populations (eg, chronic opioid-consuming patients, infants, young children) that may present some unique challenges is also discussed. As with all such efforts, there will be some overlap of information, which should help to reinforce the important aspects of postoperative pain management. We hope that our efforts will advance the management of postoperative pain.

Girish P. Joshi, MB, BS, MD, FFARSCI
Perioperative Medicine and Ambulatory Anesthesia
University of Texas Southwestern Medical Center
5323 Harry Hines Boulevard
Dallas, TX 75390-9068, USA
E-mail address: girish.joshi@utsouthwestern.edu

ELSEVIER
SAUNDERS

Anesthesiology Clin N Am
23 (2005) 1–20

ANESTHESIOLOGY
CLINICS OF
NORTH AMERICA

Mechanisms of Incisional Pain

Timothy J. Brennan, PhD, MD[a],*, Peter K. Zahn, PhD[b],
Esther M. Pogatzki-Zahn, MD, PhD[b]

[a]*Departments of Anesthesia and Pharmacology, University of Iowa College of Medicine,
200 Hawkins Drive, Iowa City, IA 52242-1079, USA*
[b]*Department of Anesthesia and Intensive Care Medicine, University of Muenster,
Albert Schweitzer Strasse 33, 48149 Muenster, Germany*

As the practice of anesthesiology extends itself into perioperative medicine, the anesthesiologist's expertise in acute pain management is highly valued. To continue to lead in the management of acute postoperative pain, basic mechanisms of postoperative pain must be explored. Because effective postoperative analgesia reduces morbidity following surgery, new treatments must continue to be investigated.

When both clinical and basic science pain models are evaluated, many novel theories and several treatments and preventative strategies for acute pain management can be developed. It is important to emphasize that the etiology of incisional pain may be different than antigen-induced inflammation, formalin injection, and capsaicin injection, and therefore, the responses to treatments also may differ. For example, the response to anti-inflammatory agents [1–3], spinal N-Methyl-D-aspartate (NMDA) receptor blockade [4–6], spinal non-NMDA receptor blockade [4,7] and parenteral ionotropic purine receptor antagonists [8] are different in incisional pain models compared with other models, particularly those that focus on antigen-induced inflammation. In an effort to differentiate between the overall research models for acute pain and those specific for postsurgical pain, the mechanisms of pain caused by incisions are being explored.

This research was supported by the Foundation for Anesthesia Education and Research, the University of Iowa Department of Anesthesia, American Society of Regional Anesthesia, and the National Institutes of Health grants GM55831 and GM 067762 to TJB, and Deutsche Forschungsgemeinschaft DFG Za 214/1-1; 1-2 to PKZ, Deutsche Forschungsgemeinschaft DFG Po 661/1-2.

* Corresponding author.

E-mail address: tim-brennan@uiowa.edu (T.J. Brennan).

Although many new discoveries are being made in several pain models, the ability to translate these directly to perioperative pain management is limited. This article evaluates studies on incisional pain mechanisms. By summarizing the incisional pain mechanisms, the authors hope that the clinician will receive a focused, concise article on the basic science of acute postoperative pain.

Sensitization and hyperalgesia

It is recognized that injury causes two changes in the responsiveness of the nociceptive system, peripheral sensitization and central sensitization [9]. Together, these changes in the processing of nociceptive and non-nociceptive information are hypothesized to contribute to acute postoperative pain.

Peripheral sensitization involves the primary afferent fibers and is characterized by lowering of response threshold, an increase in response magnitude to suprathreshold stimuli, an increase in spontaneous activity, and an increase in receptive field size (ie, the area from which stimuli can evoke action potentials in the afferent) (Fig. 1) [9,10]. Experimentally, nociceptors have been shown to sensitize to thermal stimulation. Sensitization of peripheral afferent fibers (ie, nociceptors) to mechanical stimulation (which correlates with postsurgical mechanical hyperalgesia), however, has been difficult to identify [11]. This has caused many to speculate that peripheral sensitization may not play a major role in mechanical hyperalgesia in postoperative pain. Nociceptive input, however, can enhance the responses of pain transmission neurons in the central nervous system (see Fig. 1). This phenomenon is termed as central sensitization. One example of central sensitization is increased pain responses evoked in dorsal horn neurons by stimuli from outside the area of injury.

Peripheral sensitization leads to primary hyperalgesia, defined as an exaggerated responses eliciting pain at the site of injury. Central sensitization leads to secondary hyperalgesia, defined as increased pain responses evoked by stimuli from outside the area of injury. Most studies indicate that secondary hyperalgesia to mechanical stimuli (secondary mechanical hyperalgesia), but not to thermal stimuli, occurs after injury and it is not caused by sensitization of primary afferent fibers in the uninjured tissue. Spontaneous pain from the area immediately surrounding the incision and primary mechanical hyperalgesia are perhaps most relevant to clinical acute pain and improvement in outcome in the perioperative period [12].

Clinical models of postoperative pain

After surgical procedures involving skin and deeper structures, pain occurs at rest and with stimuli such as pressure and touch, which are usually not painful [12,13]. These exaggerated responses can be measured by using pressure

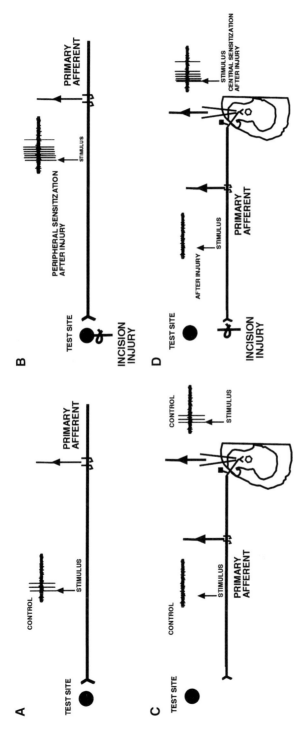

Fig. 1. Peripheral and central sensitization. (A) Responses of primary afferent fibers showing action potentials (top) and the receptive field at the fiber terminal in normal tissue. (B) Model of primary afferent (peripheral) sensitization after injury showing increased responsiveness to punctate mechanical stimulus. (C) Responses of primary afferent fibers and dorsal horn neurons showing action potentials (top) in normal tissue. The test site is located outside the area of injury. (D) Model of secondary hyperalgesia and central sensitization after injury. The responses of the primary afferents are unchanged, but the response in the dorsal horn is greater.

(eg, pressure algometry after hysterectomy [13] and thoracotomy [14]) or touch (eg, von Frey filament-induced pain after hysterectomy [12], colectomy [15], and nephrectomy [16]). Also, tenderness in an uninjured area is present after incision [12].

To understand incisional pain and mechanisms for pain caused by incisions, Kawamata et al [17] subjected volunteers to a small incision in the volar forearm, an area frequently used for sensory testing in humans. In these volunteers, pain at rest decreased and disappeared within 2 hours after the experimental incision. Pain response to mechanical stimuli at the incision (ie, primary mechanical hyperalgesia), however, was present for several days. Kawamata et al [17] found that the area of hyperalgesia (including the uninjured zone) caused by the incision was similar to that observed in postoperative patients. By examining some of the fundamental bases for incisional pain, it may be possible to develop a link between basic animal models and clinical postoperative pain.

Experimental versus clinical pain models

There are many advantages of using experimental models of postoperative pain rather than clinical studies. Clinical studies use a particular intervention to modify two or three variables such as pain scores at rest, pain scores with activity, and opioid use. Therefore, studies examining pain mechanisms and novel analgesic treatments in a clinical setting can result in a mixed and sometimes an indeterminate effect: a reduction in opioid use with the same pain score, a reduced pain score with the same opioid requirements, or an insignificant reduction in both pain scores and opioid consumption.

In addition, the degree or the extent of effort for provocative maneuvers is another variable in clinical pain measurements and analgesic trials. For example, in evaluation of a postoperative analgesic treatment, pain scores with coughing and opioid requirements may remain the same, but the cough effort may be increased markedly. It may be difficult to measure the changes in effort, however. In contrast to clinical studies, variables can be controlled more easily in experimental animal models. The authors hope that the use of translational incisional models will facilitate discoveries applicable to the clinician and the postoperative pain patient.

Laparotomy models for postoperative pain

The initial models developed to study mechanisms specific to incisional pain were laparotomy models. In rats, an ovariohysterectomy [18] is performed under general anesthesia. Mechanical nociceptive thresholds are measured using a paw pressure test, and a reduced threshold is observed after laparotomy. The importance of remote hindlimb hyperalgesia after hysterectomy, however, may be less clinically relevant than incision sensitivity. Other species also have been used to examine postoperative hysterectomy pain. In a dog model, nociception is measured using an algometer, a device used to deliver a quantifiable force, applied directly to the surgical wound [19]. The thresholds to withdrawal, vocalization, aggression, or guarding are measured. The impact of these models has been greatest to the veterinary community; however, the lack of widespread use limits the translation of these data to clinicians.

In a new rat model, subcostal incision penetrating into the peritoneal cavity is performed, and exploratory locomotor activity and conditioned operant responding are measured [20]. Laparotomy decreased ambulation and rearing by approximately 50%, 24 hours after surgery. Because the model is new, further characterization and validation are forthcoming. Mouse models of postoperative pain also have been described [21]. The behaviors caused by plantar incision in the mouse roughly parallel those in the rat.

A plantar incision model for postoperative pain

This article reviews two behaviors after plantar incision and proposes models for their transmission from the site of injury to the central nervous system. The plantar incision model that the authors have studied extensively consists of a incision that is made in the plantar aspect of the hindpaw [22]. Under halothane (or other halogenated volatile agent) anesthesia, using aseptic conditions, a 1-cm longitudinal incision is made with a scalpel blade, through skin and fascia of the paw, starting 0.5 cm from the proximal edge of the heel and extending toward the digits (Fig. 2). The underlying flexor muscle is elevated with forceps and incised longitudinally. The muscle origin and insertion are kept intact. Nylon is used for closure to minimize the inflammatory response to the suture material, which is removed late in the day on postoperative day 2. Upon emergence and recovery from anesthesia, the rats are placed in previously acclimated test cages and are reacclimated for 15 to 30 minutes and ready for behavioral testing. Many laboratories have studied this model extensively, and the behavioral responses have been used widely in many pharmacologic studies (Table 1). Hopefully, knowledge gained from behaviors caused by a simple incision could be applied to laparotomy models and human acute pain models.

Nonevoked pain

The precise pain measures in animal models that parallel clinical postoperative pain are not understood well. The authors have used several measures for pain-related behaviors in rats after plantar incision and will describe two of these in detail.

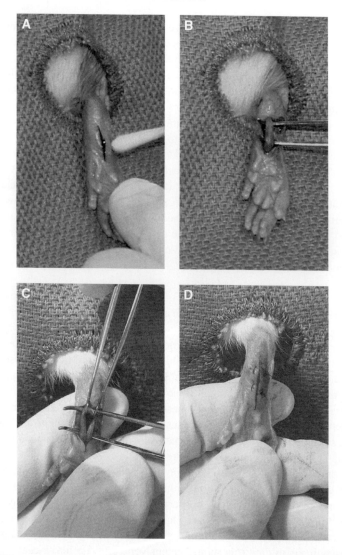

Fig. 2. Different stages of the rat plantar incision. (*A*) A 1-cm longitudinal incision is made through the skin and fascia starting 0.5 cm from the proximal edge of the heel and extending toward the middle of the paw. (*B*) The underlying flexor muscle is elevated and also incised longitudinally. (*C*) The muscle is split with a blunt dissection longitudinally. (*D*) After hemostasis, the wound is opposed with two mattress sutures of 5–0 nylon.

As rats are left undisturbed in the testing environment, the authors noted that they did not bear weight on the incised hindpaw for several days after plantar incision. A cumulative pain score was used to quantify this guarding behavior based on hindpaw position [22,23]. Two hours after plantar incision, the median pain score increased from 2 to 19 (Fig. 3). On the day after incision, the median score was 16 and then was 11 on the second day after incision. Pain scores continued to decrease at later times after the incision. In contrast to other pain models, no consistent flinching and licking behavior was observed except during emergence from general anesthesia and in the immediate recovery period. Although this behavior could not be quantified reliably, it suggests that the stimulus from incision may be less intense than that from chemical irritants.

It is recognized that the authors' pain score is a result of the position chosen by the rat after the incision rather than an evoked mechanical response; therefore, differences between these tests should be expected. This pain score, however, also may be influenced in part by mechanical sensitivity, because scoring was based on the paw touching the mesh cage floor. Of note, this cumulative pain score may correlate to pain at rest in patients after surgery.

Primary mechanical hyperalgesia

Pain in response to mechanical stimuli at the incision represents primary mechanical hyperalgesia, an exaggerated response caused by activation of injured primary afferent sensory fibers [9,24]. As mentioned previously, von Frey filament-induced touch may cause pain after a variety of surgical procedures and after experimental incisions in people. The authors have characterized the reduced withdrawal threshold to application of monofilaments adjacent to the incision, a behavioral correlate to mechanical hyperalgesia [22,23].

Unrestrained rats were placed in a clear plastic chamber on an elevated plastic mesh floor and allowed to acclimate. Withdrawal responses to mechanical stimulation were determined using calibrated monofilaments applied from underneath the cage through openings in the mesh floor to an area adjacent to the intended incision preoperatively and to the same area after incision. Each filament was applied once, starting with small force usually in the range of 10 to 15 milliNewtons (mN) and continued until a withdrawal response occurred, or a strong force (500 mN, the cutoff value) was reached. After a 5- to 10-minute test-free period, each filament again was applied, beginning with the weak filament, until a withdrawal response was elicited. This was repeated a third time 5 to 10 minutes later. The lowest force from the three tests producing a response was considered the withdrawal threshold. The test site did not vary. Rats can be tested for several days after incision. The rats were tested before incision, 2 hours afterwards, and once daily for 6 postoperative days.

The median withdrawal threshold in the incised hindpaw decreased from cutoff (522 mN) before incision to 25, 54, 61, and 119 mN at 2 hours, and 1, 2, and 3 days postincision, respectively (see Fig. 3). A gradual return toward preincision values occurred over the next 3 days. In other studies, decreased withdrawal thresholds were noted in all areas surrounding the plantar incision [22,24]. Withdrawal thresholds in sham-operated hindpaws do not decrease when tested as in the incised group. Importantly, the reduced withdrawal threshold is sustained for a greater duration than the nonevoked guarding behavior. The values and time course for the withdrawal threshold in rats are very similar to those reported by Kawamata et al [17] in healthy volunteers.

Table 1
Pharmacology of pain behaviors after plantar incision

Drug	Receptor	Route	Comments	Reference
Morphine	Mu opioid agonist	Intrathecal, parenteral	Strong inhibition of mechanical hyperalgesia and guarding behavior	[2,23]
FR140423	Delta opioid agonist	Oral	Moderate inhibition of mechanical hyperalgesia	[46]
Enadoline	Kappa-opioid receptor agonist	Parenteral	Moderate inhibition of mechanical hyperalgesia	[47]
Nociceptin	Opioid receptor-like antagonist	Intrathecal	Small inhibition of mechanical hyperalgesia	[41]
Bupivacaine	Local anesthetic	Intrathecal, local	Strong inhibition of mechanical hyperalgesia	[28,31,32]
Lidocaine	Local anesthetic	Intrathecal	Strong inhibition of mechanical hyperalgesia	[48]
MPV-2426 clonidine	α-2 adrenoceptor agonist	Intrathecal	α-2 A and non-A adrenoceptors strongly inhibit mechanical hyperalgesia	[33,34]
Adenosine	A1 agonist	Intrathecal	Moderate decrease in mechanical hyperalgesia,	[39,40]
T62	Adenosine agonist		A3 receptor agonist-increased mechanical hyperalgesia	
Ziconotide	N-type calcium Blocker	Intrathecal	Strong inhibition of heat mechanical hyperalgesia	[49]
Ketorolac	COX inhibitor	Intrathecal	Moderate inhibition of mechanical hyperalgesia	[42]
JTE522	COX-2 inhibitor	Oral, parenteral	Mild inhibition of mechanical hyperalgesia	[2,50]
L-745337 NS398 JTE522	COX-2 inhibitor	Intrathecal	No effect on mechanical hyperalgesia	[41–43]
ONO-8711	Prostaglandin EP1 receptor antagonist	Intrathecal, local	Moderate inhibition of mechanical hyperalgesia but no effect on heat hyperalgesia	[51,52]

Compound	Mechanism	Route	Effect	Reference
Gabapentin	Calcium channel antagonist	Intrathecal, parenteral	Strong inhibition of the development and maintenance of mechanical hyperalgesia	[2,53,54]
PD154075 CP 96,345 FK888	Neurokinin 1 receptor antagonist	Parenteral	Moderate prevention of the development but not the maintenance of mechanical hyperalgesia	[41,55]
Nefopam	Nonopioid analgesic	Parenteral	Moderate inhibition heat hyperalgesia	[56]
A-317491	P2X3 receptor antagonist	Parenteral	No effect on mechanical hyperalgesia	[8]
MK-801 AP-5	NMDA receptor antagonist	Intrathecal	No inhibition of mechanical hyperalgesia and guarding behavior	[6] [38]
NBQX DNQX	Non-NMDA receptor antagonist	Intrathecal	Strongly inhibited mechanical hyperalgesia and guarding behavior	[7,38]
AP3, MCPG, CPG, CPPG,	Metabotropic glutamate receptor antagonists	Intrathecal	No effect on mechanical hyperalgesia	[37]
Melatonin	Melatonin receptor antagonists	Intrathecal	No effect on mechanical hyperalgesia	[57]
TRK-A IgG fusion protein	Inhibits NGF (nerve growth factor)	Parenteral	Selective inhibition of heat but not mechanical hyperalgesia	[1]
Orexin A and B	Orexin receptor agonists	Intrathecal	Small inhibition of mechanical hyperalgesia	[58]
DALBK HOE-140	B1 receptor, B2 receptor, bradykinin antagonists	Parenteral	No effect on heat and mechanical hyperalgesia	[3]
2-PMPA	NAALADase inhibitor	Intrathecal	No effect on mechanical hyperalgesia	[44]
Sn-P	Heme-oxygenase inhibitor	Parenteral	Strongly inhibited mechanical hyperalgesia	[59]
DMPP bethanacol neostigmine	Muscarinic nicotinic cholinergic agonist cholinesterase inhibitor	Intrathecal	Strongly inhibited mechanical hyperalgesia	[39,60]

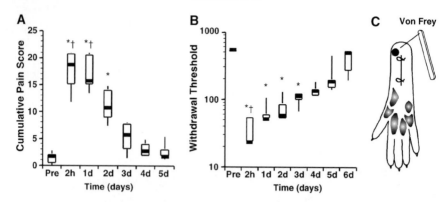

Fig. 3. Pain behaviors caused by incision. (*A*) Summary of the cumulative pain scores before and after surgery. (*B*) Summary of withdrawal thresholds in rats after skin, fascia, and muscle incision. The forces are in milliNewtons (mN) are expressed as medians (solid bold line) with first and third quartiles (box), and 10th and 90th percentiles (vertical lines). (*C*) Drawing depicts the rat paw. The filled circle adjacent to the wound near the medial heel is the testing area.
* indicates $P < 0.05$ versus preincision values. † indicates $P < 0.05$ versus skin and fascia incision.

The disappearance of pain at rest and persistence of pain with activities and in response to mechanical stimuli at the wound site are present in patients after surgery [13] and after experimental incisions.

The remainder of the article focuses on data generated from the plantar incision model, the most extensively characterized.

Primary afferent fiber sensitization

The primary afferent nociceptors are an ideal target to better understand acute pain mechanisms and hyperalgesia and direct biomedical research targeting specific receptors for management of acute pain. These mechanisms that subserve incisional pain at the level of the primary afferent terminal are not understood well, however. The characteristic features of experimentally induced peripheral sensitization of primary afferent fibers are a lowering of response threshold, an increase in response magnitude to suprathreshold stimuli, or an increase in spontaneous activity. Primary afferent fibers typically have a small receptive field. An additional mechanism for sensitization is an increase in the receptive field size (see Fig. 1) [10,11]. Most often in animal experiments, heat has been used to study nociceptors properties and enhance responsiveness, in particular the sensitization after injury. Nociceptors have been shown to sensitize to heat stimulation. Correlation of fiber sensitization with mechanical stimuli, however, has been reported only rarely despite careful testing in several peripheral injury models [9].

The authors recorded mechano-sensitive afferent fibers innervating the plantar aspect of rat hindpaw using standard teased-fiber techniques before and 45 minutes after incision (or sham procedure) [25]. The Aβ fibers did not sensitize after the incision, and only 26% of mechano-sensitive Aδ and C fibers had evidence of sensitization. In a group of mechanically insensitive Aδ and C fibers, a greater percentage of fibers (41%) was sensitized. The principal effect of an incision was an increase in receptive field size of the afferents, particularly those characterized as mechanically insensitive. The changes in response properties that occurred, however, did not totally account for the changes observed in behavioral studies.

In the second study [26], the authors examined mechanical response properties of Aδ and C fibers innervating the glabrous skin of the plantar hindpaw in rats 1 day after incision or sham procedure. Sixty-seven single afferent fibers were characterized from the left tibial nerve 1 day after sham procedure (n = 39) or incision (n = 28); electrical stimulation was used as the search stimulus to identify a representative population of Aδ and C fibers. In the incision group, 11 fibers (39%) had spontaneous activity with frequencies ranging from 0.03 to 39.3 impulses (imp) per second (Fig. 4); none were present in the sham group. The authors suggest that the ongoing activity caused by incision in primary afferent nociceptive fibers likely causes the guarding response shown (see Fig. 3) in behavioral studies.

The median response threshold of Aδ fibers was less in the incision group (56 mN, n = 13) compared with the sham group mainly because the proportion of mechanically insensitive afferents (MIAs) was less. Median C fiber response thresholds were similar between groups. The authors noted that the size of receptive fields was increased in Aδ and C fibers 1 day after incision (see Fig. 4). Spatial summation of modestly increased response magnitude may contribute

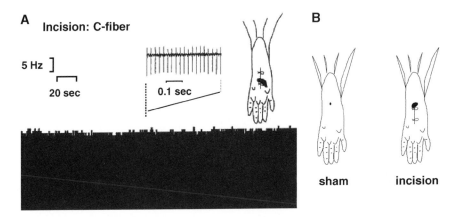

Fig. 4. Primary afferent sensitization by incision. (A) Spontaneous activity in afferent fibers 1 day after plantar incision. Peri-stimulus time histogram of spontaneous activity recorded from a C-fiber 1 day after incision (bin width 1 second). The mean firing frequency in this example was 33.2 impulses/second. Inset: Digitized oscilloscope trace from the original recording for the indicated area. The mechanical receptive field of this fiber (black area) was adjacent to and includes the incision. (B) Typical examples of receptive field from Aδ fibers; the black area depicts the receptive field determined using a von Frey filament with a force twice the response threshold of the individual fiber.

to the reduced withdrawal threshold after incision. Thus, spontaneous activity in Aδ and C fibers may not only account for nonevoked pain behavior but also may contribute to mechanical hyperalgesia by amplifying responses centrally.

Dorsal horn neuron sensitization

Because evidence that persistent pain states are in part generated from prolonged changes in the excitability of central neurons, one common strategy to decrease postoperative pain is to reduce the development of sensitization of dorsal horn neurons [27]. The response characteristics of dorsal horn neurons represent the individual components of the central sensitization process.

For these studies, the authors characterized dorsal horn neurons receiving input from the plantar aspect of the hindpaw using mechanical stimuli in anesthetized rats [28–30]. These dorsal horn neurons were characterized as wide dynamic range (WDR) and high-threshold (HT) based on their responses to brush and pinch. The WDR neurons respond to both brush and pinch, whereas the HT neurons respond only to pinch. Mechanical threshold using von Frey filaments and mechanical stimulus–response (force–activity relations) functions (SRFs) to the same filaments used in behavioral studies characterized the neurons. Changes in background activity, mechanical thresholds, force–activity relations, and receptive field were examined before and after an incision was made.

In all WDR and HT neurons, an incision increased background activity; this remained elevated in approximately 40% of neurons for at least 1 hour; both HT and WDR demonstrated this sustained ongoing activity (Fig. 5). The SRFs were enhanced in some WDR neurons and HT neurons after incision. Only the WDR neurons (see Fig. 5) were responsive to weak filaments that produced withdrawal responses after incision in behavioral experiments.

These results from dorsal horn neuron recording demonstrate that an incision caused dorsal horn cell activation and central sensitization. Both WDR and HT neurons have increased background activity that is driven by activated primary afferent fibers [28] and likely transmits evidence for nonevoked ongoing pain (eg, guarding behaviors). Because the threshold of HT neurons did not decrease to the range of the withdrawal responses in behavioral experiments, certain WDR dorsal horn neurons likely contribute to the reduced withdrawal threshold observed in behavioral experiments.

Spinal and parenteral pharmacology of incisional pain

Anesthesiologists have a particular interest in spinal pharmacology, because neuraxial, spinal, and epidural analgesia, are more effective for postoperative pain. There has been a plethora of spinal analgesic drugs administered to rats after plantar incision (see Table 1), and review of all published studies is not within the scope of this article. The importance of a preclinical model is in most cases to discover experimental treatments that have not been performed in people.

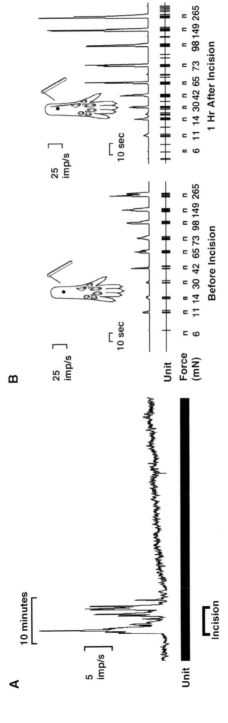

Fig. 5. Effect of an incision on background dorsal horn neuron activity and von Frey filament responses. (*A*) Example of an increase in activity produced by an incision. (*B*) Stimulus–response function of WDR neurons before and after incision. The insets depict the site of application of the von Frey filament to the low threshold area of the RF (black circle) and the incision (black line). Unit = each mark represents one action potential. *Abbreviation:* Imp/s, impulses per second.

Thus, a focus has been to discover neurotransmitters and receptors that transmit central sensitization and plasticity.

Preliminary studies with parenterally and spinally administered morphine have been performed to help validate the plantar incision model [23]. The non-evoked pain scores were decreased by parenteral and spinally injected morphine. Administration of subcutaneous or intrathecal morphine reversibly increased the withdrawal threshold. Naloxone reversed morphine's effects. This indicates that moderate doses of spinal and parenteral morphine are effective in decreasing pain behaviors. Other spinally administered drugs used in patients that are effective in reducing pain behaviors in the plantar incision model are local anesthetics like bupivacaine [28,31,32] and the α-2 agonist clonidine [33,34]. Thus, the plantar incision model also may be useful for predicting postoperative analgesic effects of investigational agents.

Because the synaptic actions of neurotransmitters released by noxious stimuli may contribute to the enhanced excitability of nociceptive pathways, recent research has focused predominantly on elucidation of those agents that mediate the hyperalgesia and sensitization induced by chemical irritation, inflammation, or thermal injury. These messengers also facilitate excitability following surgical injury. Of late, particular attention has been paid to the action of excitatory amino acids (EAAs) [35].

Excitatory amino acids like glutamate and aspartate are present in small- and large-diameter primary afferent nerve fibers and interneurons of the spinal cord are released by stimulation of sensory nerves, and activate ionotropic and metabotropic EAA receptors in the dorsal horn [36]. Ionotropic EAA receptors are subclassified into those activated by NMDA receptors and those activated by non-NMDA EAA receptors, using α-amino-3-hydroxy-5-methyl-4-isoxazole-propionic acid (AMPA) or kainate. Metabotropic EAA receptors are coupled positively or negatively to adenylate cyclase.

Several findings were derived from experiments conducted using the post-operative model of pain and spinal EAA receptor antagonists [6,7,37]. As shown in Fig. 6, an intrathecal non-NMDA receptor antagonist inhibited nonevoked pain behavior, decreasing the median pain scores for 1 hour after spinal administration [7]. The intrathecal non-NMDA receptor antagonist returned the withdrawal threshold nearly to preincision levels. Thus, unexpectedly, activation of spinal non-NMDA, AMPA-kainate receptors were found to mediate guarding behavior and the reduced withdrawal threshold that develops after an incision. Rather, both the ongoing pain behavior and mechanical hyperalgesia that occurs in this model were found not to be dependent on activation of spinal NMDA receptors [6] or spinal metabotropic EAA receptors [37]. Also, EAA receptors are not completely necessary for the development of the reduced withdrawal threshold; pain behaviors recur as the drug affect abates [38].

Other pharmacologic experiments indicate that incisional pain does not always respond similarly to other acute pain models. Some examples include the responses to intrathecal adenosine [39,40], intrathecal cyclooxygenase inhibitors [41–43], parenteral P2X receptor antagonists [8], parenteral TNF blockade [1],

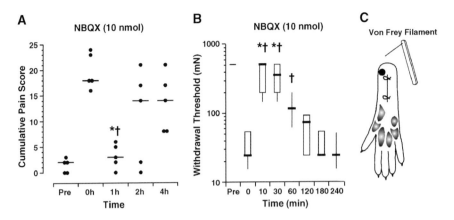

Fig. 6. Spinal Non-NMDA receptor blockade after incision. (*A*) Effect of 10 nmol NBQX (a non-NMDA receptor antagonist) on cumulative pain scores caused by an incision. Each dot is one score; the horizontal line represents the median. (*B*) Effect of 10 nmol of intrathecal NBQX on punctate mechanical hyperalgesia caused by incision. The results are expressed as median (horizontal line) with first and third quartiles (boxes), and 10th and 90th percentiles (vertical lines). (*C*) Plantar aspect of the rat foot showing site of application of von Frey filament (solid circle) *$P < 0.05$ versus 0 minutes. †$P < 0.05$ versus vehicle saline.

parenteral bradykinin receptor antagonists [3], and parenteral NAALadase inhibitors [44]. Thus, the mechanisms for maintenance of pain behaviors following an incision are different than mechanisms described for inflammatory, neurogenic, or neuropathic models of hyperalgesia. These data also suggest that models that rely on different receptor systems for the development and maintenance of pain behavior may not predict analgesia for patients with postoperative pain. A summary of pharmacologic studies in the plantar incision model is shown in Table 1.

Prevention strategies

A goal of perioperative medicine would be to discover strategies that would prevent or reduce the development of pain after surgery. Several of these prevention therapies have originated from studies in animal models [27]. The authors have undertaken several of experiments attempting to decrease the development of postoperative pain with pretreatment strategies. These include intrathecal local anesthetic and opioid administration [31] and local anesthetic infiltration and nerve block [28]. Although a reduction in pain behaviors by these drugs can be observed initially, no effect beyond the expected duration of the treatment has been noted. Even intrathecal EAA receptor antagonists have not modified the persistent pain after incision [38]. For opioids and local anesthetics, as the effects of pretreatment abate, the pain behaviors are similar to the untreated group. This may explain why clinical studies using treatments

attempting to prevent the development of postoperative pain have yielded many
negative results [45]. Perhaps long-term preventive treatment may produce positive results.

A schematic for pain caused by incision

The cell bodies of sensory A and C fibers are contained in the dorsal root
ganglia. Most low-threshold A fiber mechanoreceptors transmit responses to
innocuous stimuli (eg, touch). Small diameter Aδ and C fibers transmit several
stimuli; those which respond to painful stimuli are called nociceptors. Normally,
application of an innocuous mechanical stimulus (eg, a weak von Frey filament)
on uninjured skin activates exclusively thick myelinated A fiber mechano-

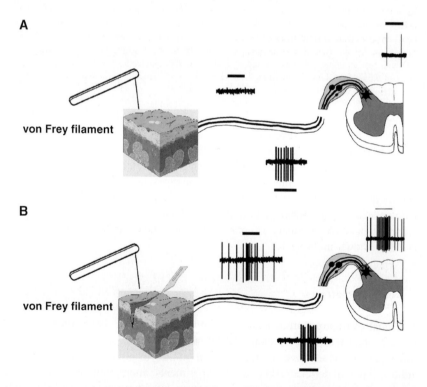

Fig. 7. A surgical incision causes activation and sensitization of peripheral and central nociceptive neurons. (*A*) Application of an innocuous mechanical stimulus (von Frey filament) on uninjured
skin activates exclusively thick myelinated mechanoreceptors (A-beta fibers) and produces a modest
increase in action potentials in spinal cord WDR neurons. Nociceptors are not excited in normal skin.
(*B*) After an incision, increased spontaneous activity of nociceptors occurs, and the same innocuous
stimulus now activates nociceptive afferent fibers. Subsequently, this continuous nociceptive barrage
and enhanced response provoke greater activity of WDR dorsal horn neurons. Black bars indicate
the time of application of von Frey filaments. Each vertical line represents a single extracellular
action potential.

receptors. Nociceptors have little or no ongoing background activity (Fig. 7) and are not affected by weak mechanical stimuli. Thus, no action potentials are evoked. The innocuous touch stimulus produces a small increase in action potentials in spinal cord WDR neurons.

After an incision, large, myelinated A fibers are not activated and do not develop an enhanced response to touch; thus they are not sensitized (see Fig. 7). In contrast, nociceptors now have spontaneous activity; therefore they are activated by the incision. The previously innocuous touch stimulus now excites nociceptive afferent fibers, indicating sensitization. Thus, after incision, ongoing activity and increased responsiveness to a touch stimulus are provoked in WDR dorsal horn neurons, which likely transmit behavioral evidence for ongoing pain and guarding after plantar incision (see Fig. 3) and pain at rest in patients after surgery. Touch is converted to evoked pain by increasing mechanical responsiveness of nociceptors, sensitization of MIA fibers, and by enlarging the receptive field of many types of nociceptors (see Fig. 4). The response of large myelinated touch fibers and touch-sensitized nociceptors together increase the response of spinal WDR neurons (see Fig. 5). This enhanced response to an innocuous stimulus likely transmits the reduced withdrawal threshold in rats (see Fig. 3) and evoked pain to previously innocuous stimuli in patients after surgery.

Clinical implications

Basic research in postoperative, incisional pain is in its early stages; thus, the direct benefits to the clinician are limited. Nevertheless, some conclusions can be made that may influence clinical care directly. First, not all clinical and experimental pain models are similar. Some analgesics may influence one modality such as pain at rest without affecting another such as evoked pain with coughing. The authors' emphasis is on mechanical hyperalgesia, because in clinical studies, it has been difficult to significantly diminish evoked pain without affecting normal sensory transmission (eg, with drugs such as local anesthetics). Finally, studies using this model indicate that administration of local anesthetics and parenteral opioids immediately before surgery begins offers little advantage to administering these drugs later during surgery.

Summary

Research on incisional pain mechanisms demonstrates that all acute pain models may not predict analgesic efficacy for postoperative pain. The authors hope that these findings direct pharmaceutical companies toward appropriate pain therapies and new drugs for postoperative pain management that may advance the armamentarium of analgesic agents for the perioperative care of surgical patients.

References

[1] Zahn PK, Subieta A, Park SS, et al. Effect of blockade of nerve growth factor and tumor necrosis factor on pain behaviors after plantar incision. J Pain 2004;5:157–63.

[2] Whiteside GT, Harrison J, Boulet J, et al. Pharmacological characterisation of a rat model of incisional pain. Br J Pharmacol 2004;141:85–91.

[3] Leonard PA, Arunkumar R, Brennan TJ. Bradykinin antagonists have no analgesic effect on incisional pain. Anesth Analg 2004;99:1166–72.

[4] Ren K, Williams GM, Hylden JLK, et al. The intrathecal administration of excitatory amino acid receptor antagonists selectively attenuated carrageenan-induced behavioral hyperalgesia in rats. Eur J Pharmacol 1992;219:235–43.

[5] Ren K, Dubner R. NMDA receptor antagonists attenuate mechanical hyperalgesia in rats with unilateral inflammation of the hindpaw. Neurosci Lett 1993;163:22–6.

[6] Zahn PK, Brennan TJ. Lack of effect of intrathecal NMDA receptor antagonists in a rat model for postoperative pain. Anesthesiology 1998;88:143–56.

[7] Zahn PK, Umali EF, Brennan TJ. Intrathecal non-NMDA excitatory amino acid receptor antagonists inhibit pain behaviors in a rat model of postoperative pain. Pain 1998;74:213–24.

[8] Jarvis MF, Burgard EC, McGaraughty S, et al. A-317491, a novel potent and selective non-nucleotide antagonist of P2X(3) and P2X(2/3) receptors, reduces chronic inflammatory and neuropathic pain in the rat. Proc Nat Acad Sci (USA) 2002;99:17179–84.

[9] Treede RD, Meyer RA, Raja SN, et al. Peripheral and central mechanisms of cutaneous hyperalgesia. Prog Neurobiol 1992;38:397–421.

[10] Handwerker HO, Reeh PW. Pain and Inflammation. In: Bond MR, Charlton JE, Woolf CJ, editors. Proceedings of the 5th World Congress of Pain. Amsterdam: Elsevier Science Publishers BV; 1991. p. 59–70.

[11] Meyer RA. Cutaneous hyperalgesia and primary afferent sensitization. Pulm Pharmacol 1995;8:187–93.

[12] Richmond CE, Bromley LM, Woolf CJ. Preoperative morphine pre-empts postoperative pain. Lancet 1993;342:73–5.

[13] Moiniche S, Dahl JB, Erichsen CJ, et al. Time course of subjective pain ratings, and wound and leg tenderness after hysterectomy. Acta Anaesthesiol Scand 1997;41:785–9.

[14] Kavanagh BP, Katz J, Sandler AN, et al. Multi-modal analgesia before thoracic surgery does not reduce postoperative pain. Br J Anaesth 1994;73:184–9.

[15] De Kock M, Lavand'homme P, Waterloos H. Balanced analgesia in the perioperative period: is there a place for ketamine? Pain 2001;92:373–80.

[16] Stubhaug A, Breivik H, Eide PK, et al. Mapping of punctate hyperalgesia around a surgical incision demonstrates that ketamine is a powerful suppressor of central sensitization to pain following surgery. Acta Anaesth Scand 1997;41:1124–32.

[17] Kawamata M, Watanabe H, Nishikawa K, et al. Different mechanisms for development and maintenance of experimental incision-induced hyperalgesia in human skin. Anesthesiology 2002;97:550–9.

[18] Lascelles BD, Waterman AE, Cripps PJ, et al. Central sensitization as a result of surgical pain: investigation of the pre-emptive value of pethidine for ovariohysterectomy in the rat. Pain 1995;62:201–12.

[19] Lascelles BDX, Cripps PJ, Jones A, et al. Postoperative central hypersensitivity and pain the pre-emptive value of pethidine for ovariohysterectomy. Pain 1997;73:461–71.

[20] Martin TJ, Buechler NL, Kahn W, et al. Effects of laparotomy on spontaneous exploratory activity and conditioned of operant responding in the rat—a model for postoperative pain. Anesthesiology 2004;101:191–203.

[21] Pogatzki EM, Raja SN. A mouse model of incisional pain. Anesthesiology 2003;99:1023–7.

[22] Brennan TJ, Vandermeulen E, Gebhart GF. Characterization of a rat model of incisional pain. Pain 1996;64:493–501.

[23] Zahn PK, Gysbers D, Brennan TJ. Effect of systemic and intrathecal morphine in a rat model of postoperative pain. Anesthesiology 1997;86:1066–77.

[24] Zahn PK, Brennan TJ. Primary and secondary hyperalgesia in a rat model for human postoperative pain. Anesthesiology 1999;90:863–72.

[25] Hamalainen MM, Gebhart GF, Brennan TJ. Acute effect of an incision on mechano-sensitive afferents in the plantar rat hindpaw. J Neurophysiology 2002;87:712–20.

[26] Pogatzki EM, Gebhart GF, Brennan TJ. Characterization of A delta and C fibers innervating the plantar rat hindpaw one day after an incision. J Neurophysiol 2002;87:721–31.

[27] Woolf CJ, Chong MS. Pre-emptive analgesia-treating postoperative pain by preventing the establishment of central sensitization. Anesth Analg 1993;77:362–79.

[28] Pogatzki EM, Vandermeulen EP, Brennan TJ. Effect of plantar local anesthetic injection on dorsal horn neuron activity and pain behaviors caused by incision. Pain 2002;97:151–61.

[29] Vandermeulen EP, Brennan TJ. Alterations in ascending dorsal horn neurons by a surgical incision in the rat foot. Anesthesiology 2000;93:1294–302.

[30] Zahn PK, Brennan TJ. Incision-induced changes in receptive field properties of rat dorsal horn neurons. Anesthesiology 1999;91:772–85.

[31] Brennan TJ, Umali EF, Zahn PK. Comparison of pre- versus postincision administration of intrathecal bupivacaine and intrathecal morphine in a rat model of postoperative pain. Anesthesiology 1997;87:1517–28.

[32] Grant GJ, Lax J, Susser L, et al. Wound infiltration with liposomal bupivacaine prolongs analgesia in rats. Acta Anaesthesiol Scand 1997;41:204–7.

[33] Onttonen T, Pertovaara A. The mechanical antihyperalgesic effect of intrathecally administered MPV-2426, a novel alpha2 -adrenoceptor agonist, in a rat model of postoperative pain. Anesthesiology 2000;92:1740–5.

[34] Duflo F, Conklin D, Li X, et al. Spinal adrenergic and cholinergic receptor interactions activated by clonidine in postincisional pain. Anesthesiology 2003;98:1237–42.

[35] Coderre TJ, Melzack R. The contribution of excitatory amino acids to central sensitization and persistent nociception after formalin-induced tissue injury. J Neurosci 1992;12:3665–70.

[36] Dougherty PM, Palacek J, Paleckova V, et al. The role of NMDA and non-NMDA excitatory amino acid receptors in the excitation of primate spinothalamic tract neurons by mechanical, chemical, thermal, and electrical stimuli. J Neurosci 1992;12:3025–41.

[37] Zahn PK, Brennan TJ. Intrathecal metabotropic glutamate receptor antagonists do not decrease mechanical hyperalgesia in a rat model of postoperative pain. Anesth Analg 1998;87:1354–9.

[38] Pogatzki EM, Zahn PK, Brennan TJ. Effect of pretreatment with intrathecal excitatory amino acid receptor antagonists on the development of pain behavior caused by plantar incision. Anesthesiology 2000;93:489–96.

[39] Chiari AI, Eisenach JC. Intrathecal adenosine—interactions with spinal clonidine and neostigmine in rat models of acute nociception and postoperative hypersensitivity. Anesthesiology 1999;90:1413–21.

[40] Obata H, Li X, Eisenach JC. Spinal adenosine receptor activation reduces hypersensitivity after surgery by a different mechanism than after nerve injury. Anesthesiology 2004;100:1258–62.

[41] Yamamoto T, Sakashita Y. The role of the spinal opioid receptor like1 receptor, the NK-1 receptor, and cyclooxygenase-2 in maintaining postoperative pain in the rat. Anesth Analg 1999;89:1203–8.

[42] Zhu X, Conklin D, Eisenach JC. Cyclooxygenase-1 in the spinal cord plays an important role in postoperative pain. Pain 2003;104:15–23.

[43] Kroin JS, Buvanendran A, McCarthy RJ, et al. Cyclooxygenase-2 inhibition potentiates morphine antinociception at the spinal level in a postoperative pain model. Reg Anesth Pain Med 2002;27:451–5.

[44] Yamamoto T, Nozaki-Taguchi N, Sakashita Y. Spinal N-acetyl-alpha-linked acidic dipeptidase (NAALADase) inhibition attenuates mechanical allodynia induced by paw carrageenan injection in the rat. Brain Res 2001;909:138–44.

[45] Moiniche S, Kehlet H, Dahl JB. A qualitative and quantitative systematic review of pre-emptive

analgesia for postoperative pain relief—the role of timing of analgesia. Anesthesiology 2002; 96:725–41.

[46] Ochi T, Ohkubo Y, Mutoh S. Effect of systemic FR140423, a new analgesic compound, in a rat model of postoperative pain: contribution of delta-opioid receptors. Neurosci Lett 2003; 350:29–32.

[47] Field MJ, Carnell AJ, Gonzalez MI, et al. Enadoline, a selective kappa-opioid receptor agonist shows potent antihyperalgesic and antiallodynic actions in a rat model of surgical pain. Pain 1999;80:383–9.

[48] Sun X, Yokoyama M, Mizobuchi S, et al. The effects of pretreatment with lidocaine or bupivacaine on the spatial and temporal expression of c-Fos protein in the spinal cord caused by plantar incision in the rat. Anesth Analg 2004;98:1093–8.

[49] Wang YX, Pettus M, Gao D, et al. Effects of intrathecal administration of ziconotide, a selective neuronal N-type calcium channel blocker, on mechanical allodynia and heat hyperalgesia in a rat model of postoperative pain. Pain 2000;84:151–8.

[50] Yamamoto T, Sakashita Y, Nozaki-Taguchi N. Antiallodynic effects of oral COX-2 selective inhibitor on postoperative pain in the rat. Can J Anaesthesiol 2000;47:354–60.

[51] Omote K, Kawamata T, Nakayama Y, et al. The effects of peripheral administration of a novel selective antagonist for prostaglandin E receptor subtype EP(1), ONO-8711, in a rat model of postoperative pain. Anesth Analg 2001;92:233–8.

[52] Omote K, Yamamoto H, Kawamata T, et al. The effects of intrathecal administration of an antagonist for prostaglandin E receptor subtype EP(1) on mechanical and thermal hyperalgesia in a rat model of postoperative pain. Anesth Analg 2002;95:1708–12.

[53] Field MJ, Holloman EF, McCleary S, et al. Evaluation of gabapentin and S-(+)-3-isobutylgaba in a rat model of postoperative pain. J Pharmacol Exp Ther 1997;282:1242–6.

[54] Cheng JK, Pan HL, Eisenach JC. Antiallodynic effect of intrathecal gabapentin and its inter- action with clonidine in a rat model of postoperative pain. Anesthesiology 2000;92:1126–31.

[55] Gonzalez M, Field MJ, Holloman EF, et al. Evaluation of pd154075, a tachykinin nk1 re- ceptor antagonist, in a rat model of postoperative pain. Eur J Pharmacol 1998;344:115–20.

[56] Girard P, Pansart Y, Coppe MC, et al. Nefopam reduces thermal hypersensitivity in acute and postoperative pain models in the rat. Pharmacol Res 2001;44:541–5.

[57] Zahn PK, Lansmann T, Berger E, et al. Expression and functional characterisation of melatonin receptors in the spinal cord of the rat: implications for pain modulation. J Pineal Res 2003; 35:24–31.

[58] Cheng JK, Chou RC, Hwang LL, et al. Antiallodynic effects of intrathecal orexins in a rat model of postoperative pain. J Pharmacol Exp Ther 2003;307:1065–71.

[59] Li X, Clark JD. The role of heme oxygenase in neuropathic and incisional pain. Anesth Analg 2000;90:677–82.

[60] Prado WA, Segalla DK. Antinociceptive effects of bethanechol or dimethylphenylpiperazinium in models of phasic or incisional pain in rats. Brain Res 2004;1018:272–82.

ELSEVIER
SAUNDERS

Anesthesiology Clin N Am
23 (2005) 21–36

ANESTHESIOLOGY
CLINICS OF
NORTH AMERICA

Consequences of Inadequate Postoperative Pain Relief and Chronic Persistent Postoperative Pain

Girish P. Joshi, MB, BS, MD, FFARCSI*, Babatunde O. Ogunnaike, MD

Perioperative Medicine and Ambulatory Anesthesia, University of Texas, Southwestern Medical Center, 5323 Harry Hines Blvd, Dallas, TX 75390-9068, USA

Postoperative pain is still inadequately relieved despite substantial improvements in the knowledge of the mechanisms and treatment of pain [1]. Evidence suggests that inadequate relief of postoperative pain may result in harmful physiologic and psychologic consequences that lead to significant morbidity and mortality [2], which may delay recovery and the return to daily living [3]. In addition, the presence of postoperative symptoms, including pain, significantly contributes to patients' dissatisfaction with their anesthesia and surgical experience [4]. Most importantly, it has been recognized that inadequately treated postoperative pain may lead to chronic pain, which is often misdiagnosed and neglected [5,6]. This article reviews the physiologic and psychologic consequences of inadequate pain relief, with an emphasis on chronic persistent postoperative pain.

Physiologic consequences

Inadequately treated pain, particularly acute pain, is associated with physiologic changes caused by endocrine, metabolic, and inflammatory responses (Table 1). This stress response activates the autonomic system, which may have adverse effects on various organ systems [2]. The somatic pathway stimulation

---

* Corresponding author.
E-mail address: girish.joshi@utsouthwestern.edu (G.P. Joshi).

0889-8537/05/$ – see front matter © 2005 Elsevier Inc. All rights reserved.
doi:10.1016/j.atc.2004.11.013   *anesthesiology.theclinics.com*

Table 1
Consequences of unrelieved pain

Organ systems	Physiologic responses
Cardiovascular	Increased heart rate, peripheral vascular resistance, arterial blood pressure, and myocardial contractility resulting in increased cardiac work, myocardial ischemia and infarction
Pulmonary	Respiratory and abdominal muscle spasm (splinting), diaphragmatic dysfunction, decreased vital capacity, impaired ventilation and ability to cough, atelectasis, increased ventilation/perfusion mismatch, hypoventilation, hypoxemia, hypercarbia, increased postoperative pulmonary infection
Gastrointestinal	Increased gastrointestinal secretions and smooth muscle sphincter tone, reduced intestinal motility, ileus, nausea, and vomiting
Renal	Oliguria, increased urinary sphincter tone, urinary retention
Coagulation	Increased platelet aggregation, venostasis, increased deep vein thrombosis, thromboembolism
Immunologic	Impaired immune function, increased infection, tumor spread or recurrence
Muscular	Muscle weakness, limitation of movement, muscle atrophy, fatigue
Psychological	Anxiety, fear, anger, depression, reduced patient satisfaction
Overall recovery	Delayed recovery, increased need for hospitalization, delayed return to normal daily living, increased health care resource utilization, increased health care costs

caused by surgical injury increases the secretion of hypothalamic-releasing hormones, which in turn stimulates the secretion of the anterior and posterior pituitary gland [2]. The autonomic overactivity results in an increased heart rate, peripheral vascular resistance, increased arterial blood pressure, and myocardial contractility, which all culminate in increased myocardial oxygen consumption from increased cardiac work [7]. In addition, intense sympathetic stimulation may also produce coronary vasoconstriction as well as atherosclerotic plaque rupture and, subsequently, decrease myocardial oxygen supply. The combination of increased myocardial oxygen demand and decreased oxygen supply can be detrimental in patients with coronary artery disease and may lead to myocardial ischemia, anginal pain, and myocardial infarction.

Inadequate pain relief, particularly after thoracic and upper abdominal surgery, may cause pulmonary dysfunction and an increase in postoperative pulmonary complications [8]. Involuntary spinal reflex responses to the noxious stimulus from the injured area result in reflex muscle spasm in the immediate region of the injury as well as the surrounding muscle groups, which prevents movement in this area (ie, splinting), with subsequent hypoventilation and hypoxemia. In addition, pain can cause diaphragmatic dysfunction, which further impairs ventilation [9]. After upper abdominal surgery, vital capacity decreases by 40% to 60%, with a greater decline in the elderly than in younger patients [9].

Increased sympathetic activity from severe pain increases gastrointestinal secretions and smooth muscle sphincter tone while also decreasing intestinal motility [10]. This partly accounts for the gastric stasis and paralytic ileus, particularly after abdominal surgery. In addition, opioid analgesics may also contribute to the decreased intestinal motility. Therefore, local anesthetic epidural blockade but not epidural opioid reduces pain-related impairment of intestinal motility [11]. Unrelieved pain can increase the incidence of postoperative nausea and vomiting. Chia et al [12] evaluated the risk factors of postoperative emesis in patients who underwent lower abdominal gyneco-logic surgery and received morphine intravenous patient-controlled analgesia (IV-PCA). They found that patients with postoperative emesis had significantly higher pain scores at rest and during coughing than those without emesis, even though the opioid consumption was similar. Logistical regression analysis further validated the fact that pain intensity is a sensitive predictor of post-operative emesis. Similar results have been documented in other studies [13,14]. Interestingly, one study [14] reported that the incidence of moderate to severe nausea was reduced from 37% to 23% with the increased use of opioids and assumed improved pain relief. It is hypothesized that the sympathetic activa-tion caused by pain results in increased firing of the area postrema, leading to emesis [15].

The increase in sympathetic activity can also lead to increased urinary sphincter tone, reflex inhibition of urinary bladder tone, and subsequent urinary retention. The metabolic response to surgical stress also leads to a hyper-coagulable state, venous stasis, and the increased risk of deep vein thrombosis and thromboembolism, which may be further exaggerated by reduced physical activity from inadequate pain relief [16]. In addition, the immune function may also be decreased, resulting in an increased incidence of infection and tumor spread or recurrence. Inadequately treated pain can also cause increased post-operative fatigue. The limitation of movement caused by pain may cause a marked impairment of muscle metabolism, muscle atrophy, muscle weakness, and delayed return to normal muscle function [17].

Psychologic and behavioral consequences

The psychologic factor related most to high levels of pain is anxiety [18]. Severe pain causes individual behavioral changes including increased sensitivity to external stimuli such as light and sound, withdrawal from interpersonal contact, and increased self-absorption and self-concern. Patients experience a loss of control over their environment if acute pain is unrelieved for prolonged periods, culminating in depression and helplessness. Prolonged and unrelieved pain can lead to the expression of anger and resentment, especially when it is believed that treatment is being withheld [19]. Premorbid tendencies for anxiety, hostility, depression, or preoccupation with health are exacerbated by severe and unrelieved acute pain. An acute psychotic reaction may occasionally result [20].

Postoperative pain has been found to be an important cause for long-lasting postoperative temper tantrums and untoward behavioral changes in children. In a prospective multicenter study, Kotiniemi et al [21] evaluated behavioral changes in children during the first month after surgery and assessed the significance of some patient-related factors on the incidence of behavioral changes. Pain on the day of surgery was found to predict the occurrence of behavioral problems up to the fourth week, which was longer than the duration of the pain itself [21].

Recovery and health care use

Uncontrolled pain has also been shown to prolong a patient's stay in the postanesthesia care unit and the hospital and to delay discharge and increase the incidence of unanticipated hospital admissions after ambulatory surgery [22–26]. Inadequate management of pain after ambulatory surgery has significant consequences (Box 1). Pavlin et al [25] reported that the three most common medical causes of delayed discharge after ambulatory surgery were pain, drowsiness, and nausea and vomiting. In a later study, Pavlin et al [26] found that pain was the most common cause of postanesthesia care unit delays, affecting 24% of patients overall. It was also a significant independent predictor of the duration of total recovery [26].

Unfortunately, after the patients are discharged, home pain management seems to be commonly ignored [27]. Numerous investigators [28–31] have reported an increased incidence of pain at home. In an analysis of studies related to postdischarge symptoms after outpatient surgery, Wu et al [31] found that the overall incidence of postdischarge pain after outpatient surgery was approximately 45%. Pain was one of the most common causes for readmission after outpatient surgery [31–34]. Poorly controlled postoperative pain may increase the incidence of postoperative delirium and cognitive dysfunction [35]. Overall pain and its consequences reduce the health-related quality of life and also delay return to normal daily activities [3,23,36,37]. Inadequate postoperative pain control was also the most frequent reason for patients to contact their family practitioner after discharge from the hospital [38].

Because pain was among the top five most undesirable outcomes after surgery [39], inadequate treatment of pain can reduce patient satisfaction [4]. A

Box 1. Consequences of inadequate pain management after ambulatory surgery

- Increased postanesthesia care unit stay
- Increased Phase II unit stay
- Delayed discharge home
- Unanticipated hospital admission
- Increased contact with family practitioner
- Delayed return to daily living function
- Decreased patient satisfaction

survey [23] intended to determine the significance of pain and other symptoms on the recovery process found that pain and analgesic side effects significantly contributed to patient dissatisfaction, distress, and delayed return to normal activity after discharge from ambulatory surgery. Inadequately treated pain may also increase the use of health care resources [3,31,40]. The economic impact of delayed recovery and delayed return to normal activities of daily living as well as unanticipated hospital admission, readmission, or lost employment time may increase health care costs [31,40].

Persistent postoperative pain

Recently, persistent pain after surgery, also referred to as chronic postsurgical pain syndrome, has been recognized as a major factor in delaying recovery and return to normal daily living [5,6]. Long-lasting pain has been reported after numerous surgical procedures including thoracotomy, mastectomy, hernia repair, and limb amputation [5,6]. Of note, all surgical procedures have the potential to develop persistent postoperative pain. The devastating consequences of persistent postoperative pain (eg, distress and disability) have led to an increased interest in its prevention [41]. With an estimated 3 million general surgical procedures performed in the United States [42], if even a small percentage of these patients develop chronic pain, it would be a significant problem. A more detailed review of the transition from acute to chronic pain has been published recently [43].

Definition

The definition of persistent postoperative pain remains controversial because it may be difficult to determine whether the pain is merely a continuum of the preoperative condition or has developed after the surgical procedure. Although chronic pain has been defined as the presence of pain that persists for longer than 3 months after surgery, such a simplistic definition has been criticized [6]. It has been suggested that the criteria for the diagnosis of persistent postoperative pain should include pain lasting for at least 2 months after a surgical procedure, with other causes for the pain excluded (Box 2). Furthermore, it is necessary to exclude the preoperative condition as the cause for persistent pain, because surgery may simply exacerbate a pre-existing painful condition [6].

Incidence

The exact incidence of persistent postoperative pain in not known. In 1992, a survey [44] of patients attending pain clinics in Scotland and northern England demonstrated that 20% of patients implicated surgery as one of the causes of their chronic pain, and in approximately half of these patients, it was the sole cause. The overall incidence varies significantly from 5% to 80% and is related

---

Box 2. Criteria for the diagnosis of chronic persistent postoperative pain

- Pain developed after a surgical procedure
  Preoperative condition as the cause of postoperative persistent pain is excluded
- Pain is of at least 2 months' duration
  Assessment of spontaneous pain intensity is not adequate
  Characteristics of chronic neuropathic pain are present
- Other causes for the pain are excluded (eg, continuing malignancy or chronic infection)
  Onset of pain from radiotherapy or infiltration is usually delayed

Modified from Macrae WA. Chronic pain after surgery. Br J Anaesth 2001;87:88–98; with permission.

---

to the type of surgical procedure [5,6,45–51]. A study [52] evaluating the incidence of persistent pain after total knee replacement surgery found that 42% of patients met the International Association on Study of Pain criteria for complex regional pain syndrome (CRPS) at 4 weeks and 3 months, whereas 19% of patients met the criteria at 6 months after surgery. Approximately 14% of patients had significant pain before surgery, including allodynia, edema, and temperature, color, and sweating asymmetry [52]. The incidence of CRPS after various orthopedic surgeries varies between 0.8% and 40% [53]. However, earlier studies had serious methodological flaws such as variable definitions of persistent pain.

Predictors of persistent postoperative pain

The predictors of chronic persistent postoperative pain can be divided into preoperative, intraoperative, and postoperative factors (Box 3). Preoperative factors include pre-existing pain at the operative site, previous surgery, and psychologic and genetic factors as well as the presence of conditions such as irritable bowel syndrome, migraine headache, fibromyalgia, and Raynaud's disease [5,6]. Preoperative pain that predicts persistent postoperative pain tends to be continuous pain of 1 month or longer [5]. The probability of phantom limb pain is increased in the presence of severe preoperative pain [54,55]. Although preoperative breast pain predicts phantom breast pain [48], preoperative breast pain did not predict chronic pain after breast surgery when evaluated prospectively [56]. Long-standing symptoms, including pain, predict chronic pain after cholecystectomy [57]. Preoperative pain sensitivity as measured by

---

Box 3. Predictors of chronic persistent postoperative pain

- Preoperative factors

Presence of preoperative pain
Repeat surgery
Psychological vulnerability (eg, neuroticism)
Work-related injury

- Surgical factors

Type of surgical procedure
Surgical approach with risk of nerve damage (eg, nerve identification, nerve
trans-section, repair technique)

- Postoperative factors

Intensity of early postoperative pain
Postoperative radiation therapy or chemotherapy
Psychologic vulnerability (eg, neuroticism)

Modified from Perkins FM, Kehlet H. Chronic pain as an outcome of surgery: a review of predictive factors. Anesthesiology 2000; 93:1123–33; with permission.

---

pressure algometry did not predict either the severity of acute pain or the probability of chronic pain after thoracotomy [45]. In contrast, Werner et al [58] observed a correlation between pain after anterior cruciate ligament reconstruction and pain during an experimental first-degree burn 6 days preoperatively. The authors did not find a correlation between postoperative pain and the extent of secondary hyperalgesia or changes in pain threshold from mechanical or thermal stimuli. However, this was a small study, and patients were not followed to evaluate the development of chronic pain.

Intraoperative factors include the type of surgical procedure performed and the probability that certain types of surgical procedures are more likely to develop chronic persistent postoperative pain. For example, patients undergoing limb amputation, thoracotomy, sternotomy, and mastectomy have a high prevalence of chronic persistent postsurgical pain. Surgical technique and incisional approach also play important roles in predicting persistent postoperative pain. The extent of tissue damage appears to be a predictor of chronic pain and the extent of acute pain (eg, phantom limb pain appears to be more common after the amputation of a leg than after toe amputation) [5]. Thoracotomy performed using a posterolateral approach is more likely to result in chronic pain than that performed using an anterolateral approach [59,60]. Similarly, chronic pain is more common after chest wall resection [61,62]. Mastectomy combined with the implantation of a prosthesis results in a higher prevalence of pain than mastectomy alone [63]. Nerve injury such as intercostobrachial nerve injury during breast surgery or intercostal nerve injury during thoracotomy also contributes to chronic pain [5,6,49,60].

Postoperative factors include the severity of postoperative pain, radiotherapy, and neurotoxic chemotherapy as well as psychologic vulnerability. Patients with a significantly greater severity of postoperative pain (particularly movement-evoked pain) are more likely to develop chronic pain [45,49,50]. However, the link between early postoperative pain and chronic pain does not necessarily imply causality. Nevertheless, adequate pain relief, particularly movement-evoked pain relief, may reduce the risk of persistent postoperative pain and deserves further investigation. There is a suggestion that certain patient personality factors may also play a role in the development of chronic pain. Psychologic vulnerability, as evaluated by a questionnaire, which appears to correlate with neuroticism and possibly somatization, has been shown to predict the post-cholecystectomy syndrome [64,65]. This contrasts with a lack of predictive power for psychologic parameters such as depression and anxiety for the development of chronic pain [45,48].

Mechanisms involved in the transition from acute to persistent postoperative pain

It has been suggested that persistent pain should be considered a disease state of the nervous system, not merely a symptom of some other disease condition [66]. Peripheral and central sensitization of the nervous system has been implicated in the development of intractable pain that potentially can become chronic. Repeated and prolonged noxious stimuli after tissue or nerve injury induce alterations in function, chemical profile, and even structure of neurons, which may increase the sensitivity to pain. Peripheral sensitization of nociceptors and the subsequent barrage of nerve impulses entering the spinal cord results in hyperexcitability in dorsal horn neurons and central sensitization (ie, metabolic activation and hyperexcitability of spinal nociceptive neurons, expansion of sensory receptive fields, and alterations in the processing of innocuous stimuli), leading to a reduced pain threshold and the amplification of the pain response. These postoperative neuroplastic changes underlie the development of "pathologic" pain, which is characterized by hyperalgesia (an increased response to a stimulus that is normally painful) and allodynia (pain caused by a stimulus that does not normally provoke pain).

De Kock et al [67] demonstrated that reducing the area of hyperalgesia after colectomy did not greatly reduce acute pain but was associated with a decrease in the number of patients who developed residual pain as late as 6 months after colectomy. Therefore, the area of secondary hyperalgesia (hyperalgesia outside of the injured area), one measure of central sensitization, could perhaps predict that patients are likely to develop persistent pain after surgery. Kawamata et al [68] subjected volunteers to a small incision in the volar forearm and mapped the area of hyperalgesia surrounding the incision. The authors noted that there was a large area of hyperalgesia, which did not develop when a local anesthetic injection was administered before the incision. Therefore, a neural blockade should significantly diminish central sensitization.

In addition to the use of local anesthetic techniques, an improved understanding of the role of cyclooxygenase (COX)-2 in pain sensitization suggests that COX-2 inhibitors should be an important consideration as a part of multimodal analgesic therapy. Recent research has advanced our understanding of the role of COX-2 and prostanoids in neural plasticity and pain sensitization [69]. Tissue injury is associated with an increased prostanoid (prostaglandin) synthesis and increased sensitivity of nociceptors (or peripheral sensitization). Peripheral inflammation also increases central prostanoid levels, which mediates more widespread changes in pain perception. Nitric oxide (NO) also has a possible role in the development and persistence of hyperalgesia [70]. Proposed mechanisms for the role of NO-induced nociceptor sensitization include enhancement of the release of an algesic substance (prostaglandin E_2), inhibition of the action of an endogenous antinociceptive substance acting on peripheral nociceptors, and a direct action of NO on nociceptors [71]. In addition, central sensitization may be partially mediated by the activation of N-methyl-D-aspartate (NMDA) receptors with subsequent NO production. Recent animal research suggests that in the periphery, NO modulates the response to a noxious stimulus. A new class of NO-releasing nonsteroidal anti-inflammatory drugs (NSAIDs) is being developed that releases nitric oxide in relatively small amounts over a prolonged period of time (6–12 h) [70]. Furthermore, the plasma concentration of stable NO products may be a useful predictor of subsequent development of chronic postoperative pain.

Prevention of persistent postoperative pain

The first step in prevention is to recognize that pain can occur after surgery. Of the number of interventions that have been identified to reduce chronic pain after surgery, the surgical approach is of great importance. A surgical approach that minimizes tissue and nerve damage should be used whenever possible. Because the classical posterolateral approach for thoracotomy is associated with greater tissue damage and a higher probability of nerve injury resulting in greater acute pain and a higher probability of chronic pain, it should be avoided, and an anterolateral approach should be used instead. The skill or finesse of the surgical team appears to be critical, as suggested by a low prevalence of chronic pain in specialized surgical centers [5,72–74]. The type of anesthesia (ie, general versus regional) by itself does not appear to be a significant factor.

Recent evidence suggests that achieving pain relief only at rest is not adequate and that movement-evoked (dynamic) pain relief is necessary to prevent postoperative physiologic impairment. It seems that the specific modality of pain relief is not as important as the degree of dynamic pain relief achieved. The use of multimodal analgesia techniques, which has been shown to provide optimal dynamic pain relief with minimal side effects, may prevent persistent postoperative pain. Although opioids have potent analgesic effects for spontaneous pain, they are inadequate for the treatment of movement-evoked pain. Thus, opioids may have only minimal effects in modifying neuronal plasticity and reversing established central sensitization. In contrast, local anesthetic techniques, COX-2 inhibitors, α_2 agonists, and NMDA receptor antagonists may be important for controlling movement-evoked pain and preventing central sensitization.

Conduction blockade with local anesthetics (eg, epidural analgesia and continuous peripheral nerve blockade) provides superior dynamic pain relief. When appropriate, the use of an epidural anesthesia with local anesthetics (both intraoperatively and postoperatively) may be beneficial. Because it has been theorized that persistent postsurgical pain results from sensitization, the blockade of sensitization may help with prevention. Obata et al [75] reported a significantly reduced incidence of post-thoracotomy pain at 6 months (67%–33%) when epidural analgesia with local anesthetics was administered both during and after surgery. Senturk et al [76] compared the effects of thoracic epidural analgesia with bupivacaine and morphine (initiated either preoperatively or postoperatively) or IV-PCA morphine. Patients receiving preoperative thoracic epidural analgesia experienced a significantly lower incidence of pain at 6 months (78% versus 45%) compared with IV-PCA. However, randomized controlled trials have not validated these reports [54,77,78].

Although regional analgesic techniques form the basis of postoperative pain management, current evidence suggests that combing them with COX-2 inhibitors (ie, NSAIDs and COX-2–specific inhibitors) may be more effective [79]. A combination of NSAIDs with preoperative opioids, preincisional regional block, and postoperative continuous paravertebral block or epidural block has been promoted as ideal for nearly total analgesia [60]. Several studies [80] have suggested that small doses of ketamine (an NMDA antagonist) enhance opioid analgesia, prevent tolerance to opioids, and improve pain relief as well as reduce hyperalgesia. However, at this time, the treatment recommendations are nonspecific. It is also suggested that the early use of tricyclics and anticonvulsants may be of benefit in the prevention of the neuropathic component of chronic pain. Recent studies [81] have suggested that gabapentin and pregabalin reduce postoperative morphine requirements and movement-related pain and thus may provide a "protective" effect that may diminish the hyperalgesic response to surgery. Recently, Reuben [53] reviewed various novel therapies for the prevention and treatment of chronic persistent postoperative pain, with an emphasis on CRPS. These therapies include free radical scavengers such as dimethylsulfoxide [82–86], *N*-acetylcysteine [86], vita-

min C [87,88], mannitol [89], and carnitine [90], with only dimetylsulfoxide and
N-acetylcysteine showing some promise. The basis for the trial of these free
radical scavengers is that CRPS is induced by an exaggerated inflammatory
response to tissue injury caused by excessive toxic oxygen radical production
[87,88]. Calcitonin [91,92] and kentanserin [93,94] have also been tried with
variable but marginal success.

Summary

It is now well accepted that inadequately treated pain and associated stress
response have significant physiologic and psychologic consequences, which
may lead to organ dysfunction and increase postoperative mortality and
morbidity. In addition, unrelieved postoperative pain reduces the ability to
participate in rehabilitation programs, leading to poor postoperative outcomes.
Furthermore, poorly controlled pain can potentially increase the incidence of
chronic persistent postoperative pain. Thus, pain delays recovery and discharge
home and reduces quality of life and patient satisfaction. Overall, inadequately
treated pain increases resource use and health care costs. Therefore, an
improvement in perioperative analgesia is not only desirable for humanitarian
reasons but is also essential for the potential reduction in postoperative
morbidity, improved health-related quality of life, and reduced health care costs.

Chronic persistent postoperative pain is common but often under-recognized
or misdiagnosed. The first step in preventing persistent postoperative pain is to
accept that it can occur after surgery. Despite numerous reports of persistent
postoperative pain resulting in distress and disability, it has been ignored. The
prevalence of chronic persistent postoperative pain appears to vary with the type
of surgery as well as the surgical approach. Therefore, the use of a surgical
approach that minimizes tissue trauma is crucial. However, it is not clear why
some patients develop persistent pain, whereas others undergoing the same
surgical procedure do not. Other risk factors include pre-existing pain, the extent
of acute pain, and certain personality factors (psychologic vulnerability).

It appears that the intensity of acute postoperative pain (particularly
movement-evoked pain) is an important predictor of persistent postoperative
pain. Therefore, it is necessary to provide effective and rational early interventions, which reduce postoperative pain not only at rest but also on movement. Multimodal analgesia techniques, including regional analgesia (epidural
analgesia or continuous peripheral nerve blocks), COX-2 inhibitors (NSAIDs
and COX-2 specific inhibitors), and opioids have been recommended for
providing dynamic pain relief with a lower incidence of side effects. In addition,
NMDA antagonists (eg, ketamine), α_2 agonists (eg, clonidine and dexmedetomidine), and anticonvulsants (eg, gabapentin and pregabalin) have been investigated. However, the use of these adjunct analgesics remains controversial and
needs to be evaluated in larger studies.

It is imperative that future acute pain studies collect appropriate data, including preoperative pain intensity and physiologic and psychologic risk factors. In addition, data regarding the location and length of surgical incisions and handling of nerves and muscles should also be obtained. Furthermore, postoperative follow-up, including quantitative and descriptive pain assessment, patient function, and physical signs and symptoms as well as postoperative interventions (eg, radiation therapy and chemotherapy), should be collected for at least 1 year. Areas of interest include identifying high-risk individuals, because focused interventions may be beneficial for these patient populations. In addition, the determination and adoption of surgical techniques that will minimize the incidence of chronic postoperative pain are imperative. It is necessary to assess the relationship between the intensity and time course of postoperative pain and the occurrence of persistent postoperative pain. Finally, prospective randomized, controlled studies are needed to determine how different pain management strategies influence the incidence of persistent postoperative pain.

References

[1] Apfelbaum JL, Chen C, Mehta SS, et al. Postoperative pain experience: results from a national survey suggest postoperative pain continues to be undermanaged. Anesth Analg 2003; 97:534–40.
[2] Liu SS, Carpenter RL, Mackey DC, et al. Effects of perioperative analgesic technique on rate of recovery after colon surgery. Anesthesiology 1995;83:757–65.
[3] Wu CL, Naqibuddin M, Rowlingson AJ, et al. The effect of pain on health-related quality of life in the immediate postoperative period. Anesth Analg 2003;97:1078–85.
[4] Tong D, Chung F, Wong D. Predictive factors in global and anesthesia satisfaction in ambulatory surgical patients. Anesthesiology 1997;87:856–64.
[5] Perkins FM, Kehlet H. Chronic pain as an outcome of surgery: a review of predictive factors. Anesthesiology 2000;93:1123–33.
[6] Macrae WA. Chronic pain after surgery. Br J Anaesth 2001;87:88–98.
[7] Liu SS, Block BM, Wu CL. Effects of perioperative central neuraxial analgesia on outcome after coronary artery bypass surgery: a meta-analysis. Anesthesiology 2004;101:153–61.
[8] Ballantyne JC, Carr DB, de Ferranti S, et al. The comparative effects of postoperative analgesic therapies on pulmonary outcome: cumulative meta-analyses of randomized, controlled trials. Anesth Analg 1998;86:598–612.
[9] Desai PM. Pain management and pulmonary dysfunction. Crit Care Clin 1999;15:151–66.
[10] Fotiadis RJ, Badvie S, Weston MD, et al. Epidural analgesia in gastrointestinal surgery. Br J Surg 2004;91:828–41.
[11] Baig MK, Wexner SD. Postoperative ileus: a review. Dis Colon Rectum 2004;47:516–26.
[12] Chia YY, Kuo MC, Liu K, et al. Does postoperative pain induce emesis? Clin J Pain 2002;18:317–23.
[13] Palazzo MGA, Strunin L. Anaesthesia and emesis I: aetiology. Can Anaesth Soc J 1984; 31:178–87.
[14] Harmer M, Davies KA. The effect of education, assessment, and standardized prescription on postoperative pain management: the value of clinical audit in the establishment of acute pain services. Anaesthesia 1998;53:424–30.
[15] Carpenter DO. Neural mechanisms in emesis. Can J Physiol Pharmacol 1990;68:230–6.

[16] Rosenfeld BA, Faraday N, Campbell D, et al. Hemostatic effects of stress hormone infusion. Anesthesiology 1994;81:1116–26.

[17] Gonzalez-Alegre P, Recober A, Kelkar P. Idiopathic brachial neuritis. Iowa Orthop J 2002; 22:81–5.

[18] Feeney SL. The relationship between pain and negative affect in older adults: anxiety as a predictor of pain. J Anxiety Disord 2004;18:733–44.

[19] Janssen SA, Spihoven P, Arntz A. The effects of failing to control pain: an experimental investigation. Pain 2004;107:227–33.

[20] Koivisto K, Janhonen S, Vaisanen L. Patients' experiences of psychosis in an inpatient setting. J Psychiatr Ment Health Nurs 2003;10:221–9.

[21] Kotiniemi LH, Ryhanen PT, Moilanen IK. Behavioral changes in children following day-case surgery: a 4-week follow-up of 551 children. Anaesthesia 1997;52:970–6.

[22] Tong D, Chung F. Postoperative pain control in ambulatory surgery. Surg Clin North Am 1999;79:401–30.

[23] Pavlin DJ, Chen C, Penaloza DA, et al. A survey of pain and other symptoms that affect the recovery process after discharge from an ambulatory surgery unit. J Clin Anesth 2004;16: 200–6.

[24] Fortier J, Chung F, Su J. Unanticipated admission after ambulatory surgery – a prospective study. Can J Anaesth 1998;45:612–9.

[25] Pavlin DJ, Rapp SE, Polissar NL, et al. Factors affecting discharge time in adult outpatients. Anesth Analg 1998;87:816–26.

[26] Pavlin DJ, Chen C, Penaloza DA, et al. Pain as a factor complicating recovery and discharge after ambulatory surgery. Anesth Analg 2002;95:627–34.

[27] Marley RA, Swanson J. Patient care after discharge from the ambulatory surgical center. J Perianesth Nurs 2001;16:399–419.

[28] Rawal N, Hylander J, Nydahl P-A, et al. Survey of postoperative analgesia following ambulatory surgery. Acta Anaesthesiol Scand 1997;41:1017–22.

[29] Chung F, Ritchie E, Su J. Postoperative pain in ambulatory surgery. Anesth Analg 1997; 85:808–16.

[30] McHugh GA, Thomas GMM. The management of pain following day-case surgery. Anaesthesia 2002;57:266–83.

[31] Wu CL, Berenholtz SM, Pronovost PJ, et al. Systematic review and analysis of postdischarge symptoms after outpatient surgery. Anesthesiology 2002;96:994–1003.

[32] Gold BS, Kitz DS, Lecky JH, et al. Unanticipated admissions to the hospital following ambulatory surgery. JAMA 1989;262:3008–10.

[33] Fancourt-Smith PF, Hornstein J, Jenkins LC. Hospital admissions from the surgical day care center of Vancouver General Hospital 1977–1987. Can J Anaesth 1990;37:699–704.

[34] Twersky R, Fishman D, Homel P. What happens after discharge: return hospital visits after ambulatory surgery. Anesth Analg 1977;84:319–24.

[35] Morrison RS, Siu AL. A comparison of pain and its treatment in advanced dementia and cognitively intact patients with hip fracture. J Pain Symptom Manage 2000;19:240–8.

[36] Swan BA, Maislin G, Traber KB. Symptom distress and functional status changes during the first seven days after ambulatory surgery. Anesth Analg 1998;86:739–45.

[37] Fraser RA, Hotz SB, Hurtig JB, et al. The prevalence and impact of pain after day-care tubal ligation surgery. Pain 1989;39:189–210.

[38] Ghosh S, Sallam S. Patient satisfaction and postoperative demands on hospital and community services after day surgery. Br J Surg 1995;82:1635–8.

[39] Macario A, Winger M, Carney S, et al. Which clinical anesthesia outcomes are important to avoid: the perspective of patients. Anesth Analg 1999;89:652–8.

[40] Strassels SA, Chen C, Carr DB. Postoperative analgesia: economics, resource use, and patient satisfaction in an urban teaching hospital. Anesth Analg 2002;94:130–7.

[41] Chapman CR, Gavrin J. Suffering: the contributions of persistent pain. Lancet 1999;353: 2233–7.

[42] Liu JH, Etzioni DA, O'Connell JB, et al. The increasing workload of general surgery. Arch Surg 2004;139:423–8.

[43] Poleschuck EL, Dworkin RH. Risk factors for chronic pain in patients with acute pain and their implications for prevention. In: Dworkin RH, Breitbart WS, editors. Psychosocial aspects of pain: a handbook for health care providers. Seattle (WA): IASP Press; 2003. p. 589–606.

[44] Davis HTO, Crombie IK, Macrea WA, et al. Pain clinic patients in northern Britain. Pain Clin 1992;5:129–35.

[45] Katz J, Jackson M, Kavanagh BP, et al. Acute pain after thoracic surgery persists: long-term post-thoracotomy pain. Clin J Pain 1996;12:50–5.

[46] Meyerson J, Thelin S, Gordh T, et al. The incidence of chronic post-sternotomy pain after cardiac surgery–a prospective study. Acta Anaesthesiol Scand 2001;45:940–4.

[47] Nikolajsen L, Ilkjaer S, Kroner K, et al. The influence of preamputation pain on postamputation stump and phantom pain. Pain 1997;72:393–405.

[48] Kroner K, Kerbs B, Skov J, et al. Immediate and long-term phantom breast syndrome after mastectomy: incidence, clinical characteristics, and relationship to pre-mastectomy breast pain. Pain 1989;36:327–34.

[49] Tasmuth T, Kataja M, Blomqvist C, et al. Treatment-related factors predisposing to chronic pain in patients with breast cancer–a multivariate approach. Acta Oncol (Madr) 1997;36:625–30.

[50] Callesen B, Kehlet H. Prospective study of chronic pain after hernia repair. Br J Surg 1999;86: 1528–31.

[51] Gehling M, Scheidt CE, Niebergall H, et al. Persistent pain after elective trauma surgery. Acute Pain 1999;2:110–4.

[52] Stanos SP, Harden RH, Wagner-Raphael R, et al. A prospective clinical model for investigating the development of CRPS. In: Harden RN, Baaron R, Jianig W, editors. Complex regional pain syndrome, progress in pain research and management. Seattle (WA): IASP Press; 2001. p. 151–64.

[53] Reuben SS. Preventing the development of complex regional pain syndrome after surgery. Anesthesiology 2004;101:1215–24.

[54] Nikolajsen L, Ilkjaer S, Christensen JH, et al. Randomised trial of epidural bupivacaine and morphine in prevention of stump and phantom pain in lower limb amputation. Lancet 1997;350:1353–7.

[55] Krane EJ, Heller LB. The prevalence of phantom limb sensation and pain in pediatric amputees. J Pain Symptom Manage 1995;10:21–9.

[56] Tasmuth T, Estlanderb AM, Kalso E. Effect of present pain and mood on the memory of past postoperative pain in women treated surgically for breast cancer. Pain 1996;68:343–7.

[57] Bates T, Ebbs SR, Harrison M, et al. Influence of cholecystectomy on symptoms. Br J Surg 1991;78:964–7.

[58] Werner MU, Duun P, Kehlet H. Prediction of postoperative pain by preoperative nociceptive responses to heat stimuli. Anesthesiology 2004;100:115–9.

[59] Nomori H, Horio H, Fuyuno G, et al. Non serratus-sparing antero-axillary thoracotomy with disconnection of anterior rib cartilage: improvement in postoperative pulmonary function and pain in comparison to posterolateral thoracotomy. Chest 1997;11:572–6.

[60] Benedetti F, Vighetti S, Ricco C, et al. Neuroradiologic assessment of nerve impairment in posterolateral and muscle-sparing thoracotomy. J Thorac Cardiovasc Surg 1998;115:841–7.

[61] Keller SM, Carp NZ, Levy MN, et al. Chronic post thoracotomy pain. J Cardiovasc Surg 1994;35:161–4.

[62] Burgess FW, Anderson DM, Colonna D, et al. Thoracic epidural analgesia with bupivacaine and fentanyl for postoperative thoracotomy pain. J Cardiothorac Vasc Anesth 1994;8:420–4.

[63] Wallace MS, Wallace AM, Lee J, et al. Pain after breast surgery: a survey of 282 women. Pain 1996;66:195–205.

[64] Jørgensen T, Teglbjerg JS, Wille-Jørgensen P, et al. Persisting pain after cholecystectomy: a prospective investigation. Scand J Gastroenterol 1991;26:124–8.

[65] Jess P, Jess T, Beck H, et al. Neuroticism in relation to recovery and persisting pain after laparoscopic cholecystectomy. Scand J Gastroenterol 1998;33:550–3.

[66] Basbaum AI. Spinal mechanisms of acute and persistent pain. Reg Anesth 1999;24:59–67.

[67] De Kock M, Lavand'homme P, Waterloos H. "Balanced analgesia" in the perioperative period: is there a place for ketamine? Pain 2001;92:373–80.

[68] Kawamata M, Watanabe H, Nishikawa K, et al. Different mechanisms of development and maintenance of experimental incision-induced hyperalgesia in human skin. Anesthesiology 2002;97:550–9.

[69] Woolf CJ. Pain: moving from symptom control toward mechanism-specific pharmacologic management. Ann Intern Med 2004;140:442–51.

[70] Salter M, Strijbos PJ, Neale S, et al. The nitric oxide-cyclic GMP pathway is required for nociceptive signaling at specific loci within the somatosensory pathway. Neuroscience 1996; 73:649–55.

[71] Anbar M, Gratt BM. Role of nitric oxide in the physiopathology of pain. J Pain Symptom Manage 1997;14:225–54.

[72] Rutkow IM, Robbins AW. The mesh plug technique for recurrent groin herniorrhaphy: a nine-year experience of 407 repairs. Surgery 1998;124:844–7.

[73] Amid PK, Lichtenstein IL. Long-term result and current status of the Lichtenstein open tension-free hernioplasty. Hernia 1998;2:89–94.

[74] Deysine M, Grimson RC, Soroff HS. Inguinal herniorrhaphy: reduced morbidity by service standardization. Arch Surg 1991;126:628–30.

[75] Obata H, Saito S, Fujita N, et al. Epidural block with mepivacaine before surgery reduces long-term post-thoracotomy pain. Can J Anaesth 1999;46:1127–32.

[76] Senturk M, Ozcan PE, Talu GK, et al. The effects of three different analgesia techniques on long-term postthoracotomy pain. Anesth Analg 2002;94:11–5.

[77] Bach S, Noreng MF, Tjellden NU. Phantom limb pain in amputees during the first 12 months following limb amputation, after preoperative lumbar epidural blockade. Pain 1988;33:297–301.

[78] Jahangiri M, Bradley JWP, Jayatunga AP, et al. Prevention of phantom pain after major lower limb amputation by epidural infusion of diamorphine, clonidine and bupivacaine. Ann R Coll Surg Engl 1994;76:324–6.

[79] Buvanendran A, Kroin JS, Tuman KJ, et al. Effects of perioperative administration of a selective cyclooxygenase 2 inhibitor on pain management and recovery of function after knee replacement: a randomized control trial. JAMA 2003;290:2411–8.

[80] Schmid RI, Sandler AN, Katz J. Use and efficacy of low-dose ketamine in the management of acute postoperative pain: a review of current techniques and outcomes. Pain 1999;82: 111–25.

[81] Gilron I. Is gabapentin a broad-spectrum analgesic? Anesthesiology 2002;97:537–9.

[82] Goris RJA, Dongen LMV, Winters HAH. Are toxic oxygen radicals involved in the pathogenesis of reflex sympathetic dystrophy? Free Radic Res Commun 1987;3:13–8.

[83] Zuurmond WW, Langendijk PN, Bezemer PD, et al. Treatment of acute reflex sympathetic dystrophy with DMSO 50% in a fatty cream. Acta Anaesthesiol Scand 1996;40:364–7.

[84] Geertzen JHB, de Bruijn H, de Bruijn-Kofman AT, et al. Reflex sympathetic dystrophy: early treatment and psychological aspects. Arch Phys Med Rehabil 1994;75:442–6.

[85] Zurmond WWA, Langendijk PHJ, Bezemer PD, et al. Treatment of acute reflex sympathetic dystrophy with DMSO 50% in a fatty cream. Acta Anaesthesiol Scand 1996;40:364–7.

[86] Perez RS, Zuurmond WW, Bezemer PD, et al. The treatment of complex regional pain syndrome type I with free radical scavengers: a randomized controlled study. Pain 2003;102: 297–307.

[87] Zollinger PE, Tuinebreijer WE, Kreis RW, et al. Effect of vitamin C on frequency of reflex sympathetic dystrophy in wrist fractures: a randomized trial. Lancet 1999;354:2025–8.

[88] Cazenueve JF, Leborgne JM, Kermad K, et al. Vitamin C and prevention of reflex sympathetic dystrophy following surgical management of distal radius fractures. Acta Orthop Belg 2002; 68:481–4.

[89] Veldman PH, Goris RJ. Multiple reflex sympathetic dystrophy: which patients are at risk for developing recurrence of reflex sympathetic dystrophy in the same or another limb. Pain 2003;103:199–207.

[90] Moesker A. Complex regional pain syndrome, formerly called reflex sympathetic dystrophy, treatment with ketanserin and carnitine [thesis]. Rotterdam: Erasmus University; 2000. p. 1–147.

[91] Braga PC. Calcitonin and its antinoceceptive activity: animal and human investigations 1975–1992. Agents Actions 1994;41:121–31.

[92] Yoshimura M. Analgesic mechanism of calcitonin. J Bone Miner Metab 2000;18:230–3.

[93] Moesker A. The purpose of a serotonin antagonist in reflex sympathetic dystrophy. Pain Clin 1995;8:31–7.

[94] Burnstock J. Autonomic neurotransmitters and trophic factors. J Auton Nerv Syst 1983;7: 213–7.

ELSEVIER
SAUNDERS

Anesthesiology Clin N Am
23 (2005) 37–48

ANESTHESIOLOGY
CLINICS OF
NORTH AMERICA

Postoperative Care of the Chronic Opioid-Consuming Patient

Jeffrey D. Swenson, MD[a,b,*], Jennifer J. Davis, MD[a],
Ken B. Johnson, MD[a]

[a]Department of Anesthesiology, University of Utah School of Health Sciences, 30 North 1900 East,
Salt Lake City, UT 84132, USA
[b]Acute Pain Service, University of Utah School of Health Sciences, 30 North 1900 East,
Salt Lake City, UT 84132, USA

Historically, opioids have been used for the transient management of acute pain, whereas chronic administration has been reserved for patients with malignancy or terminal disease. Recently, however, a greater emphasis has been placed on pain as an important health problem. As a result, opioids now play a greater role in the treatment of chronic pain of various causes [1,2]. This has resulted in a rapid increase in the annual sales of opioid analgesics. For example, between 1999 and 2003, the annual sales of outpatient opioid analgesics in the United States increased by approximately 130%, more than doubling the sales recorded in the previous decade [3]. Because more patients are treated chronically with opioids, every anesthesiologist is likely to be confronted with acute pain management issues in these patients. Chronic opioid-consuming patients can experience significant postoperative pain given that health care professionals are not accustomed to their markedly increased opioid requirements [4]. Therefore, anesthesiologists must acquire the necessary skills and understanding to effectively treat these patients.

This article describes a technique based on pharmacokinetic models that can be used to provide analgesia safely when opioids must be used as the primary form of pain control. In addition, a discussion of the adjuvant agents and

* Corresponding author. Department of Anesthesiology, University of Utah School of Health Sciences, 30 North 1900 East, Salt Lake City, UT 84132.

E-mail address: jeff.swenson@hsc.utah.edu (J.D. Swenson).

0889-8537/05/$ – see front matter © 2005 Elsevier Inc. All rights reserved.
doi:10.1016/j.atc.2004.11.006   *anesthesiology.theclinics.com*

procedures for providing superior analgesia while reducing opioid requirements is included.

Opioid tolerance

Despite extensive publications about the classifications and mechanisms of opioid tolerance [5–8], there is little practical guidance on how to safely and effectively use opioids when treating acute postoperative pain in chronic opioid-consuming patients. Discussions of various types of "associative" and "non-associative" tolerance are useful with respect to long-term management; however, because this review focuses on acute postoperative management, the reader is referred to other publications on this topic [9,10]. For the purposes of this discussion, the broad group of "chronic opioid-consuming patients" encompasses all patients who have been consuming opioids on a daily basis before surgery. Although many arbitrary time intervals have been used to define what constitutes "chronic opioid use," the most recent data suggest that physiologic changes occur much earlier than suggested previously and that clinically relevant tolerance can be detected within hours or days of use [11–13]. Therefore, the clinician must recognize that a unique set of skills is required to manage patients with a history of regular preoperative opioid use in comparison with skills required to manage opioid-naive patients.

Preoperative plan

It is important to identify chronic opioid-consuming patients preoperatively and involve them in the plan for postoperative pain control. The optimal strategy for analgesia will vary according to the surgical site and may include various regional anesthesia procedures as well as adjuvant pharmacologic agents. Because opioids will likely comprise a significant component of most analgesic regimens, it is important to establish clear criteria with the patient for opioid dosing. Despite a predicted tolerance to common side effects associated with opioids such as nausea and pruritis, chronic opioid-consuming patients are not immune to the catastrophic consequences of opioids such as respiratory depression. Comparing the incidence of postoperative sedation, Rapp et al [14] found moderate to severe sedation in 50% of chronic opioid-consuming patients compared with 19% in opioid-naive patients. In the same study, postoperative pain scores for patients who were chronically receiving opioids before surgery tended to be higher at rest and with stimulation (visual analog scores of 5 and 8, respectively) than opioid-naive controls (visual analog scores of 3 and 7, respectively). This seemingly paradoxical rate of sedation in chronically consuming patients may be explained by a narrowing in the ratio of analgesia-to-respiratory depression in response to opioid for chronic opioid-consuming patients compared with naive populations. Indeed this theory has been proposed as a mechanism for lethal overdose in chronic opioid users [15]. With this in mind, it is important to explain to the patient and family that changes in opioid dosing must be based on objective criteria. Importantly, the respiratory rate and level of sedation take precedence over trying to achieve an arbitrary value on the pain scale.

Regional analgesia techniques and nonopioid analgesics

Although parenteral opioids may be the only viable mode of analgesia for some patients, a multitude of other procedures and pharmacologic options are available in many cases. The anesthesiologist caring for these challenging patients must be knowledgeable about adjunctive pharmacologic agents and skilled in regional analgesia procedures that can ameliorate postoperative pain. The use of regional analgesia techniques and adjunctive analgesics are discussed only briefly because they have been discussed elsewhere in this issue.

Epidural analgesia and peripheral nerve blocks

Epidural analgesia is well established in providing excellent pain relief for a variety of surgical procedures. Thoracic epidural analgesia is particularly well suited for providing pain control after thoracic or upper abdominal surgery. A combination of local anesthetic and lipid soluble opioid provides segmental analgesia while sparing motor and sensory function in the lower extremities and thereby preserving ambulation. The most commonly used epidural solution is bupivacaine (0.1%–0.125%) in combination with a lipid soluble opioid such as fentanyl (2–6 µg/ml). A number of studies have demonstrated the superiority of peripheral nerve blocks in comparison with opioid analgesia.

Most importantly, despite having undergone a successful epidural analgesia or peripheral nerve block, the patient who chronically receives opioids will require supplemental opioid to prevent symptoms of acute withdrawal. An initial dose of approximately 40% to 50% of baseline consumption is usually adequate to prevent acute withdrawal symptoms [16]. Doses may then be tapered at a rate of 10% to 15% per day as tolerated in patients with physical dependence. Note that the use of local anesthetic only (opioid-free) solutions should be considered when significant doses of parenteral opioids are used in conjunction with epidural analgesia.

Nonopioid analgesics

Recent trials show a 30% to 40% reduction in opioid requirements with the use of nonselective nonsteroidal anti-inflammatory drugs and cyclooxygenase-2 specific inhibitors in the perioperative period. These drugs are particularly appealing in the management of opioid-tolerant patient because they are not associated with sedation or respiratory depression.

The potential of ketamine as an adjuvant to opioid analgesia is substantial, and its unique receptor activity has been studied for nearly 40 years [17]. Ketamine induces analgesia at subanesthetic doses; however, its mechanism of action is not entirely understood. It is an attractive addition to opioids because the effects produced by ketamine are mediated by a variety of non-μ receptor actions including muscarinic receptors [18], monoaminergic pain pathways [19], and calcium channels [20]. Additionally, ketamine has N-methyl-D-aspartate (NMDA) receptor antagonist properties. A number of authors [21–23] have suggested that NMDA receptor activation plays an important role in the development of opioid-induced tolerance. This combination of non-μ receptor-mediated analgesia and NMDA antagonist action has led to the performance of numerous clinical trials of ketamine as an adjunct to opioid analgesia [24]. Clinical trials evaluating the combination of opioids with ketamine have demonstrated improvements in comparison with opioids alone; however, its use has been associated with some undesirable psychomimetic effects. The role of ketamine in pain management is discussed elsewhere in this issue.

Clonidine and dexmedetomidine are the α_2-adrenergic agonists that have been used most extensively in clinical practice. These drugs may be useful in opioid-tolerant patients because they produce analgesia, which is not μ receptor-dependent [25]. However, treatment with clonidine may be associated with decreases in blood pressure, heart rate, and varying degrees of sedation. Of note, clonidine has also been used effectively to treat symptoms of opioid withdrawal [26]. Dexmedetomidine is the short-acting specific α_2-adrenergic agonist currently approved for sedation in humans. It has been anticipated as an analgesic agent as well. In a comparison with opioids, it lacked broad analgesic activity even at doses resulting in significant sedation [27]. The role of α_2-agonists in pain management is discussed elsewhere in this issue.

Intravenous patient-controlled analgesia with opioid as the primary mode of analgesia

Despite the many adjunctive analgesic agents and local anesthetic blocks available for postoperative pain control, there are a number of patients who must rely primarily on opioids for analgesia after surgery. When parenteral opioids must be used as the primary form of analgesia, it is useful to define dose-response relationships for clinical endpoints such as analgesia and respiratory depression. In chronic opioid-consuming patients, this is especially important because doses causing respiratory depression and analgesia may vary dramatically compared with opioid-naive patients. This discussion focuses on a method of providing postoperative opioid analgesia for chronic opioid-consuming patients by using pharmacokinetic applications rather than experimenting with escalating opioid doses.

Because most clinicians are justifiably concerned about excessive sedation and respiratory depression when administering large doses of opioid, objective information with respect to an individual patient's ventilatory response to opioid should be valuable. Existing methods of predicting the postoperative analgesic requirements in chronic opioid-consuming patients are imperfect. Considering the pharmacokinetic and pharmacodynamic variability among opioids, attempts to predict postoperative requirements based on estimates of preoperative "morphine equivalent" usage are difficult. In addition, patients may be inconsistent in their opioid consumption from day to day as well as inaccurate in their reporting of daily opioid consumption. Ideally, patients should be tested for their individual ventilatory response to the same drug that is anticipated for postoperative analgesia.

Preoperative "fentanyl challenge" defines individual response to opioid

Fentanyl is a logical choice for testing an individual's clinical response to an opioid and is also well suited for intravenous patient-controlled analgesia (IV-PCA) use during the postoperative period. Its rapid onset makes it easily titratable in the operating room. In addition, fentanyl has no active metabolites, and its pharmacokinetic and pharmacodynamic characteristics are well defined. Although pharmacokinetic data are available for other synthetic phenylpiperidines such as sufentanil, alfentanil, and remifentanil, fentanyl has achieved more widespread acceptance among health care providers.

Defining the threshold for respiratory depression

Drug titration has been used to determine an individual's response to opioids [28,29]. The clinical response to drug titration, however, must be interpreted with caution. During the initial drug administration (bolus or infusion), there is a disparity between the concentrations in the plasma and the site of drug action or the effect site concentration (Ce). This problem can be addressed by predicting the Ce, which approximates steady state concentration at the site of drug effect. Stanpump simulation software (Stanpump, Stanford, California, available at no charge: anesthesia.stanford.edu/pkpd/) provides tools to predict the fentanyl Ce following a fentanyl bolus or continuous infusion at the moment respiratory depression occurs. This software combines pharmacokinetic parameters for fentanyl described by Shafer et al [30] and a first-order rate constant that describes the temporal equilibration of fentanyl between the plasma concentration and Ce.

The present authors routinely use pharmacokinetic simulation and a preoperative fentanyl infusion in chronic opioid-consuming patients before anesthetic induction. All patients are instructed to stop opioid medications after midnight on the evening before surgery, and no preoperative sedation is used. In the operating room, an intravenous infusion of fentanyl, 2 μg · kg^{-1} · min^{-1} (based on ideal body weight), is begun. During the fentanyl infusion, no adjunctive agents are administered, and no tactile or verbal stimulation is allowed. The fentanyl infusion is continued until the patient demonstrates depression of spontaneous ventilation (defined as a respiratory rate of less than 5 breaths per minute as measured by capnography). At that point, the fentanyl infusion is withdrawn, and general anesthesia is induced. The duration of the fentanyl infusion is recorded for each patient. Fig. 1 displays the predicted fentanyl Ce over 30 minutes for a continuous infusion of 2 μg · kg^{-1} · min^{-1}. By using this graph, clinicians can determine the predicted Ce for an individual patient at the time respiratory depression occurs.

Predicting intravenous patient-controlled analgesia settings

Existing data for fentanyl suggest that concentrations that produce analgesia are approximately 30% of those associated with respiratory depression [31,32]. Fig. 2 presents a series of simulated fentanyl infusions that yield a fentanyl Ce

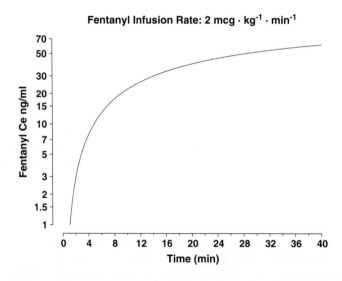

Fig. 1. Simulation of fentanyl Ce versus time for a sample patient. In this example, the patient received a preoperative fentanyl infusion (fentanyl challenge) of 2 μg · kg^{-1} · min^{-1} for 10 minutes. The estimated peak fentanyl Ce at the end of the fentanyl challenge was 20 ng/ml. Intraoperatively, a continuous fentanyl infusion was maintained at 5 μg · kg^{-1} · hr^{-1}. Postoperatively, patient-controlled analgesia was initiated with a demand dose of 0.6 mL (31.25 μg) every 10 minutes and a basal infusion of 2.5 μg · kg^{-1} · hr^{-1} (3.75 mL/h).

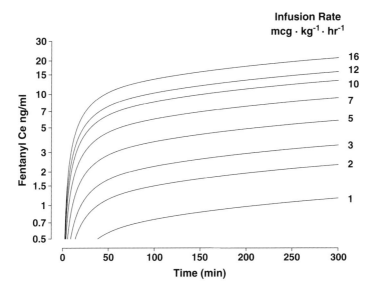

Fig. 2. Pharmacokinetic simulation to predict fentanyl Ce during an infusion of 2 $\mu g \cdot kg^{-1} \cdot min^{-1}$.

ranging from 0.2 to 20 ng/ml. These simulated fentanyl infusions are used to determine an hourly infusion rate that will provide a fentanyl Ce that is 30% of that associated with respiratory depression for each individual. The target analgesic infusion rate of fentanyl is maintained intraoperatively as well as in the recovery room. Postoperatively, patients receive IV-PCA programmed to deliver 50% of the target fentanyl infusion rate as a basal infusion, with the remaining 50% administered as demand doses with a 10- to 15-minute lockout interval (Box 1). At 4-hour intervals, the basal infusion rate is increased or decreased to maintain a demand rate of 2 to 3 doses per hour. For example, in patients using less than 1 interval dose per hour, the basal infusion is decreased by 20%. Alternatively, for those patients using greater than 3 doses per hour, the basal infusion is increased by 20%. The basal infusion is withdrawn for any patient with a respiratory rate of less than 10 breaths per minute. All patients should be monitored with hourly respiratory rate and continuous pulse oximetry. All patients receive supplemental oxygen.

Using this protocol in a series of 20 chronic opioid-consuming patients who underwent multilevel spine fusion [33], only 16% of the patients required more than a single adjustment to their initial IV-PCA settings. Despite continuing fentanyl infusions until completion of surgery, there were no cases of delayed awakening. Each subject was monitored continuously for the initial 24 hours after surgery by one of the investigators. There were no episodes of hypoxia, respiratory depression, or excessive sedation. No patient required naloxone or verbal prompting to breath.

Box 1. Sample fentanyl challenge

1. A patient with an ideal body weight of 75 kg (see Fig. 1)
2. Infusion rate of 2 $\mu g \cdot kg^{-1} \cdot min^{-1}$ (150 μg/min)
3. Respiratory depression at 10 min (see Fig. 2); Ce, 20 ng/ml
4. Target analgesic Ce is 0.30 × 20 ng/ml or 6 ng/ml
5. Total hourly infusion rate to achieve Ce of 6 ng/ml is approximately 5 $\mu g \cdot kg^{-1} \cdot h^{-1}$ (see Fig. 3)
6. Intraoperative fentanyl infusion of 5 $\mu g \cdot kg^{-1} \cdot h^{-1}$ (approximately 375 μg/h)
7. Postoperative PCA settings
   Administer 50% of the total hourly requirement as a basal infusion of 375 μg/h × 0.5 = 187.5 μg/h (3.75 cc/h)
   The remaining 50% of the hourly requirement in divided demand doses
   Lockout of 10 minutes = 6 demand doses/h
   187.5 μg/6 doses = 31.25 μg per dose or approximately 0.6 cc per dose

Initial PCA settings

Basal rate = 3.75 cc/h
Lockout interval = 10 minutes
Demand dose = 0.6 cc

8. Adjust basal rate according to the average demand dose use (respiratory rate and sedation should be carefully assessed before any adjustment)
   For patients using ≤1 demand dose/h, the basal rate is decreased by 20%
   For patients using ≥3 demand doses/h, the basal rate is increased by 20%

Practical considerations for intravenous patient-controlled analgesia

1. Chronic opioid-consuming patients should have surgery scheduled early in the day. This allows the patients to arrive in the recovery room with sufficient time to be observed on the planned analgesic regimen by the anesthesiologist coordinating their care.
2. Discuss the planned analgesic regimen in detail with the patient and family before surgery. Special emphasis should be placed on the criteria for adjusting IV-PCA settings. Specifically, it should be explained to the patient

and family that changes will be made according to the number of demand doses used, the respiratory rate, and the level of consciousness. If the family and patient understand that safety is a primary concern, they are more likely to work in conjunction with caregivers postoperatively.

3. Use caution in trying to achieve a specific "pain score." Previous reports [14] suggest that chronic opioid-consuming patients typically report higher pain scores at rest and with movement despite having higher rates of sedation. At least one author [15] has explained this paradox by suggesting that the ratio of intoxicating or lethal dose may be higher in chronically consuming individuals compared with opioid-naive subjects. A safer approach to IV-PCA management is to make changes in the dose based on objective criteria such as demand dose use and respiratory rate.

4. These patients require careful monitoring. Supplemental oxygen, continuous pulse oximetry, and hourly documentation of the respiratory rate are advisable. Patients with a history of sleep apnea are of particular concern because there are few data regarding their risk of perioperative respiratory depression. Patients with unusually large opioid requirements or severe sleep apnea may be managed most effectively in an intensive care setting during the early postoperative period.

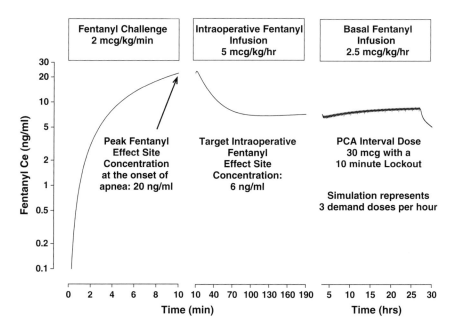

Fig. 3. Pharmacokinetic simulation to predict fentanyl Ce for infusion rates ranging from 0.5 to 16 $\mu g \cdot kg^{-1} \cdot h^{-1}$.

Transition to oral opioids

When the patient makes the transition to oral medication, it is important to remember that after a prolonged infusion of fentanyl several hours are required to achieve significant reductions in Ce [34]. For example, the time required to achieve a 50% reduction in fentanyl Ce after a 24-hour infusion may be as long as 5 to 7 hours. With this in mind, it is advisable to transit patients in the morning. This allows the clinician to monitor the patient carefully throughout the day and treat sedation or inadequate analgesia as needed. Most patients will require a combination of long-acting opioid equal to their basal infusion rate and interval doses at 3 to 4 hours for breakthrough pain.

The interest in methadone has recently increased as a result of its NMDA receptor antagonist activity demonstrated in animals [35,36]. The use of methadone may attenuate problems related to tolerance, which are thought to be NMDA-mediated [37]. These NMDA antagonist properties of methadone in addition to its long (although less predictable) half-life may make it an attractive alternative to other extended release opioids in patients who undergo an early transition to oral analgesics. Many practitioners have avoided using methadone as an analgesic because dosing more than once per day may result in dangerous plasma levels [38]. Although this is a risk for opioid-naive patients, respiratory depression in patients who are opioid-tolerant is unlikely, and these concerns have resulted in the under-use of this drug. Methadone has also been suggested as an ideal drug to be used for "opioid rotation" [39]. The concept of opioid rotation is based on the theory of incomplete cross-tolerance of various opioids working at μ and κ receptors. Based on incomplete cross-tolerance, it has been suggested that when changing from other opioids to methadone, the equivalent dose of methadone may be decreased by as much as 50% [39].

Summary

Chronic opioid-consuming patients present a challenge in management that requires a unique set of skills for the anesthesiologist. To provide safe and effective analgesia for these patients, adjunctive pharmacologic agents and regional techniques should be used where appropriate to provide multimodal analgesia. However, a significant number of these patients require parenteral opioids as the primary mode of analgesia. Despite a tolerance to many of the untoward effects of opioids such as nausea and pruritis, chronic opioid-consuming patients are still at risk for catastrophic effects such as respiratory depression. When using opioids as the primary analgesic technique, clinical endpoints for dosing such as respiratory depression and analgesia should be clearly identified. As is the case with many clinical scenarios, vigilance is essential to balance the need for effective analgesia with patient safety.

References

[1] Collett BJ. Chronic opioid therapy for non-cancer pain. Br J Anaesth 2001;87:133–43.

[2] Nissen LM, Tett SE, Cranoud T, et al. Opioid analgesic prescribing: use of an audit of analgesic prescribing by general practioners and the multidisciplinary pain center at Royal Brisbane Hospital. Br J Clin Pharmacol 2001;52:693–8.

[3] IMS H. IMS National sales perspective. 2004.

[4] Davis JJ, Johnson KB, Egan TD, et al. Preoperative fentanyl infusion with pharmacokinetic simulation for anesthetic and perioperative management of an opioid tolerant patient. Anesth Analg 2003;97(6):1661–2.

[5] Ballantyne JC, Mao J. Opioid therapy for chronic pain. N Engl J Med 2003;349:1943–53.

[6] He L, Fong J, von Zastrow M, et al. Regulation of opioid receptor trafficking and morphine tolerance by receptor oligomerization. Cell 2002;108:271–82.

[7] Kieffer BL, Evans CJ. Opioid tolerance-in search of the holy grail. Cell 2002;108:587–90.

[8] Mayer DJ, Mao J, Price DD. The development of morphine tolerance and dependence is associated with translocation of protein kinase C. Pain 1995;61:365–74.

[9] Mitchell JM, Basbaum AI, Fields HL. A locus and mechanism of action for associative morphine tolerance. Nat Neurosci 2000;3:47–52.

[10] O'Brien CP. Drug addiction and drug abuse. In: Hardman JG, Limbird LE, Gilman AG, editors. Goodman and Gilman's the pharmacologic basis of therapeutics. 10th edition. New York: McGraw-Hill; 2001. p. 621–42.

[11] Chia YY, Liu K, Wang JJ, et al. Intraoperative high dose fentanyl induces postoperative fentanyl tolerance. Can J Anaesth 1999;46:872–7.

[12] Guignard B, Bossard AE, Coste C, et al. Acute opioid tolerance: intraoperative remifentanil increases postoperative pain and morphine requirement. Anesthesiology 2000;93:409–17.

[13] Vinik HR, Kissin I. Rapid development of tolerance to analgesia during remifentanil infusion in humans. Anesth Analg 1998;86:1307–11.

[14] Rapp SE, Ready LB, Nessly ML. Acute pain management in patients with prior opioid consumption: a case-controlled retrospective review. Pain 1995;61:195–201.

[15] White JM, Irvine RJ. Mechanisms of fatal opioid overdose. Addiction 1999;94:961–72.

[16] Miyoshi HR, Leckband SG. Systemic opioid analgesics. In: Loeser JD, Butler SH, Chapman CR, et al, editors. Bonica's management of pain. 3rd edition. Philadelphia: Lippincott Williams & Wilkins; 2001. p. 1682–709.

[17] Reich DL, Silvay G. Ketamine: an update on the first twenty-five years of clinical experience. Can J Anaesth 1989;36:186–97.

[18] Hustveit O, Maurset A, Oye I. Interaction of the chiral forms of ketamine with opioid, phencyclidine, sigma and muscarinic receptors. Pharmacol Toxicol 1995;77:355–9.

[19] Crisp T, Perrotti JM, Smith DL, et al. The local monoaminergic dependency of spinal ketamine. Eur J Pharmacol 1991;194:167–72.

[20] Yamakage M, Hirshman CA, Croxton TL. Inhibitory effects of thiopental, ketamine, and propofol on voltage-dependent Ca2 + channels in porcine tracheal smooth muscle cells. Anesthesiology 1995;83:1274–82.

[21] Liu JG, Anand KJ. Protein kinases modulate the cellular adaptations associated with opioid tolerance and dependence. Brain Res Brain Res Rev 2001;38:1–19.

[22] Mao J. NMDA and opioid receptors: their interactions in antinociception, tolerance and neuroplasticity. Brain Res Brain Res Rev 1999;30:289–304.

[23] Williams JT, Christie MJ, Manzoni O. Cellular and synaptic adaptations mediating opioid dependence. Physiol Rev 2001;81:299–343.

[24] Subramaniam K, Subramaniam B, Steinbrook RA. Ketamine as adjuvant analgesic to opioids: a quantitative and qualitative systematic review. Anesth Analg 2004;99:482–95.

[25] Unnerstall JR, Kopajtic TA, Kuhar MJ. Distribution of alpha 2 agonist binding sites in the rat and human central nervous system: analysis of some functional, anatomic correlates of the pharmacologic effects of clonidine and related adrenergic agents. Brain Res Brain Res Rev 1984;7:69–101.

[26] Gold MS, Pottash AC, Sweeney DR, et al. Opiate withdrawal using clonidine: a safe, effective and rapid nonopiate treatment. JAMA 1980;242:343–6.

[27] Angst MS, Ramaswamy B, Davies MF, et al. Comparative analgesic and mental effects of increasing plasma concentrations of dexmedetomidine and alfentanil in humans. Anesthesiology 2004;101:744–52.

[28] Butscher K, Mazoit JX, Samii K. Can immediate opioid requirements in the post-anaesthesia care unit be used to determine analgesic requirements on the ward? Can J Anaesth 1995;42: 461–6.

[29] Stamer UM, Grond S, Maier C. Responders and non-responders to post-operative pain treatment: the loading dose predicts analgesic needs. Eur J Anaesthesiol 1999;16:103–9.

[30] Shafer SL, Varvel JR, Aziz N, et al. Pharmacokinetics of fentanyl administered by computer-controlled infusion pump. Anesthesiology 1990;73:1091–102.

[31] Gourlay GK, Kowalski SR, Plummer JL, et al. Fentanyl blood concentration-analgesic response relationship in the treatment of postoperative pain. Anesth Analg 1988;67:329–37.

[32] Peng PW, Sandler AN. A review of the use of fentanyl analgesia in the management of acute pain in adults. Anesthesiology 1999;90:576–99.

[33] Davis JJ, Swenson JD, Hall RH, et al. Preoperative "fentanyl challenge" as a tool to estimate postoperative opioid dosing in chronic opioid consuming patients. Anaesth Analg 2004 [in press].

[34] Shafer SL, Varvel JR. Pharmacokinetics, pharmacodynamics, and rational opioid selection. Anesthesiology 1991;74:53–63.

[35] Bulka A, Plesan A, Xu XJ, et al. Reduced tolerance to the anti-hyperalgesic effect of methadone in comparison with morphine in a rat model of mononeuropathy. Pain 2002;95:103–9.

[36] Davis AM, Inturrisi CE. d-Methadone blocks morphine tolerance and N-methyl-D-aspartate-induced hyperalgesia. J Pharmacol Exp Ther 1999;289:1048–53.

[37] Scimeca MM, Savage SR, Portenoy R, et al. Treatment of pain in methadone-maintained patients. Mt Sinai J Med 2000;67:412–22.

[38] Fishman SM, Wisley B, Mahajan G, et al. Methadone reincarnated: novel clinical applications with related concerns. Pain Med 2002;3:339–48.

[39] Ballantyne JC, Mao J. Opioid therapy for chronic pain. N Engl J Med 2003;349:1943–53.

ELSEVIER
SAUNDERS

Anesthesiology Clin N Am
23 (2005) 49–72

ANESTHESIOLOGY
CLINICS OF
NORTH AMERICA

Role of Cyclooxygenase-2 Inhibitors in Postoperative Pain Management

Noor M. Gajraj, MD, FRCA, DABPM[a,*], Girish P. Joshi, MB, BS, MD, FFARCSI[b]

[a]Baylor Center for Pain Management, Baylor University Medical Center, 5575 Warren Parkway # 220, Frisco, TX 75034, USA
[b]Perioperative Medicine and Ambulatory Anesthesia, University of Texas Southwestern Medical Center, 5323 Harry Hines Blvd, Dallas, TX 75390-9068, USA

The acceptance of the concept of multimodal analgesia and the availability of parenteral preparations of nonsteroidal anti-inflammatory drugs (NSAIDs) have increased the popularity of NSAIDs in the management of perioperative pain. The potential advantages of NSAIDs include opioid sparing and possibly reduced opioid-related side effects, improved analgesia, particularly when combined with other analgesics, reduced sensitization of nociceptors, attenuation of the inflammatory pain response, and prevention of central sensitization. Therefore, NSAIDs are valuable adjuvants to opioids and local anesthetics for the management of postoperative pain. However, concerns have been raised regarding the potential side effects of NSAIDs such as impaired coagulation, gastrointestinal (GI) complications, and renal dysfunction. These may be reasons why NSAIDs are often avoided in the perioperative period, even when they may be indicated.

Cyclooxygenase (COX)-2–specific inhibitors, which selectively target COX-2 while sparing COX-1, were developed in an attempt to obtain the therapeutic benefits of NSAIDs while overcoming their limitations. Until recently, three COX-2–specific inhibitors, celecoxib (Celebrex), rofecoxib (Vioxx) and valdecoxib (Bextra), were available in the United States. However, rofecoxib was recently removed from the market because of concerns over its association with

* Corresponding author.
 E-mail address: noorgajraj@aol.com (N.M. Gajraj).

0889-8537/05/$ – see front matter © 2005 Elsevier Inc. All rights reserved.
doi:10.1016/j.atc.2004.11.011　　　　　　　　　　　　*anesthesiology.theclinics.com*

an increased risk of cardiovascular events. With the withdrawal of rofecoxib from the market, there are increasing concerns of the safety of COX-2–specific inhibitors [1]. This article focuses on the efficacy and safety of currently available coxibs (ie, celecoxib and valdecoxib) as well as parecoxib, which is an injectable prodrug of valdecoxib that has yet to be approved by the US Food and Drug Administration (FDA).

Cyclooxygenase expression and function

Nonselective NSAIDs were discovered to act by inhibiting the enzyme cyclo-oxygenase, which catalyzes the synthesis of prostaglandins from arachidonic acid [2]. The COX gene was cloned by three separate research groups in 1988 [3–5], and two isoforms of cyclooxygenase have since been identified, COX-1 and COX-2. COX-1 is expressed constitutively throughout the body [6] and is only slightly up-regulated (two to fourfold) in some cells in response to hormones or growth factors [7]. It plays an essential role in homeostatic processes such as platelet aggregation, gastric protection, and renal function. In contrast, COX-2 is expressed predominantly in inflammatory cells and is involved in the synthesis of prostaglandins that mediate pathologic processes such as pain [8], inflammation, angiogenesis [9], fever, and carcinogenesis [10–12]. The expression of COX-2 may facilitate several oncogenic processes including tumor invasion, angiogene-sis, and metastasis [13]. However, COX-2 has also been detected in the brain, testes, kidney, [14] and trachea [15].

Both COX-1 and COX-2 are expressed constitutively in dorsal root ganglia and spinal dorsal and ventral gray matter [16]. In the spinal cord, COX-2 immunoreactivity is present in neurons of all lamina, particularly in the super-ficial layers. A COX-1 selective inhibitor is effective when applied systemically but not spinally against carrageenan-evoked thermal hyperalgesia and is in-effective against spinal hyperalgesia [17]. The intraspinal administration of a COX-2 inhibitor decreases inflammation-induced central prostaglandin E_2 levels and mechanical hyperalgesia [18]. COX-2 induction within the spinal cord may play an important role in central sensitization [19–26]. Indeed, the acute anti-hyperalgesic action of NSAIDs has been shown to be mediated by the inhibition of constitutive spinal COX-2 [27]. Blocking constitutive spinal COX-2 before tissue injury may reduce the initial peripheral and central sensitization that occurs after tissue injury [28]. In response to inflammation and other stressors, COX-2 expression is markedly up-regulated (10- to 20-fold) by a variety of mediators [29].

These distinct expression patterns have led to the theory that COX-1–derived prostaglandins are largely responsible for physiologic ("housekeeping") func-tions [30], whereas COX-2–derived prostaglandins mediate pathophysiologic and inflammatory processes, including pain (Fig. 1). Conventional NSAIDs in-hibit both COX-1 and COX-2. It was hypothesized that the development of selective COX-2 inhibitors would have the advantages of conventional NSAIDs

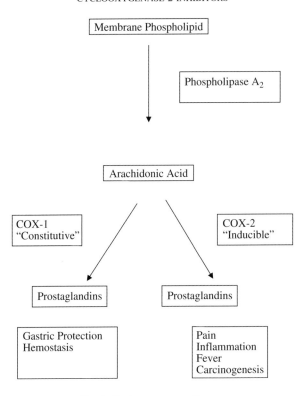

Fig. 1. Cyclooxygenase pathways.

but would not interfere with gastric protection or hemostasis [31–34], but the simplicity of this concept has been challenged [35,36]. Studies [37] have shown that mice that lack the COX-1 enzyme have only 1% to 3% of the GI mucosal prostaglandin levels as wild-type animals, yet they do not spontaneously develop GI lesions. It may be overly simplistic to view the efficacy and safety of NSAIDs only in terms of their effects on prostaglandin synthesis [38]. Physicochemical and pharmacokinetic factors may also be important [39–41], as well as the relationship with other mediators such as nitric oxide [42]. Interestingly, the existence of a COX-3 enzyme has been postulated [43,44]. COX-3 has been proposed as a possible site of action for acetaminophen [45–48].

Efficacy in the management of postoperative pain

The efficacy of COX-2–specific inhibitors for the management of post-operative pain has been evaluated in numerous controlled clinical trials (Table 1). It must be emphasized that the efficacy of the COX-2–specific inhibitors is similar to that of nonselective NSAIDs.

Table 1
Postoperative pain studies

Author/study population	Groups	Efficacy
Celecoxib		
Gimbel et al [52]	Placebo	Celecoxib 200 mg
418 patients undergoing	Celecoxib 200 mg TID	> hydrocodone 10/1000
ambulatory orthopedic	Hydrocodone 10/1000 TID	> placebo
surgery	(10mg/APAP 1000 mg)	
Reuben et al. [53]	Placebo	Rofecoxib 50 mg
60 patients undergoing	Rofecoxib 50 mg	> celecoxib 200 mg
spinal fusion	Celecoxib 200 mg	> placebo
Issioui et al [54]	Placebo	Celecoxib 200 mg/APAP 2 g
112 patients undergoing	Acetaminophen 2 g	> celebrex 200 mg = APAP
ear, nose, throat surgery	Celecoxib 200 mg	2g = placebo
	Celecoxib	
	200 mg/acetaminophen 2 g	
Valdecoxib		
Oral surgery studies		
Daniels et al [58]	Placebo	Valdecoxib 40 mg
406 patients undergoing	Valdecoxib 20 mg	> valdecoxib 20 mg
oral surgery	Valdecoxib 40 mg	> oxycodone 10/1000 > placebo
	Oxycodone 40 mg/	
	acetaminophen 1000 mg	
Fricke et al [59]	Placebo	Valdecoxib 40 mg
203 patients undergoing	Valdecoxib 40 mg	> rofecoxib 50 mg > placebo
oral surgery	Rofecoxib 50 mg	
Christensen and	Placebo	Valdecoxib 40 mg
Cawkwell [60]	Valdecoxib 40 mg	> rofecoxib 50 mg > placebo
119 patients undergoing	Rofecoxib 50 mg	
oral surgery		
Other surgical studies		
Dejardins et al [61]	Placebo	Valdecoxib 80mg
223 patients undergoing	Valdecoxib 20 mg	= valdecoxib 40 mg
bunionectomy	Valdecoxib 40 mg	> valdecoxib 20 mg > placebo
	Valdecoxib 80 mg	
Camu et al [62]	Valdecoxib 20 mg BID	Valdecoxib 40 mg BID
217 patients undergoing	Valdecoxib 40 mg BID	= 20 mg BID
hip arthroplasty	Placebo	> placebo (morphine
		requirement decreased 40%)
Reynolds et al [63]	Placebo	Valdecoxib 80 mg
20 patients undergoing	Valdecoxib 40 mg/d	> valdecoxib 40 mg > placebo
total knee arthroplasty	Valdecoxib 80 mg/d	
Parecoxib		
Oral surgery studies		
Daniels et al [67]	Parecoxib 20 mg IM	Parecoxib 20 and 40 mg
304 patients undergoing	Parecoxib 20 mg IV	= ketorolac 60 mg
oral surgery	Parecoxib 40 mg IM	
	Parecoxib 40 mg IV	
	Ketorolac 60 mg IM	
	Placebo IM/IV	

(continued on next page)

Table 1 (*continued*)

Author/study population	Groups	Efficacy
Desjardins et al [79] 214 patients undergoing oral surgery	Parecoxib 20 mg IV Parecoxib 40 mg IV Parecoxib 80 mg IV Placebo IV	Parecoxib 40 mg = 80 mg > 20 mg > placebo
Mehlisch et al [69] 199 patients undergoing oral surgery	Parecoxib 20 mg IV Parecoxib 50 mg IV Ketorolac 30 mg IV Placebo IV	Parecoxib 50 mg > parecoxib 20 mg = ketolorac 30 mg > placebo
Other surgical studies		
Barton et al [70] 202 patients undergoing gynecological surgery	Parecoxib 20 mg IV Parecoxib 40 mg IV Ketorolac 30 mg IV Morphine 4 mg IV Placebo IV	Parecoxib 40 mg = parecoxib 40 mg = ketolorac 30 mg > morphine 4 mg > placebo
Tang et al [71] 60 patients undergoing gynecological surgery	Parecoxib 20 mg IV Parecoxib 40 mg IV Placebo IV	Parecoxib 20 and 40 reduced opioid requirements but no difference in opioid side effects and pain scores
Ng et al [72] 35 patients undergoing laparoscopic sterilization	Parecoxib 40 mg IV Ketorolac 30 mg IV	Pareccoxib 40 mg = ketorolac 30 mg
Rasmussen et al [73] 208 patients undergoing total knee replacement	Parecoxib 20 mg IV Parecoxib 40 mg IV Ketorolac 30 mg IV Morphine 4 mg IV Placebo IV	Parecoxib 40 mg = ketorolac 30 mg Parecoxib 40 mg > morphine 4 mg
Hubbard et al [74] 195 patients undergoing total knee arthroplasty	Parecoxib 20 mg BID IV Parecoxib 40 mg BID IV Placebo BID IV	Parecoxib 40 mg BID = parecoxib 20 mg BID > placebo
Malan et al [75] 201 patients undergoing total hip arthroplasty	Parecoxib 20 mg BID IV Parecoxib 40 mg BID IV Placebo BID IV	Parecoxib 40 mg BID = parecoxib 20 mg BID > placebo
Joshi et al [76] 201 patients undergoing laparoscopic cholecystectomy	Parecoxib 40 IV/ valdecoxib 40 mg OD Placebo IV then oral	Parecoxib group had lower pain scores and less opiod side effects
Ott et al [78] 462 patients undergoing coronary artery bypass grafting surgery	Parecoxib 40 mg BID IV Placebo IV	Parecoxib group required less morphine

Abbreviations: APAP, acetaminophen; BID, twice per day; IM, intramuscular; IV, intravenous; OD, once per day; TID, three times per day.

Celecoxib

Celecoxib is an oral COX-2–specific inhibitor, which has a 22% to 40% bioavailability, an analgesic onset of 30 to 60 minutes, and a time to peak concentration of 2 hours after oral administration [49]. It is eliminated predominantly by hepatic metabolism and has no active metabolites. The elimination half-life of celecoxib is approximately 11 hours. The initial oral dose of celecoxib, 400 mg, has been shown to be more effective than 200 mg in reducing both severe postoperative pain and the need for rescue medication in the postoperative period [50]. The need for a loading dose of celecoxib is related to its large volume of distribution. Also, peak blood levels of celecoxib occur within 2 hours after oral administration on an empty stomach, so adequate time must be given to achieve analgesic blood levels [51].

Gimbel et al [52] studied the efficacy and tolerability of celecoxib versus hydrocodone-acetaminophen in the treatment of pain after ambulatory orthopedic surgery. Patients were randomly allocated to receive celecoxib 200 mg, hydro-codone 10 mg/acetaminophen 1000 mg, or placebo within 24 hours after the end the surgery, with pain assessments made for 8 hours after the first dose of medication. During the subsequent 5 days, patients received either celecoxib, 200 mg three times per day as needed, or hydrocodone 10 mg/acetaminophen 1000 mg, three times per day as needed. During the first 8 hours after surgery, patients with moderate to severe pain after orthopedic surgery experienced com-parable analgesia with single doses of celecoxib and hydrocodone. During the 5-day period, patients in the celecoxib group experienced superior analgesia and tolerability compared with patients in the hydrocodone/acetaminophen group. Most patients required no more than two daily doses of celecoxib, 200 mg, for control of their postoperative orthopedic surgery pain.

Reuben et al [53] studied the analgesic efficacy of a single dose of rofecoxib, 50 mg, celecoxib, 200 mg, or placebo given 1 hour before spinal fusion surgery. Patients given placebo required an average of 117 mg of morphine per day postoperatively, celecoxib patients required 107 mg (a 9% reduction), and rofe-coxib patients required 71 mg (a 39% reduction). Although both rofecoxib and celecoxib produced similar analgesic effects in the first 4 hours after surgery, rofecoxib demonstrated an extended analgesic effect that lasted throughout the 24-hour study period. It must be noted that this study did not compare equi-analgesic doses of the two COX-2–specific inhibitors (celecoxib, 400 mg, is equal to rofecoxib, 50 mg); also, for postoperative pain management, celecoxib should be administered twice per day rather than once daily. In another study [54], patients undergoing elective ear-nose-throat surgery were allocated to receive placebo, acetaminophen, 2 g, celecoxib, 200 mg, or celecoxib, 200 mg, together with acetaminophen 2 g. Only the combination of celecoxib and acetaminophen was significantly more effective than placebo. Again, in this study, the dose of celecoxib was inappropriate because the recommended dosage of celecoxib for postoperative pain management is 400 mg, initially, followed by 200 mg twice per day.

By performing a systematic review, Barden et al [55] assessed the analgesic efficacy and adverse effects of a single oral dose of celecoxib for moderate to severe postoperative pain. A single dose of oral celecoxib was found to be an effective means of postoperative pain relief, similar in efficacy to aspirin, 600 to 650 mg, and paracetamol, 1000 mg. The two trials included the use of celecoxib, 200 mg, a dose that is 50% less than that recommended for acute pain.

Valdecoxib

Valdecoxib is a new COX-2–specific inhibitor that is more highly selective for COX-2 than COX-1 [56,57]. The elimination half-life of valdecoxib is approximately 11 to 13 hours. Early clinical trials have reported effective postoperative analgesia with valdecoxib dosages of 40 mg once daily or in two divided doses. Of note, the FDA has not yet approved valdecoxib for acute pain management.

A study [58] compared the efficacy of a single dose of valdecoxib, 20 mg or 40 mg, a combination of oxycodone 10 mg/APAP (acetaminophen) 1000 mg, or placebo for the treatment of postoperative oral surgery pain. The efficacy of valdecoxib, 40 mg, was comparable to oxycodone/APAP. Both doses of valdecoxib had a significantly longer duration of action than oxycodone/APAP and had a tolerability profile similar to that of placebo. Another study [59] assessed patients undergoing extraction of two or more third molars (at least one of which was impacted), requiring bone removal. Patients were allocated to receive valdecoxib, 40 mg, rofecoxib, 50 mg, or placebo. Patients receiving valdecoxib, 40 mg, experienced a significantly faster onset of analgesia, significantly improved pain relief, and lower pain intensity compared with patients receiving rofecoxib, 50 mg, or placebo. The median time to perceptible pain relief was 34 minutes in the valdecoxib, 40 mg, group, 55 minutes in the rofecoxib, 50 mg, group, and more than 24 hours in the placebo group. Cristensen and Cawkwell [60] compared the analgesic efficacy of valdecoxib and rofecoxib in patients after they underwent oral surgery. The onset of action was significantly faster with valdecoxib, 40 mg (30 minutes), compared with rofecoxib, 50 mg (45 minutes), as measured by pain intensity difference and pain relief scores. Both agents were well tolerated.

In a dose range study [61] patients undergoing bunionectomy were randomly allocated to receive either valdecoxib, 20, 40, or 80 mg, or placebo 45 to 75 minutes before surgery. Paients in the valdecoxib groups experienced superior analgesia compared with the placebo group and required less rescue medication. Time to use of rescue medication was significantly longer in the valdecoxib, 40 and 80 mg, groups relative to the valdecoxib, 20 mg, and placebo groups.

In a more recent study [62] of patients undergoing hip arthroplasty, subjects received either placebo, valdecoxib, 20 mg twice per day, or valdecoxib, 40 mg twice per day. Study medication was first given 1 to 2 hours preoperatively, and the surgery was performed under spinal anesthesia. After surgery, patients received intravenous patient-controlled analgesia using morphine. Patients receiving valdecoxib, 20 or 40 mg twice per day, required an average of 40% less morphine than those receiving the placebo. Pain intensity levels and patient satisfaction were significantly improved in both valdecoxib groups compared with placebo.

A multicenter, randomized, double-blind, placebo-controlled study [63] evaluated the analgesic efficacy and opioid-sparing effects of valdecoxib in patients undergoing knee replacement surgery. Patients received morphine by intravenous patient-controlled analgesia, valdecoxib, 40 or 80 mg daily, or placebo, for up to 2 days. Morphine consumption over 48 hours by patients receiving valdecoxib, 40 or 80 mg daily plus morphine, was 83.7% and 75.8%, respectively, of the total amount consumed by patients receiving morphine alone. On the first postoperative day, valdecoxib, 80 mg/d, gave superior analagesia compared with valdecoxib, 40 mg/d; however on day 2, the analgesic efficacy was comparable.

Parecoxib

Parecoxib (SC-69124A) is a water-soluble prodrug of valdecoxib developed for parenteral administration [64,65]. It is the first injectable COX-2–specific inhibitor approved in Europe for the short-term treatment of moderate to severe postoperative pain. It is currently undergoing Phase III clinical trials for approval by the FDA.

Parecoxib is rapidly hydrolyzed by the liver to valdecoxib [66]. The mean plasma elimination half-life of single- or multiple-dose parecoxib, 20 mg intravenous (IV) or intramuscular (IM), is 20 to 30 minutes. The mean time to the peak plasma concentration of parecoxib after IV administration is approximately 5 minutes and after IM administration is 20 minutes. The peak plasma concentration (C_{max}) of parecoxib after IM administration (1–1.25 mg/L) is approximately 73% lower than that after IV administration (3.8–4.7 mg/L). However, this difference is not clinically significant because the C_{max} and the area under the plasma concentration time curve (AUC) to valdecoxib (the active form of parecoxib) is independent of the route of parecoxib administration. The C_{max} of valdecoxib is reached approximately 30 minutes after IV administration and in 1 to 2.5 hours after the IM administration of parecoxib, 20 mg. The mean AUC to 24 hours, and the C_{max} of valdecoxib increases proportionately with the dose of parecoxib after IV and IM administration. The plasma concentration of valdecoxib reaches a steady state within 4 days of twice daily dosing. Both parecoxib and valdecoxib do not accumulate after multiple dosing. Parecoxib is almost completely converted to valdecoxib and is undetectable in the urine, with only traces being detected in the feces.

Parecoxib has been evaluated for the treatment of pain after dental, gynecological, orthopedic, general, and coronary artery bypass grafting surgery [67–79]. The efficacy and duration of analgesia of parecoxib appears to be dose-dependent but is not significantly affected by the route of administration (ie, IV versus IM). The time to onset of analgesia occurs 7 to 14 minutes after IV or IM administration of parecoxib, 40 mg. Clinically meaningful pain relief (ie, 50% reduction in pain) occurs within 17 minutes after 40 mg IV and 26 to 37 minutes after 20 mg IV and IM. The peak analgesic effect occurs within 2 hours, and the duration of analgesia is 5 to 22 hours. Collectively, these studies demonstrate that parecoxib significantly reduces morphine requirements, with a concomitant reduction in the incidence of clinically meaningful opioid-related adverse events. The analgesic efficacy of parecoxib, 20 and 40 mg, IV or IM, has been found to be similar to that of ketorolac, 15 to 30 mg IV or 30 to 60 mg IM, and morphine, 12 mg IV.

Kranke et al [80] performed a systematic review of randomized controlled trials comparing parecoxib with other analgesics to evaluate the patients' global satisfaction with their analgesic regimen. The study found that the overall adverse effects of parecoxib, 20 and 40 mg, were similar to those for placebo, morphine, or ketorolac. Parecoxib, 20 and 40 mg, significantly improved patients' global satisfaction of analgesic regimen compared with the placebo. Parecoxib, 40 mg, appeared to be more effective than 20 mg without the additional side effects. Parecoxib, 40 mg, was equally effective compared with ketorolac, 30 to 60 mg, from the patients' point of view.

In Europe, the recommended dosages of parecoxib are 40 mg IV or IM, initially, followed by 20 to 40 mg every 6 to 12 hours, to a maximum daily dose of 80 mg. Dosage adjustments are not necessary in the elderly or in patients with mild hepatic or renal impairment. However, in elderly patients weighing less than 50 kg, the dosage should be reduced by 50%.

Safety and tolerability

Overall COX-2–specific inhibitors are well tolerated when used for peri-operative pain management. In postoperative studies [57,81], the most commonly occurring adverse events reported by patients were headache, dizziness, and fever. The incidence of these adverse events was comparable with patients taking the placebo. The overall incidence, type, and severity of adverse events with parecoxib were similar to that of placebo, ketorolac, and morphine [65]. The incidence of adverse events was similar with parecoxib, 20 and 40 mg doses, as well as with IV and IM administration. Because COX-2–specific inhibitors do not inhibit the COX-1 isoform at therapeutic concentrations, the associated risk of antiplatelet and GI adverse effects is reduced; however, the cardiorenal effects of these drugs remain controversial [1].

Hematologic effects

Platelet aggregation and hemostasis depend on the ability of platelets to generate thromboxane A_2 from prostaglandin H_2. Because platelets do not contain COX-2, all synthesis of thromboxane A_2 in the platelet is mediated by COX-1. By inhibiting COX-1, conventional NSAIDs impair the ability of platelets to aggregate [82]. COX-2 inhibitors have no effect on platelet function at therapeutic dosages [83–86]. In contrast to ketorolac, 15 to 30 mg IV administered for 5 days, parecoxib, 40 mg twice per day administered for 7, days did not affect platelet function in healthy adults or elderly volunteers [87]. Similarly, ketorolac significantly reduced thromboxane B_2 levels compared with the placebo and parecoxib [88]. Although the total number of patients evaluated in clinical studies is relatively smaller, the bleeding-related complications with COX-2–specific inhibitors do not differ from placebo or nonselective NSAIDs.

Gastrointestinal toxicity

NSAID-induced GI toxicity is one of the most common drug-related serious adverse events in industrialized countries [89,90]. It has been estimated that more than 100,000 patients are hospitalized and 16,500 die each year in the United States as a result of NSAID-associated GI events. Symptomatic ulcers and ulcer complications associated with the use of conventional NSAIDs may occur in approximately 1% of patients treated for 3 to 6 months and 2% to 4% of patients treated for 1 year [91–93]. It has been shown that most ulcers and ulcer complications in patients treated with traditional NSAIDs occur in patients with a low number, or no-risk factors [94], and 80% of patients may have no preceding symptoms [95].

Because prostaglandins are involved in the maintenance of GI mucosal integrity and only COX-1 is present in the normal GI mucosa, the GI toxicity of NSAIDs has been proposed to result largely from the inhibition of COX-1 activity [96,97]. Indeed, selective COX-2 inhibitors have been shown to cause less GI side effects than conventional NSAIDs [98–108].

Recent studies [109] suggest that even with short-term use, nonselective NSAIDs are associated with a higher incidence of GI ulcers compared with a placebo and COX-2–specific inhibitors. In healthy volunteers, valdecoxib, 40 mg twice per day for 6 days, was associated with a lower incidence of GI ulcers compared with naproxen, 500 mg twice per day, but similar to the placebo group. Parecoxib, 40 mg, was associated with a lower incidence of GI adverse effects (ie, ulcers or lesions) in healthy adults and elderly compared with ketorolac, 30 mg, and naproxen, 500 mg twice per day [110].

Cardiorenal effects

Prostaglandins have a critical role in renal function by affecting blood flow, glomerular filtration, natriuresis, and antidiuretic hormone secretion [111]. It is well known that conventional NSAIDs cause hypertension and edema [112] and nephrotoxicity in patients who are at risk [113]. Angiotensin-converting enzyme (ACE) inhibitors and β-blockers stimulate vasodilator prostaglandins, whereas nonselective NSAIDs inhibit the production of such prostaglandins and thereby de-stabilize blood pressure control. The intrarenal distribution and regulation of renal COX-2 by sodium intake suggests a role for this enzyme in renal physi-ology and in the renal effects of NSAIDs [114,115]. The renal [116,117] and cardiovascular effects of the selective COX-2 inhibitors are similar to nonselec-tive NSAIDs [118]. COX-2 metabolites have been implicated in the maintenance of renal blood flow, the mediation of renin release, and the regulation of sodium excretion [119]. COX-2 inhibition may transiently decrease urine sodium excretion in some subjects and induce mild to moderate elevation of blood pressure. Furthermore, in conditions of relative intravascular volume depletion or renal hypoperfusion, interference with COX-2 activity can have deleterious effects on the maintenance of renal blood flow and glomerular filtration rate. In addition to physiologic regulation of COX-2 expression in the kidney, increased renal cortical COX-2 expression is seen in experimental models associated with altered renal hemodynamics and progressive renal injury (decreased renal mass, poorly controlled diabetes), and long-term treatment with selective COX-2 inhibitors ameliorates functional and structural renal damage in these conditions. In patients with severe, preexisting renal impairment, the use of a COX-2 inhibitor should be closely monitored, as is required for nonselective NSAIDs. It has been hypothesized that, like other sulphonamides, celecoxib and valdecoxib may inhibit carbonic anhydrase, resulting in a diuretic effect [120,121].

Studies of celecoxib and rofecoxib [122,123] in elderly cohorts have evaluated the stability of renal function as measured by glomerular filtration rate. These studies have identified a pattern of modest systemic sodium retention (100–150 mmol) during the fist few days of administration [124]. Within approximately 5 to 7 days of treatment, the typical individual returned to a pretreatment state of sodium balance through renal elimination of the retained sodium using homeostatic mechanisms that are independent of renal prostaglandin.

In a 6-week study [125], patients of 65 years or older with osteoarthritis who were undergoing antihypertensive therapy were randomly allocated to receive either celecoxib, 200 mg daily, or rofecoxib, 25 mg daily. The incidence of increased systolic blood pressure was significantly greater in the rofecoxib group compared with the celecoxib group (17% versus 11%, respectively). At week 6, the mean systolic blood pressure change from baseline was +2.6 mm Hg for the rofecoxib group compared with −0.5 mm Hg for the celecoxib group. Small elevations in systolic blood pressure are now known to be both measurable and important determinants of cardiovascular risk [126–128] .The incidence of edema was also significantly greater in the rofecoxib group compared with the celecoxib group (9.5% versus 4.9%, respectively). Patients undergoing antihypertensive therapy and receiving COX-2 inhibitors should be monitored for the development of cardiorenal events.

More recently, in a 6-week study, Whelton et al [129] assessed the effects of celecoxib, 200 mg/day, and rofecoxib, 25 mg/day, on blood pressure and edema in 1092 patients 65 years of age or older with systemic hypertension and osteoarthritis. Significantly more patients in the rofecoxib compared with the celecoxib group developed increased systolic blood pressure (change ≥ 20 mm Hg plus absolute value ≥ 140 mm Hg) at any time (14.9% versus 6.9%, respectively, $P \leq 0.01$). Rofecoxib caused the greatest increase in systolic blood pressure in patients receiving angiotensin-converting enzyme inhibitors or β-blockers, whereas those taking calcium channel antagonists or diuretic montherapy receiving either celecoxib or rofecoxib showed no significant increases in blood pressure. Clinically significant new onset or worsening edema associated with weight gain developed in a greater percentage of patients in the rofecoxib group (7.7%) compared with the celecoxib group (4.7%). More of the patients in the rofecoxib group were taking calcium channel antagonist (36.6% versus 32.6%), which can cause edema. This underlies the importance of controlling the groups for differences in concurrent medication usage. A recent retrospective study [130] of the Tennessee Medicaid program found that the use of rofecoxib at doses higher than 25 mg was associated with an increased incidence of congestive heart failure. The cost of blood pressure destabilization and edema associated with COX-2 therapy requires consideration [131].

Cho et al [132] compared the difference between the effect of celecoxib and rofecoxib on blood pressure change. A retrospective review of medical records in which the mean blood pressure in a 90-day period before and after the start of the COX-2 inhibitors celecoxib and rofecoxib was compared. The average total daily dose of COX-2 inhibitor was 219.2 mg for celecoxib and 25.23 mg for rofecoxib. A post hoc analysis of patients aged 65 years and older showed that the mean systolic blood pressure in the rofecoxib group increased by 7.37 mm Hg ($P = 0.016$), whereas there was an insignificant decrease for the celecoxib group (-1.94 mm Hg). This study showed that there were no significant changes in blood pressure after the initiation of celecoxib, whereas in the rofecoxib group, there was a significant increase in systolic blood pressure, with an even greater increase for patients aged 65 years and older.

Solomon et al [133] recently examined the risk of new onset hypertension in a retrospective case-controlled study involving 17,844 subjects aged 65 years or older. Multivariable logistic models were examined to assess the relative risk of new onset hypertension requiring treatment in patients who used celecoxib or rofecoxib compared with patients taking either the other COX-2–specific inhibitor, a nonspecific NSAID, or no NSAID. In this retrospective case-controlled study of patients aged 65 years or older, the use of rofecoxib was associated with an increased relative risk of new onset hypertension, which was not seen in patients taking celecoxib. A recent meta-analysis [134] found increased cardiovascular risk with COX-2 inhibitors. However, such analyses have been criticized for combining results from different studies with differing patient populations, cardiovascular risk factors, protocols, and study drug comparators and differing use of concomitant medications. In the Vioxx GI Outcome Research study [134a], the incidence of myocardial infarction was 0.1% in the naproxen group and 0.4% in the rofecoxib group. The reason for this difference remains controversial [135,136]. In another study, Solomon et al [137] studied the relative risk of acute myocardial infarction among users of celecoxib, rofecoxib, and NSAIDs in Medicare beneficiaries with a comprehensive drug benefit. The matched case-controlled study included 54,475 patients 65 years of age or older who received their medications through two state-sponsored pharmaceutical benefits programs in the United States. The current use of rofecoxib was associated with an elevated relative risk of acute myocardial infarction compared with celecoxib. Celecoxib was not associated with an increased relative risk of acute myocardial infarction in these comparisons.

White et al [138] analyzed the incidence of cardiovascular events for celecoxib, placebo, and NSAIDs in the entire controlled, arthritis clinical trial database for celecoxib. In clinical arthritis trials involving more than 31,000 patients, no significant increase in cardiovascular events (myocardial infarction, stroke, or cardiovascular death) was found when patients treated with celecoxib were compared with patients who received nonselective NSAIDs or placebo. In a similar analysis of the available data for valdecoxib, short- and intermediate-term treatment with therapeutic (10 or 20 mg daily) and supratherapeutic (40 or 80 mg daily) valdecoxib dosages were not associated with an increased incidence of thrombotic events relative to nonselective NSAIDs or placebo in osteoarthritis and rheumatoid arthritis patients in controlled clinical trials [139]. Other studies have failed to show that celecoxib increases the risk of myocardial infarction or congestive heart failure relative to nonselective NSAIDs [140,141].

The decision to withdraw rofecoxib from the market on September 30, 2004 was based on 3-year data from a prospective, randomized, placebo-controlled clinical trial, the Adenomatous Polyp Prevention on VIOXX trial [142]. The trial, which was stopped, was designed to evaluate the efficacy of rofecoxib, 25 mg, in preventing the recurrence of colorectal polyps in patients with a history of colorectal adenomas. In this study, there was an increased relative risk for confirmed cardiovascular events, such as heart attack and stroke, beginning after 18 months of treatment in the patients taking rofecoxib compared with those taking placebo.

A possible mechanism for increased cardiovascular risk associated with COX-2 inhibitors is the alteration in the balance between of prostacyclin I_2 and throboxane A_2 [1]. Prostacyclin I_2 has been shown to be the predominant cyclooxygenase product in endothelium, inhibiting platelet aggregation, causing vasodilatation, and preventing the proliferation of vascular smooth muscle cells in vitro. These effects contrast with thromboxane A_2, the major product of platelets, which causes platelet aggregation, vasoconstriction, and vascular proliferation. Whereas nonselective NSAIDs inhibit both throboxane A_2 and prostacyclin I_2, the COX-2 inhibitors leave throboxane A_2 unaffected. Thus, the selective depression of prostacyclin I_2 might be expected to elevate blood pressure and accelerate therogenesis. Interestingly, in a rabbit model, the damage after temporary coronary artery ligation was increased by treatment with celecoxib, which completely blocked the cardioprotective effects of the COX-2 enzyme [143]. The authors concluded that the COX-2 enzyme is a "cardioprotective protein," suggesting that COX-2 inhibitors may neutralize these protective effects. The cardiovascular risks associated with the use of COX-2 inhibitors, especially in high-risk patients, will likely continue to be a very controversial issue.

Hepatic effects

Borderline elevations of one or more liver tests may occur in up to 15% of patients taking NSAIDs, and notable elevations of alanine transaminase or aspartate transaminase (approximately three or more times the upper limit of normal) have been reported in approximately 1% of patients in clinical trials with NSAIDs. These laboratory abnormalities may progress, remain unchanged, or may be transient with continuing therapy. Rare cases of severe hepatic reactions, including jaundice and fatal fulminant hepatitis, liver necrosis, and hepatic failure (some with fatal outcome), have been reported with NSAIDs. A patient with symptoms or signs suggesting liver dysfunction or in whom an abnormal liver test has occurred should be monitored carefully for evidence of the development of a more severe hepatic reaction while undergoing therapy with COX-2 inhibitors. If clinical signs and symptoms consistent with liver disease develop or if systemic manifestations occur, COX-2 therapy should be discontinued. It should be noted that in the Vioxx GI Outcome Research study [134a], patients treated with rofecoxib showed increased numbers of liver-related adverse events compared with naproxen (10 versus 3, respectively).

Effects on bone and wound healing

NSAID compounds are known to affect bone osteogenesis during bone repair [144–146]. A retrospective study by Deguchi et al [147] found that patients who continued to take NSAIDs for more than 3 months postoperatively showed lower bone fusion success rates than control subjects (44% versus 37%, respectively) after posterolateral fusion for isthmic spondylolisthesis. In a rat model of posterior spine fusion, Dimar et al [148] demonstrated a fusion rate of 10% if indomethacin was given for 12 weeks postoperatively versus 45% in control subjects. Glassman et al [149] further demonstrated that even short-term administration of NSAIDs can significantly affect spinal fusion. This retrospective study of 288 patients showed that non-union was five times more likely to occur if ketorolac was administered postoperatively compared with no use of NSAIDS. Recently it has been demonstrated that COX-2 inhibitors do not have significant deleterious effects on the healing of intertransverse process fusions in the rabbit model [150]. In this study, rabbits were randomly allocated to receive celecoxib (10 mg/kg), indomethacin (10 mg/kg), or placebo for 8 weeks after undergoing single level intertransverse posterolateral fusions using autogenous iliac crest bone. Gross inspection and palpation revealed that 64% of the 22 control spines and 45% of the 22 spines in the rabbits treated with celecoxib were fused. This difference was not statistically significant. Of the 22 spines in the indomethacin-treated rabbits, 18% were fused, and this percentage was significantly different from the control value. On radiographic assessment, the spine segment was judged to be fused in 82% of the 22 control subjects, 86% of the 22 rabbits treated with celecoxib, and 41% of the 22 indomethacin-treated animals. Only the difference between the indomethacin-treated and control groups was significant. A study [151] in mice has suggested that selective inhibition of COX-2 may prevent or reduce bone loss in inflammation-induced bone disease. Using a rat closed femur fracture model, Simon et al [152] showed that COX-2 inhibitors can affect normal fracture healing, resulting in incomplete unions and non-unions. These findings cannot be extrapolated to the short-term perioperative use of COX-2 inhibitors in humans. There are no data from prospective randomized trials in humans. More recently, Bakker et al [153] studied loading-induced prostaglandin production in primary bone cells in vitro. They concluded that COX-2 is the mechanosensitive form of COX that determines the response of bone tissue to mechanical loading. The effect of COX-2 inhibitors on bone healing continues to be controversial [154–157].

It has been suggested that COX-2–mediated prostaglandins may have a role in wound healing [158,159]. Although there is some evidence for impaired ligament healing in the rat [160], the effects of COX-2 inhibitors on human wound healing has not been fully studied.

Drug interactions

NSAIDs may diminish the antihypertensive effect of ACE inhibitors and the natriuretic effect of furosemide and thiazides in some patients. Concomitant administration of fluconazole may result in an increase in plasma levels of celecoxib and valdecoxib [51]. Concomitant administration of aspirin and COX-2 inhibitors increases the risk of GI ulceration, thus diminishing the beneficial effects of COX-2 inhibitor. However, the combination of COX-2 inhibitors and aspirin is probably associated with less GI side effects than combinations of nonselective NSAIDs and aspirin [108,161].

All of the currently available COX-2 inhibitors may increase serum warfarin levels, and therefore anticoagulant therapy should be monitored, particularly in the first few days of initiating or changing therapy [162]. Lithium levels may also increase with administration of celecoxib and valdecoxib [163].

Contraindications

NSAIDs and COX-2 inhibitors should not be given to patients who have a known hypersensitivity to the medication or to patients who have experienced asthma, urticaria, or allergic-type reactions (the aspirin triad) after taking aspirin or other NSAIDs [164]. Depletion of prostaglandin E_2, which is usually generated by COX-1, appears to be an important event in the generation of this reaction. However, COX-2 inhibitors have been given to such patients without deleterious results [165–167]. Interestingly, in a mouse model, data suggested that a genetic deficiency of COX-1 but not COX-2 modulates T cell recruitment, T helper type-2 cytokine secretion, and lung function in the allergic airway [168]. Celecoxib and valdecoxib should not be given to patients who have demonstrated allergic-type reactions to sulphonamides. The overall incidence of sulphonamide hypersensitivity in the general population is low, approximately 3% [169]. All sulphonamides can be regarded as belonging to one of two main biochemical categories, arylamines or non-arylamines [170]. The key to sulphonamide allergenicity is thought to be related to the formation of a hydroxylamine metabolite that is unique to the aryalamine structure. Celecoxib and valdecoxib belong to the non-aryalamine group of medications and are contraindicated in patients who are allergic to sulphonamides.

Summary

COX-2 inhibitors represent a significant therapeutic development because of their improved side-effect profile compared with nonselective NSAIDs [81]. Although the analgesic efficacy of the COX-2 inhibitors is similar to that of nonselective NSAIDs, the use of COX-2 inhibitors in the perioperative period is associated with several potential advantages (Box 1). Because of the lack of antiplatelet effects, the COX-2 inhibitor therapy may be continued throughout the perioperative period thus avoiding an exacerbation of postoperative pain. This may be important because the intensity of preoperative pain has been shown to correlate directly with the severity of postoperative pain and opioid requirements [171].

However, questions remain regarding the use of COX-2 inhibitors, such as the restriction of their use to patients at high risk for complications, the impact on postoperative outcomes [172], adverse events [173], cost effectiveness [174], effectiveness compared with nonselective NSAIDs plus prostaglandin replacement or acid reduction therapy, efficacy compared with and in combination

---

Box 1. Potential advantages of using COX-2 inhibitors perioperatively

Improved quality of analgesia
Reduced incidence of GI side effects versus
   conventional NSAIDs
May be given preoperatively on an empty stomach
No platelet inhibition
Opioid sparing effect (20%–50%)
   Avoidance of opioid side effects
   Sedation
   Pruritis
   Nausea and vomiting
   Cardiovascular side effects
Decreased postoperative ileus
Probable synergistic effects with opioids
Long duration of action; provide continuous round-the-
   clock regimen

with other analgesics [175], and safety in patients also taking aspirin for platelet inhibition [176,177]. Future studies as well as post-marketing surveillance should provide more information regarding the safety of COX-2–specific inhibitors, particularly in high-risk populations.

References

[1] FitzGerald GA. Coxibs and cardiovascular disease. N Engl J Med 2004;351:1709–11.

[2] Vane J. Inhibition of prostaglandin synthesis as a mechanism of action for the aspirin-like drugs. Nature 1971;231:232–5.

[3] Dewitt DL, Smith WL. Primary structure of prostaglandin G/H synthase from sheep vesicular gland determined from the complementary DNA sequence. Proc Natl Acad Sci U S A 1998; 85:1412–6.

[4] Merlie J, Fagan D, Mudd J, et al. Isolation and characterization of the complimentary DNA for sheep seminal vesicle prostaglandin endoperoxide synthase (cyclooxygenase). J Biol Chem 1998;263:3550–3.

[5] Yokoyama C, Takai T, Tanabe T. Primary structure of sheep seminal vesicle prostaglandin endoperoxide synthase deduced from cDNA sequence. FEBS Lett 1988;231:347–51.

[6] Seibert K, Masferrer J. Role of inducible cyclooxygenase in inflammation. Receptor 1994;4: 17–23.

[7] Dewitt D. Prostaglandin endoperoxide synthase: regulation of enzyme expression. Biochim Biophys Acta 1991;1083:121–34.

[8] Camu F, Shi L, Vanlersberghe C. The role of COX-2 inhibitors in pain modulation. Drugs 2003;63(Suppl 1):S1–7.

[9] Gately S, Li W. Multiple roles of COX-2 in tumor angiogenesis: a target for antiangiogenic therapy. Semin Oncol 2004;31:2–11.

[10] Fosslien E. Adverse effects of nonsteroidal anti-inflammatory drugs on the gastrointestinal system. Ann Clin Lab Sci 1998;28:67–81.

[11] Schwartz J, Chan C, Mukhopadhyay S, et al. Cyclooxygenase-2 inhibition by rofecoxib reverses naturally occurring fever in humans. Clin Pharmacol Ther 1999;65:653–60.

[12] Lee S, Soyoola E, Chanmugam P, et al. Selective expression of mitogeninducible cyclooxygenase in macrophages stimulated with lipopolysaccharide. J Biol Chem 1992;267:25934–8.

[13] Soslow R, Dannenberg A, Rush D, et al. COX-2 is expressed in human pulmonary, colonic and mammary tumors. Cancer 2000;89:2637–45.

[14] Kramer B, Kammerl M, Komhoff M. Renal cyclooxygenase-2 (Cox-2): physiological, pathophysiological, and clinical implications. Kidney Blood Press Res 2004;27:43–62.

[15] Walenga R, Kester M, Coroneos E, et al. Constitututive expression of prostaglandin G/H synthetase (PGHS)-2 not PGHS-1 in human tracheal epithelial call in vitro. Prostaglandins 1996;52:341–59.

[16] Svensson CI, Yaksh TL. The spinal phospholipase-cyclooxygenase-prostanoid cascade in nociceptive processing. Annu Rev Pharmacol Toxicol 2002;42:553–83.

[17] Yaksh TL, Dirig DM, Conway CM, et al. The acute antihyperalgesic action of nonsteroidal, anti-inflammatory drugs and release of spinal prostaglandin E2 Is mediated by the inhibition of constitutive spinal cyclooxygenase-2 (COX-2) but not COX-1. J Neurosci 2001; 21:5847–53.

[18] Samad TA, Moore KA, Sapirstein A, et al. Interleukin-1[beta]-mediated induction of Cox-2 in the CNS contributes to inflammatory pain hypersensitivity. Nature 2001;410:471–5.

[19] Hay C, de Belleroche J. Carrageenan-induced hyperalgesia is associated with increased-cyclooxgenase-2nexpression in the spinal cord. Neuroreport 1997;8:1249–51.

[20] Beiche F, Scheuerer S, Brune K, et al. Up-regulation of cyclooxygenase-2 mRNA in the rat spinal cord following peripheral inflammation. FEBS Lett 1996;390:165–9.

[21] Ibuki T, Matsumura K, Yamazaki Y, et al. Cyclooxygenase-2 is induced in the endothelial cells throughout the central nervous system during carrageenan-induced hind paw inflammation; its possible role in hyperalgesia. J Neurochem 2003;86:318–28.

[22] McCrory C, Fitzgerald D. Spinal prostaglandin formation and pain perception following thoracotomy: a role for cyclooxygenase-2. Chest 2004;125:1321–7.

[23] Guay J, Bateman K, Gordon R, et al. Carrageenan-induced paw edema in rat elicits a predominant prostaglandin E2 (PGE2) response in the central nervous system associated with the induction of microsomal PGE2 synthase-1. J Biol Chem 2004;279:24866–72.

[24] Lee K, Kang B, Lee H, et al. Spinal NF-kB activation induces COX-2 upregulation and contributes to inflammatory pain hypersensitivity. Eur J Neurosci 2004;19:3375–81.

[25] Kroin JS, Buvanendran A, McCarthy RJ, et al. Cyclooxygenase-2 inhibition potentiates morphine antinociception at the spinal level in a postoperative pain model. Reg Anesth Pain Med 2002;27:451–5.

[26] Dirig D, Isakson P, Yaksh T. Effect of COX-1 and COX-2 inhibition on induction and maintenance of carrageenan-evoked thermal hyperalgesia in rats. J Pharmacol Exp Ther 1998; 285:1031–8.

[27] Yaksh T, Dirig D, Conway C, et al. The acute antihyperalgeisc action of nonsteroidal, anti-inflammatory drugs and release of spinal prostaglandin E2 is mediated by the inhibition of constitutive spinal cyclooxygenase-2 (COX-2) but not COX-1. J Neurosci 2001;21:5847–53.

[28] Ghilardi JR, Svensson CI, Rogers SD, et al. Constitutive spinal cyclooxygenase-2 participates in the initiation of tissue injury-induced hyperalgesia. J Neurosci 2004;24:2727–32.

[29] Mitchell J, Akarasereenont P, Thiemermann C, et al. Selectivity of nonsteroidal anti-inflammatory drugs as inhibitors of constitutive and inducible cyclo-oxygenase. Proc Natl Acad Sci U S A 1993;90:11693–7.

[30] Meade E, Smith W, DeWitt D. Differential inhibition of prostaglandin endoperoxide sythase (cyclooxygenase) isoenzymes by aspirin and other non-steroidal anti-inflammatory drugs. J Biol Chem 1993;268:6610–4.

[31] Prasit P, Wang Z, Brideau C, et al. The discovery of rofecoxib, [MK 966, VIIOXX, 4-(4'-methylsulfonylphenyl)-3-phenyl-2(5H)-furanone], an orally active cyclo-oxygenase-2- inhibitor. Bioorg Med Chem Lett 1999;9:1773–8.

[32] DeWitt D. COX-2 selective inhibitors: The new super aspirins. Mol Pharmacol 1999;55: 625–31.

[33] Warner TD, Mitchell JA. Cyclooxygenases: new forms, new inhibitors, and lessons from the clinic. FASEB J 2004;18:790–804.

[34] Simmons DL, Botting RM, Hla T. Cyclooxygenase isozymes: the biology of prostaglandin synthesis and inhibition. Pharmacol Rev 2004;56:387–437.

[35] Bjarnason I, Takeuchi K, Simpson R. NSAIDs: the emperor's new dogma? Gut 2003;52: 1376–8.

[36] Whittle BJR. New dogmas or old? Gut 2003;52:1379–81.

[37] Langenbach R, Morham S, Tiano H, et al. Disruption of the mouse cyclooxygenase 1 gene: characteristics of the mutant and areas of future study. Adv Exp Med Biol 1997;407:87–92.

[38] Spangler R. Cyclooxygenase 1 and 2 in rheumatic disease: implications for nonsteroidal anti-inflammatory drug therapy. Semin Arthritis Rheum 1996;26:436–47.

[39] Wallace J. Selective cyclooxygenase-2 inhibitors: after the smoke has cleared. Dig Liver Dis 2002;34:89–94.

[40] Rainsford K. Profile and mechanisms of gastrointestinal and other side-effects of nonsteroidal anti-inflammatory drugs (NSAID's). Am J Med 1999;107:27S–35S.

[41] Rainsford K. The ever-emerging anti-inflammatories: have there been any real advances? J Physiol Paris 2001;95:11–9.

[42] Boje KMK, Jaworowicz Jr D, Raybon JJ. Neuroinflammatory role of prostaglandins during experimental meningitis: evidence suggestive of an in vivo relationship between nitric oxide and prostaglandins. J Pharmacol Exp Ther 2003;304:319–25.

[43] Schwab J, Beiter T, Linder JU, et al. COX-3–a virtual pain target in humans? FASEB J 2003;17:2174–5.

[44] Shaftel S, Olschowka J, Hurley S, et al. COX-3: a splice variant of cyclooxygenase-1 in mouse neural tissue and cells. Brain Res Mol Brain Res 2003;119:213–5.

[45] Chandrasekharan NV, Dai H, Roos KLT, et al. COX-3, a cyclooxygenase-1 variant inhibited by acetaminophen and other analgesic/antipyretic drugs: cloning, structure, and expression. Proc Natl Acad Sci U S A 2002;15:13926–31.

[46] Warner TD, Mitchell JA. Cyclooxygenase-3 (COX-3): filling in the gaps toward a COX continuum? Proc Natl Acad Sci U S A 2002;99:13371–3.

[47] Wickelgren I. Pain research: enzyme might relieve research headache. Science 2002; 297:1976a.

[48] Swierkosz T, Jordan L, McBride M, et al. Actions of paracetamol on cyclooxygenases in tissue and cell homogenates of mouse and rabbit. Med Sci Monit 2002;8:496–503.

[49] Paulson SK, Hribar JD, Liu NWK, et al. Metabolism and excretion of [14C]celecoxib in healthy male volunteers. Drug Metab Dispos 2000;28:308–14.

[50] Recart A, Issioui T, White PF, et al. The efficacy of celecoxib premedication on postoperative pain and recovery times after ambulatory surgery: a dose-ranging study. Anesth Analg 2003;96:1631–5.

[51] Davies N, McLachlan A, Day R, et al. Clinical pharmacokinetics and pharmacodynamics of celecoxib: a selective cyclo-oxygenase-2 inhibitor. Clin Pharmacokinet 2000;38:225–42.

[52] Gimbel J, Brugger A, Zhao W, et al. Efficacy and tolerability of celecoxib versus hydrocodone/acetaminophen in the treatment of pain after ambulatory orthopedic surgery in adults. Clin Ther 2001;23:228–41.

[53] Reuben SS, Connelly NR. Postoperative analgesic effects of celecoxib or rofecoxib after spinal fusion surgery. Anesth Analg 2000;91:1221–5.

[54] Issioui T, Klein K, White P, et al. The efficacy of premedication with celecoxib and acetaminophen in preventing pain after otolaryngologic surgery. Anesth Analg 2002;94: 1188–93.

[55] Barden J, Edwards J, McQuay H, et al. Single dose oral celecoxib for postoperative pain. Cochrane Database Syst Rev 2003;2:CD004233.

[56] Ormrod D, Wellington K, Wagstaff A. Valdecoxib: new drug profile. Drugs 2002;62:2059–71.

[57] Joshi GP. Valdecoxib for the management of chronic and acute pain. Expert Rev Neurotherapeutics 2005;5:11–24.

[58] Daniels S, Desjardins P, Talwalker S, et al. The analgesic efficacy of valdecoxib vs. oxycodone/acetaminophen after oral surgery. Journal of the American Dental Association 2002;133:611–21.

[59] Fricke J, Varkalis J, Zwillich S, et al. Valdecoxib is more efficacious than rofecoxib in relieving pain associated with oral surgery. Am J Ther 2002;9:89–97.

[60] Christensen KS, Cawkwell GD. Valdecoxib versus rofecoxib in acute postsurgical pain: results of a randomized controlled trial. J Pain Symptom Manage 2004;27:460–70.

[61] Desjardins P, Shu V, Recker D, et al. A single preoperative oral dose of valdecoxib, a new cyclooxygenase-2 specific inhibitor, relieves post-oral surgery or bunionectomy pain. Anesthesiology 2002;97:565–73.

[62] Camu F, Beecher T, Recker D, et al. Valdecoxib, a COX-2-specific inhibitor, is an efficacious, opioid-sparing analgesic in patients undergoing hip arthroplasty. Am J Ther 2002;9:43–51.

[63] Reynolds LW, Hoo RK, Brill RJ, et al. The COX-2 specific inhibitor, valdecoxib, is an effective, opioid-sparing analgesic in patients undergoing total knee arthroplasty. J Pain Symptom Manage 2003;25:133–41.

[64] Talley J, Bertenshaw S, Brown D, et al. N-[[(5-methyl-3-phenylisoxazol-4-yl)-phenyl] sulfonyl]propanamide, sodium salt, parecoxib sodium: a potent and selective inhibitor of COX-2 for parenteral administration. J Med Chem 2000;43:1661–3.

[65] Cheer S, Gao K. Parecoxib (parecoxib sodium). Drugs 2001;61:1133–41.

[66] Karim A, Laurent A, Slater M, et al. A pharmacokinetic study of intramuscular (i.m.) parecoxib sodium in normal subjects. J Clin Pharmacol 2001;41:1111–9.

[67] Daniels SE, Grossman EH, Kuss ME, et al. A double-blind, randomized comparison of intramuscularly and intravenously administered parecoxib sodium versus ketorolac and placebo in a post–oral surgery pain model. Clin Ther 2001;23:1018–31.

[68] Desjardins P, Grossman E, Kuss M, et al. The injectable cyclooxygenase-2-specific inhibitor paracoxib sodium has analgesic efficacy when administered preoperatively. Anesth Analg 2001;93:721–7.

[69] Mehlisch DR, Desjardins PJ, Daniels S, et al. Single doses of parecoxib sodium intravenously are as effective as ketorolac in reducing pain after oral surgery. J Oral Maxillofac Surg 2003;61:1030–7.

[70] Barton S, Langeland F, Snabes M, et al. Efficacy and safety of intravenous parecoxib sodium in relieving acute postoperative pain following gynecologic laparotomy surgery. Anesthesioloy 2002;97:306–14.

[71] Tang J, Li S, White P, et al. Effect of parecoxib, a novel intravenous cyclooxygenase type-2 inhibitor, on the postoperative opioid requirement and quality of pain control. Anesthesioloy 2002;96:1305–9.

[72] Ng A, Smith G, Davidson AC. Analgesic effects of parecoxib following total abdominal hysterectomy. Br J Anaesth 2003;90:746–9.

[73] Rasmussen G, Steckner K, Hogue C, et al. Intravenous parecoxib sodium for acute pain after orthopedic knee surgery. Am J Orthop 2002;31:336–43.

[74] Hubbard RC, Naumann TM, Traylor L, et al. Parecoxib sodium has opioid-sparing effects in patients undergoing total knee arthroplasty under spinal anaesthesia. Br J Anaesth 2003; 90:166–72.

[75] Malan TJ, Marsh G, Hakki S, et al. Parecoxib sodium, a parenteral cyclooxygenase 2 selective inhibitor, improves morphine analgesia and is opioid-sparing following total hip arthroplasty. Anesthesioloy 2003;98:950–6.

[76] Joshi GP, Viscusi ER, Gan TJ, et al. Effective treatment of laparoscopic cholecystectomy pain with intravenous followed by oral COX-2 specific inhibitor. Anesth Analg 2004;98:336–42.

[77] Gan TJ, Joshi GP, Zhao SZ, et al. Presurgical intravenous parecoxib sodium and follow-up oral valdecoxib for pain management after laparoscopic cholecystectomy surgery reduces opioid requirements and opioid-related adverse effects. Acta Anaesthesiol Scand 2004;48: 1194–207.

[78] Ott E, Nussmeier NA, Duke PC, et al. Efficacy and safety of the cyclooxygenase 2 inhibitors parecoxib and valdecoxib in patients undergoing coronary artery bypass surgery. J Thorac Cardiovasc Surg 2003;125:1481–92.

[79] Desjardins PJ, Grossman EH, Kuss ME, et al. The injectable cyclooxygenase-2-specific inhibitor parecoxib sodium has analgesic efficacy when administered preoperatively. Anesth Analg 2001;93:721–7.

[80] Kranke P, Morin AM, Roewer N, et al. Patients' global evaluation of analgesia and safety of injected parecoxib for postoperative pain: a quantitative systematic review. Anesth Analg 2004;99:797–806.

[81] Gajraj NM. Cyclooxygenase-2 inhibitors. Anesth Analg 2003;96:1720–38.

[82] Schafer A. Effects of nonsteroidal antiinflammatory drugs on platelet function and systemic hemostasis. J Clin Pharmacol 1995;35:209–19.

[83] Leese PT, Recker DP, Kent JD. The COX-2 selective inhibitor, valdecoxib, does not impair platelet function in the elderly: results of a randomized controlled trial. J Clin Pharmacol 2003;43:504–13.

[84] Leese PT, Talwalker S, Kent JD, et al. Valdecoxib does not impair platelet function. Am J Emerg Med 2002;20:275–81.

[85] Leese P, Hubbard R, Karim A, et al. Effects of celecoxib, a novel cyclooxygenase-2 inhibitor, on platelet function in healthy adults: a randomized, controlled trial. J Clin Pharmacol 2000; 40:124–32.

[86] Silverman DG, Halaszynski T, Sinatra R, et al. Rofecoxib does not compromise platelet aggregation during anesthesia and surgery [Le rofecoxib n'altere pas l'agregation plaquettaire pendant l'anesthesie et la chirurgie]. Can J Anesth 2003;50:1004–8.

[87] Noveck R, Laurent A, Kuss M, et al. The COX-2 specific inhibitor, parecoxib sodium, does not impair platelet function in healthy elderly and non-elderly individuals. Clin Drug Invest 2001;21:465–76.

[88] Noveck RJ, Hubbard RC. Parecoxib sodium, an injectable COX-2-specific inhibitor, does not affect unfractionated heparin-regulated blood coagulation parameters. J Clin Pharmacol 2004;44:474–80.

[89] Fries J. NSAID gastropathy: the second most deadly rheumatic disease: epidemiology and risk appraisal. J Rheumatol 1991;28:6–10.

[90] Wolfe M, Lichtenstein D, Singh D. Gastrointestinal toxicity of nonsteroidal ani-inflammatory drugs. N Engl J Med 1993;340:1888–99.

[91] Paulus H. FDA arthritis advisory committee meeting: postmarketing surveillance of nonsteroidal antiinflammatory drugs. Arthritis Rheum 1985;28:1168–9.

[92] Silverstein F, Graham D, Senior J, et al. Misoprostol reduces serious gastrointestinal complications in patients with rheumatoid arthritis receiving nonsteroidal anti-inflammatory drugs. Ann Intern Med 1995;123:241–9.

[93] Singh G, Rosen Ramey D. NSAID induced gastrointestinal complications: the ARAMIS perspective-1997. J Rheumatol 1998;51:8–16.

[94] Goldstein J. Lack of utility of risk factors in predicting symptomatic ulcers and ulcer complications on non-steroidal anti-inflammatory drugs (NSAIDs): analysis from the celecoxib long-term assessment of safety study (CLASS) [abstract]. Arthritis Rheum 2000;43:A481.

[95] Singh G, Ramey D, Morfeld D, et al. Gastrointestinal tract complications of nonsteroidal anti-inflammatory drug treatment in rheumatoid arthritis. Arch Intern Med 1996;156:1530–6.

[96] Langman M, Weil J, Wainwright P, et al. Risks of bleeding peptic ulcer associated with individual non-steroidal anti-inflammatory drugs. Lancet 1994;343:1075–8.

[97] Gabriel S, Jaakkimainen L, Bombardier C. Risk for serious gastrointestinal complications related to the use of nonsteroidal anti-inflammatory drugs: a meta-analysis. Ann Intern Med 1991;115:787–96.

[98] Griswold D, Adams J. Constitutive cyclooxygenase (COX-1) and inducible cyclooxygenase (COX-2): rationale for selective inhibition and progress to date. Med Res Rev 1996;16:181–206.

[99] Prasit P, Riendeau D. Selective cyclooxygenase 2 inhibitors. Annual Reports in Medicinal Chemistry 1997;30:179–88.

[100] Simon L, Lanza F, Lipsky P, et al. Preliminary study of the safety and efficacy of SC-58635, a novel cyclooxygenase 2 inhibitor: efficacy and safety in two placebo-controlled trials in osteoarthritis, and studies of gastrointestinal and platelet effects. Arthritis Rheum 1998;41:1591–602.

[101] Lanza F, Rack M, Simon T, et al. Specific inhibition of cyclooxgenase-2 with MK-0966 is associated with less gastroduodenal damage than either aspirin or ibuprofen. Aliment Pharmacol Ther 1999;13:761–7.

[102] Harris S, Kuss M, Hubbard R, et al. Upper gastrointestinal safety evaluation of paracoxib sodium, a new parenteral cyclooxygenase-2-specific inhibitor, compared with ketorolac, naproxen, and placebo. Clin Ther 2001;23:1422–8.

[103] Wolfe F, Anderson J, Burke T, et al. Gastroprotective therapy and risk of gastrointestinal ulcers: risk reduction by COX-2 therapy. J Rheumatol 2002;29:467–73.

[104] Bombardier C. An evidence-based evaluation of the gastrointestinal safety of coxibs. Am J Cardiol 2002;89:3–9.

[105] Goldstein J, Silverstein F, Agraval N, et al. Reduced risk of upper gastrointestinal ulcer complications with celecoxib, a novel COX-2 inhibitor. Am J Gastroenterol 2000;95:1681–90.

[106] Masferrer J, Zweifel B, Manning P, et al. Selective inhibition of inducible cyclooxygenase-2 in vivo is antiinflammatory and nonulcerogenic. Pro Natl Acad Sci U S A 1994;91:3228–32.

[107] Jacobsen RB, Phillips BB. Reducing clinically significant gastrointestinal toxicity associated with nonsteroidal antiinflammatory drugs. Ann Pharmacother 2004;38:1469–81.

[108] Silverstein F, Faich G, Goldstein J, et al. Gastrointestinal toxicity with celecoxib vs nonsteroidal anti-inflammatory drugs for osteoarthritis and rheumatoid arthritis; the CLASS study: a randomized controlled trial. JAMA 2000;284:1247–55.

[109] Goldstein J, Kivitz A, Verburg K, et al. A comparison of the upper gastrointestinal mucosal effects of valdecoxib, naproxen and placebo in healthy elderly subjects. Aliment Pharmacol Ther 2003;18:125–32.

[110] Harris S, Kuss M, Hubbard R, et al. Upper gastrointestinal safety evaluation of parecoxib sodium, a new parenteral cyclooxygenase-2-specific inhibitor, compared with ketorolac, naproxen, and placebo. Clin Ther 2001;23:1422–8.

[111] Johnson A. NSAIDs and increased blood pressure: what is the clinical significance? Drug Saf 1997;17:277–89.

[112] Frishman W. Effects of nonsteroidal anti-inflammatory drug therapy on blood pressure and peripheral edema. Am J Cardiol 2002;89:18–25.

[113] Perazella M, Tray K. Selective cyclooxygenase-2 inhibitors: a pattern of nephrotoxicity similar to traditional nonsteroidal anti-inflammatory drugs. Am J Med 2001;111:64–9.

[114] Guan Y, Chang M, Cho W, et al. Cloning, expression, and regulation of rabbit cyclo-ooxygenase-2 in renal medullary interstitial cells. Am J Physiol 1997;273:F18–26.

[115] Harris R, Breyer M. Physiologic regulation of cyclooxygenase-2 in the kidney. Am J Renal Physiol 2001;281:F1–11.

[116] Heyneman CA, Sandhu GK. Nephrotoxic potential of selective cyclooxygenase-2 inhibitors. Ann Pharmacother 2004;38:700–4.

[117] Barkin R, Buvanendran A. Focus on the COX-1 and COX-2 agents: renal events of nonsteroidal and anti-inflammatory drugs-NSAIDs. Am J Ther 2004;11:124–9.

[118] Komers R, Anderson S, Epstein M. Renal and cardiovascular effects of selective cyclo-oxygenase-2-inhibitors. Am J Kidney Dis 2001;38:1145–57.

[119] Cheng HF, Harris RC. Cyclooxygenases, the kidney, and hypertension. Hypertension 2004;43: 525–30.

[120] Weber A, Casini A, Heine A, et al. Unexpected nanomolar inhibition of carbonic anhydrase by COX-2-selective celecoxib: new pharmacological opportunities due to related binding site recognition. J Med Chem 2004;47:550–7.

[121] Supuran C, Casini A, Mastrolorenzo A, et al. COX-2 selective inhibitors, carbonic anhydrase inhibition and anticancer properties of sulfonamides belonging to this class of pharmacological agents. Mini Rev Med Chem 2004;4:625–32.

[122] Whelton A, Schulman G, Wallemark C, et al. Effects of celecoxib and naproxen on renal function in the elderly. Arch Intern Med 2000;160:1465–70.

[123] Swan S, Rudy D, Lasseter K, et al. Effect of cyclooxygenase-2 inhibition on renal function in elderly persons receiving a low-salt diet: a randomized controlled trial. Ann Intern Med 2000;133:1–9.

[124] Catella-Lawson F, McAdam B, Morrison B, et al. Effects of specific inhibition of cyclooxygenase-2 on sodium balance, hemodynamics, and vasoactive eicosanoids. J Pharmacol Exp Ther 1999;289:735–41.

[125] Whelton A, Fort J, Puma J, et al. Cyclo-oxygenase-2-specific inhibitors and cardiorenal function: a randomized, controlled trial of celecoxib and rofecoxib in older hypertensive osteoarthritis patients. Am J Ther 2001;8:85–95.

[126] Yusuf S, Sleight P, Pogue J, et al. Effects of an angiotensin-converting-enzyme inhibitor, ramipril, on cardiovascular events in high-risk patients. N Engl J Med 2000;342:145–53.

[127] ALLHAT Collaborative Research Group. Major cardiovascular events in hypertensive patients randomized to doxazosin vs chlorthalidone: the antihypertensive and lipid-lowering treatment to prevent heart attack trial (ALLHAT). JAMA 2000;283:1967–75.

[128] SHEP Cooperative Research Group. Prevention of stroke by antihypertensive drug treatment in older persons with isolated systolic hypertension: final results of the systolic hypertension in the elderly program (SHEP). JAMA 1991;265:3255–64.

[129] Whelton A, White W, Bello A, et al. Effects of celecoxib and rofecoxib on blood pressure and edema in patients $\geq$ 65 years of age with systemic hypertension and osteoarthritis. Am J Cardiol 2002;90:959–63.

[130] Ray WA, Stein CM, Daugherty JR, et al. COX-2 selective non-steroidal anti-inflammatory drugs and risk of serious coronary heart disease. Lancet 2002;360:1071–3.

[131] Becker R, Burke T, McCoy M, et al. A model analysis of costs of blood pressure destabilization and edema associated with rofecoxib and celecoxib among older patients with osteoarthritis and hypertension in a medicare choice population. Clin Ther 2003;25:647–62.

[132] Cho J, Cooke C, Proveaux W. A retrospective review of the effect of COX-2 inhibitors on blood pressure change. Am J Ther 2003;10:311–7.

[133] Solomon DH, Schneeweiss S, Levin R, et al. Relationship between COX-2 specific inhibitors and hypertension. Hypertension 2004;44:140–5.

[134] Mukherjee D, Nissen S, Topol E. Risk of cardiovascular events associated with selective COX-2 inhibitors. JAMA 2001;286:954–9.

[134a] Food and Drug Administration. Vioxx gastrointestinal outcome research (VIGOR) Arthritis Advisory Committee meeting, February 8, 2001. Available at: http://www.fda.gov/ohrms/dockets/ac/01/slides/3677s2_02_villalba/. Accessed December 22, 2004.

[135] Fitzgerald G. Cardiovascular pharmacology of nonselective nonsteroidal anti-inflammatory drugs and coxibs: clinical considerations. Am J Cardiol 2002;89:26–32.

[136] Konstam MA, Weir MR, Reicin A, et al. Cardiovascular thrombotic events in controlled, clinical trials of rofecoxib. Circulation 2001;104:2280–8.

[137] Solomon DH, Schneeweiss S, Glynn RJ, et al. Relationship between selective cyclooxygenase-2 inhibitors and acute myocardial infarction in older adults. Circulation 2004;109: 2068–73.

[138] White WB, Faich G, Borer JS, et al. Cardiovascular thrombotic events in arthritis trials of the cyclooxygenase-2 inhibitor celecoxib. Am J Cardiol 2003;92:411–8.

[139] White W, Strand V, Roberts R, et al. Effects of the cyclooxygenase-2 specific inhibitor valdecoxib versus nonsteroidal antiinflammatory agents and placebo on cardiovascular thrombotic events in patients with arthritis. Am J Ther 2004;11:244–50.

[140] Mamdani M, Juurlink DN, Lee DS, et al. Cyclo-oxygenase-2 inhibitors versus non-selective non-steroidal anti-inflammatory drugs and congestive heart failure outcomes in elderly patients: a population-based cohort study. Lancet 2004;363:1751–6.

[141] Mamdani M, Rochon P, Juurlink DN, et al. Effect of selective cyclooxygenase 2 inhibitors and naproxen on short-term risk of acute myocardial infarction in the elderly. Arch Intern Med 2003;163:481–6.

[142] Rofecoxib APPROVE study results and their implications. Presented at the 68th Annual Meeting of the American College of Rheumatology. 2004.

[143] Shinmura K, Tang X-L, Wang Y, et al. Cyclooxygenase-2 mediates the cardioprotective effects of the late phase of ischemic preconditioning in conscious rabbits. Proc Natl Acad Sci U S A 2000;97:10197–202.

[144] Ho M, Chang J, Wang G. Anti-inflammatory drug effects on bone repair and remodeling in rabbits. Clin Orthop 1995;13:270–8.

[145] Maxy R, Glassman S. The effect of nonsteroidal anti-inflammatory drugs on osteogenesis and spinal fusion. Reg Anesth Pain Med 2001;26:156–8.

[146] Endo K, Sairyo K, Komatsubara S. Cyclooxygenase-2 Inhibitor inhibits the fracture healing. J Physiol Anthropol 2002;21:235–8.

[147] Deguchi M, Rapoff A, Zdeblick T. Posterolateral fusion for isthmic spondylolisthesis in adults: a study of fusion rate and clinical results. J Spinal Disord 1998;11:459–64.

[148] Dimar J, Ante W, Zhang Y, et al. The effects of nonsteroidal anti-inflammatory drugs on posterior spinal fusions in the rat. Spine 1996;21:1870–6.

[149] Glassman S, Rose S, Dimar J, et al. The effect of postoperative nonsteroidal anti-inflammatory drug administration on spinal fusion. Spine 1998;23:834–8.

[150] Long J, Lewis S, Kuklo T, et al. The effect of cyclooxygenase-2 inhibitors on spinal fusion. J Bone Joint Surg Am 2002;84:1763–8.

[151] Zhang X, Morham S, Langenbach R, et al. Evidence for a direct role of cyclo-oxygenase 2 in implant wear debris-induced osteolysis. J Bone Miner Res 2001;16:660–70.

[152] Simon A, Manigrasso M, O'Connor J. Cyclo-oxygenase 2 function is essential for bone fracture healing. J Bone Miner Res 2002;17:963–76.

[153] Bakker AD, Klein-Nulend J, Burger EH. Mechanotransduction in bone cells proceeds via activation of COX-2, but not COX-1. Biochem Biophys Res Commun 2003;305:677–83.

[154] Seidenberg A, An Y. Is there an inhibitory effect of COX-2 inhibitors on bone healing? Pharmacol Res 2004;50:151–6.

[155] Allami M, Giannoudis P. Cox inhibitors and bone healing. Acta Orthop Scand 2003;74: 771–2.

[156] Aspenberg P. Avoid cox inhibitors after skeletal surgery! Acta Orthop Scand 2002;73:489–90.

[157] Gajraj NM. The effect of cyclooxygenase-2 inhibitors on bone healing. Reg Anesth Pain Med 2003;28:456–65.

[158] Stenson W. Cyclooxygenase 2 and wound healing in the stomach. Gastroenterology 1997;112: 645–8.

[159] Sato T, Kirimura Y, Mori Y. The co-culture of dermal fibroblasts with human epidermal keratinocytes induces increased prostaglandin E2 production and cyclooxygenase 2 activity in fibroblasts. J Invest Dermatol 1997;109:334–9.

[160] Elder C, Dahners L, Weinhold P. A cyclooxygenase-2 inhibitor impairs ligament healing in the rat. Am J Sports Med 2001;29:801–5.

[161] Geba G, Polis A, Skalky C, et al. Gastrointestinal tolerability among patients receiving low dose aspirin in combination with rofecoxib or naproxen. Arthritis & Rheumatism 2002;46:S462.

[162] Mersfelder T, Stewart L. Warfarin and celecoxib interaction. Ann Pharmacother 2000;34: 325–7.

[163] Slordal L, Samstad S, Bathen J, et al. A life-threatening interaction between lithium and celecoxib. Br J Clin Pharmacol 2003;55:413.

[164] Kruse R, Ruzicka T, Grewe M, et al. Intolerance reactions due to the selective cyclooxygenase type II inhibitors rofecoxib and celecoxib: results of oral provocation tests in patients with NSAID hypersensitivity. Acta Derm Venereol 2003;83:183–5.

[165] Martin-Garcia C, Hinojosa M, Berges P, et al. Safety of a cyclooxygenase-2 inhibitor in patients with aspirin sensitive asthma. Chest 2002;121:1812–7.

[166] Stevenson D, Simon R. Lack of cross-reactivity between rofecoxib and aspirin-sensitive patients with asthma. J Allergy Clin Immunol 2001;108:47–51.

[167] West P, Fernandez C. Safety of COX-2 inhibitors in asthma patients with aspirin hypersensitivity. Ann Pharmacother 2003;37:1497–501.

[168] Carey MA, Germolec DR, Bradbury JA, et al. Accentuated T helper type 2 airway response after allergen challenge in cyclooxygenase-1$^{-/-}$ but not cyclooxygenase-2$^{-/-}$ mice. Am J Respir Crit Care Med 2003;167:1509–15.

[169] Walley T, Coleman J. Allergic drug reactions: incidence and avoidance. Clinical Immunotherapy 1994;1:101–9.

[170] Cribb A, Lee B, Trepanler L, et al. Adverse reactions to sulphonamide and sulphonamide-trimethoprim antimicrobials: clinical syndromes and pathogenesis. Adverse Drug Reactions and Toxicological Reviews 1996;15:9–50.

[171] Slappendel R, Weber E, Bugter M, et al. The intensity of preoperaive pain is directly correlated with the amount of morphine needed for postoperative analgesia. Anesth Analg 1999;88:146–8.

[172] Stephens J, Laskin B, Pashos C, et al. The burden of acute postoperative pain and the potential role of the COX-2-specific inhibitors. Rheumatology 2003;42:40–52.

[173] Verrico M, Weber R, McKaveney T, et al. Adverse drug events involving COX-2 inhibitors. Ann Pharmacother 2003;37:1203–13.

[174] Cox E, Motheral B, Frisse M, et al. Prescribing COX-2s for patients new to cyclooxygenase inhibition therapy. Am J Manag Care 2003;9:735–42.

[175] Sunshine A. A comparison of the newer COX-2 drugs and older nonnarcotic oral analgesics. J Pain 2000;1:10–3.

[176] Lipsky P, Brooks P, Crofford L, et al. Unresolved issues in the role of cyclooxygenase-2 in normal physiologic processes and disease. Arch Intern Med 2000;160:913–30.

[177] Bannwarth B. Selective COX-2 inhibitors: do they retain any gastroduodenal toxicity. Gastroenterol Clin Biol 2004;28:C90–5.

ELSEVIER
SAUNDERS

Anesthesiology Clin N Am
23 (2005) 73–84

ANESTHESIOLOGY
CLINICS OF
NORTH AMERICA

Clinical Pharmacology of Local Anesthetics

J. Lee White, MD, Marcel E. Durieux, MD, PhD*

*Department of Anesthesiology, University of Virginia Health System, Box 800710,
Charlottesville, VA 22908, USA*

Local anesthetics have for many years served an essential function in post-operative pain management. The development, several decades ago, of a range of compounds with varying durations made flexible clinical application possible. Lidocaine and bupivacaine came to the forefront as the most useful of these drugs and firmly established themselves in the anesthesiologist's armamentarium. Their mechanism of action, the sodium (Na) channel blockade, was clearly defined [1]. For quite some time, therefore, most practitioners were convinced that not only did we know all about local anesthetics, which we needed to know for safe clinical practice, but also that the clinically available local anesthetics were sufficiently flexible; no new compounds would be required. In short, local anesthetic pharmacology was complete. However, this viewpoint has turned out to be wrong.

Unexpected local anesthetic toxicity

Almost 20 years ago, a series of unsuccessful resuscitations after cardiac arrest associated with the use of bupivacaine in pregnant women made it abundantly clear that the compounds were not as innocuous as we believed them to be. Although the toxicity of bupivacaine was largely resolved by adjusting the concentrations used in clinical practice, these issues led to studies that identified a stereoselective action of the drug on the heart and, subsequently, to two new local anesthetics, ropivacaine and levobupivacaine [2]. At the end of the 1990s, another alarm sounded about lidocaine, the prototypical local anesthetic, which

* Corresponding author.
E-mail address: med2p@virginia.edu (M.E. Durieux).

0889-8537/05/$ – see front matter © 2005 Elsevier Inc. All rights reserved.
doi:10.1016/j.atc.2004.11.005
anesthesiology.theclinics.com

was shown to have neurotoxic properties. A disturbingly frequent rate of transient radicular irritation was reported as well as the, luckily, much rarer occurrence of cauda equina syndrome [3]. This issue is presently far from resolved. The affect of lidocaine is not altered by changing concentrations or doses, and no new drugs are on the horizon that can effectively fill the niche currently occupied by lidocaine. Hence, most practitioners continue to use the drug, although it is debatable if this is truly in the best interest of our patients.

Interestingly, the two issues were not anticipated. These drugs had been used and studied for decades without any clear indication that they carried such significant risks. This, of course, immediately begs the question whether more toxicity issues may be lurking in the shadows. Such may indeed be the case. For example, the myotoxic effects of bupivacaine are probably underestimated and are presently being investigated [4].

Nonetheless, currently, we observe a mindset similar to that of 20 years ago. Most practitioners feel that we have an adequate diversity of local anesthetics and that we understand their mechanisms of action and their side effects sufficiently well that no further drugs are needed. The pharmaceutical industry appears to feel the same way, and no new drugs are "in the pipeline."

These authors, however, believe this viewpoint is incorrect. We do need new drugs, and we will be facing potential safety issues that will require great vigilance and a major scientific effort to confront. This article attempts to project trends in the use and development of local anesthetics and explain why this is not the moment for us to believe that our local anesthetic drawer in the anesthesia cart is essentially complete.

The shift to outpatient surgery

We are in the midst of a major shift in surgical practice. For a variety of reasons ranging from patient preference to cost [5], surgery is changing from an inpatient to an outpatient activity. In the United States, more than 70% of all surgical procedures are being performed on an outpatient basis. The type of procedures that can be performed on an outpatient basis depends more on the postoperative requirements for specialized care, pain relief, and the risk of postoperative complications than on intraoperative factors. In clinical practice, it has become clear that the reasons for unplanned hospital admission or readmission are pain and nausea (and the two are probably closely related). Thus, it is now recognized that anesthesia-related rather than surgically related factors influence the ability to perform more invasive procedures on an outpatient basis. Therefore, we will need to respond to this challenge and develop methodologies that allow us to provide several days of effective and safe relief of moderate to severe pain for the unmonitored patients at home. It is clear that local anesthetic techniques, particularly peripheral nerve blockade, will be one of the cornerstones of postoperative pain management.

The approaches for local anesthetic techniques are divided into two approaches. One approach is the use of novel delivery techniques for existing drugs. For example, liposome encapsulation of local anesthetics [6] or catheter techniques that can be safely used at home [7]. The second approach is the development of novel, extremely long-acting local anesthetics [8]. However, it is likely that the most effective techniques may combine both approaches. The following sections discuss these new concepts for local anesthetic techniques.

Novel delivery techniques for currently available local anesthetics

It is likely that further modification of the molecular structure of currently available local anesthetics will not lead to a safe and ultra-long-lasting agent. However, two novel drug delivery vehicles that will allow clinicians to "stretch out" the duration of analgesia with local anesthetics already in clinical use show great promise. One method involves the continuous infusion of a local anesthetic through a peripheral nerve catheter, which presently is the only method available to provide prolonged analgesia. The other delivery vehicle, under development and investigation, involves loading local anesthetics into either a liposome or a microcapsule glycoprotein matrix [6].

Encapsulated drugs

Liposomal drug delivery techniques are currently being used for a variety of medications, including chemotherapeutic drugs and antifungal agents [9–13]. Although the use of epidural liposomal bupivacaine has been reported in human cancer and surgical patients, no commercial product is presently available on the market [14,15]. Liposomes are similar in structure to animal cell membranes and are formed when amphipathic lipid molecules are dissolved in an aqueous medium and form a lipid bilayer surrounding an aqueous compartment. Local anesthetics can be loaded into either the aqueous or lipid phases for later release after being injected into biological tissue. The release of the local anesthetic is in turn affected by a number of factors including the size of the vesicle (small vesicles, less than 120 nm, tend to be rapidly redistributed from the site of injection), the structure of the vesicle, which is characterized by the number of lipid bilayers present (single bilayer [unilamellar] or multiple bilayers [multilamellar]), as well as the composition of the lipid layer. For instance, the presence of cholesterol in the membrane layer influences the permeability of the lipid membrane layer, which in turn will influence the release rate of the encapsulated drug. Multilamellar vesicles as well as multivesicular vesicles (vesicles within vesicles) will also tend to favor a slower drug release than unilamellar or single vesicle solutions.

Of importance is the drug to lipid ratio (D:PL) within the liposome that determines the volume of drug to be injected. Lower D:PL ratios necessitate a larger volume of drug to achieve the desired effect. A very low D:PL ratio would make the use of the compound impractical in certain clinical situations because the volume of the lipid-anesthetic solution would be too large. It is possible that this can be overcome through the use of a novel formulation process that achieves higher D:PL ratios than conventional methods by concentrating bupivacaine into multivesicular liposomes within large aqueous compartments [16].

Animal studies showing a lack of histopathologic neural lesions after the injection of liposomal bupivacaine must be tempered by other studies showing that certain products formed during the manufacture and metabolism of liposomes are potentially neurotoxic [17–19]. Of concern also are the stability of the liposome once injected and the subsequent rate at which the liposome releases the drug. Obviously, too slow a release will result in inadequate analgesia. Of greater concern, however, is the sudden release of a large amount of local anesthetic that could result in systemic and local toxicity. Additional research will be needed to confirm the safety of these compounds before they can be adapted for a broad range of clinical uses in regional anesthesia.

Microcapsules composed of biodegradable polymers and serving as a matrix for the loading of local anesthetics have produced prolonged periods of analgesia after subcutaneous injection and intercostal nerve blockade [20,21]. Pedersen et al [22] recently demonstrated a dose-dependent duration of analgesia up to 96 hours in human volunteers after a subcutaneous injection of bupivacaine and dexamethasone loaded into microspheres made of polymers of polylactic-co-glycolic acid (PLGA).

The biocompatibility of microspheres is achieved with the use of naturally occurring polymers and monomers such as cellulose and glycolic acid. Drug release is affected by the physical structure and chemical properties of the microsphere and encapsulated drug. With degradation of the microcapsule polymer and diffusion of drug through the pores of the capsule being the major determinants of the rate of release of drug from the device. Other factors that affect drug release from the microcapsule include the molecular weight of the polymer, blends of different polymers within the capsule, porosity, size distribution, and crystallinity [23].

The use of PLGA has already been approved for in vivo degradation, and at least one animal study [24] (rat sciatic nerve) using PLGA microspheres containing bupivacaine to produce prolonged analgesia has shown plasma bupivacaine levels to be well below the toxic threshold. However, as with liposomal preparations, the results of additional studies examining the safety of these compounds, as well as their adaptability from laboratory formulation to large scale manufacturing processes, will ultimately determine the clinical fate of these novel drug preparations.

Catheter techniques

Presently, a continuous infusion of a local anesthetic through a peripheral nerve catheter is the only available method to deliver prolonged postoperative analgesia. Indeed, the use of peripheral nerve catheters is increasing both in the hospital and the outpatient setting as new technology makes the placement and management of these catheters more reliable and safe [7]. However, not all patients need a peripheral nerve catheter for postoperative pain control, and it is the identification of patients who will benefit most from prolonged infusions of local anesthetics that is the subject of debate and study. It would seem logical that patients undergoing surgeries that are characterized by extensive postoperative pain and rehabilitation requirements would benefit the most from a continuous catheter technique. This was the finding of one study [25] that showed that not only was hospital stay shortened, but, more importantly, the total number of days spent in rehabilitation was substantially reduced.

Just as catheter techniques are not appropriate for every patient, these devices are also not suited for every anesthesiologist or practice situation. Current catheter techniques are cumbersome, labor intensive, require additional training, and are time consuming. The recent introduction of a catheter (Stimucath, Arrow International, Reading, Pennsylvania) that can be attached to a nerve stimulator to guide its placement is receiving increasing acceptance. Studies are now beginning to appear showing that these catheters have an advantage over blindly inserted catheters in the ease and accuracy of placement [26]. It can be expected that the number of physicians who use this technique will increase as the clinical advantages of peripheral nerve catheters become more apparent and the technical aspects of insertion become less daunting.

What will the future bring? The intuitive appeal of a single injection of a long-acting local anesthetic that is safe and provides a predictable period of analgesia with little or no motor block is obvious; a quick and efficient method for providing prolonged postoperative analgesia that does not require a significant investment in training, manpower, time, and precious facility resources. In such a case, the simple and familiar steps involved in performing a peripheral nerve block remain unaltered. Are catheters merely a bridge between the local anesthetic agents of today and the ultra-long–acting agent of tomorrow? Maybe, but one distinct advantage that a catheter has over any single injection technique is its flexibility: the infusion can be stopped, increased, or decreased at any time. Undoubtedly, the knowledge we gain from the use of peripheral nerve catheters will guide our use of that elusive ultra-long–acting agent whenever it should arrive. Until then, we will have to continue to use a combination of single injection and catheter techniques to optimally care for our patients.

Long-lasting local anesthetics

Presently, although a number of compounds are under investigation, there is no drug that appears likely to make it to market as a truly ultra-long–acting local anesthetic. It is of little benefit, therefore, to discuss the specifics of the chemistry involved. Instead, discussion will focus on some general concepts of importance in the development and clinical testing of such drugs.

Historically, local anesthetic techniques focused on short and relatively limited types of surgical procedures. Office-based procedures and dentistry, in which the operator performs the anesthesia using local anesthetic, are typical examples. Subarachnoid anesthesia is limited in duration to a few hours at most and is not the preferred technique for procedures with anticipated major physiologic trespass. The introduction of epidural catheter techniques allowed anesthesia of essentially unlimited duration, but even then anesthesiologists were hesitant to use epidural local anesthesia as the sole technique for procedures of more than several hours duration.

A major change in practice occurred when postoperative analgesia using epidural techniques was introduced. Now patients were exposed to local anesthetics for days. The pharmacologic effects of this change in practice have, in the authors' opinion, been insufficiently investigated, and this becomes particularly pertinent when dealing with extremely long-lasting drugs. In this section we will discuss separately the potential toxicity issues and the potential beneficial effects related to prolonged nerve blockade.

A key point in this discussion is the concept that many of the relevant actions that will be discussed depend not on the blockade of Na channels, the classic local anesthetic action, but instead on interactions at other sites (ie, non-Na channel actions [NNCA]). The NNCA are likely to become more relevant in drugs with very long duration of action, as explained below.

Toxicity issues

Although scientists have tried for decades to synthesize a longer-acting local anesthetic or to modify existing drugs and their pharmaceutical preparations to the same end, toxicity often paralleled the duration of effect of these newly developed compounds such that a compromise had to be struck between the duration of neural blockade and the potential for systemic and local toxicity. For example, a procaine-peanut oil preparation—while prolonging analgesia—was also found to be a potent allergen, a local tissue irritant, and extremely neurotoxic causing transverse myelitis after the peanut oil was transported centrally along the nerve [27].

For several reasons, the safety of the local anesthetics will be a major issue, particularly with compounds that remain active for several days. First, although most Na channel actions are not time-dependent, NNCA effects can have pronounced time-dependent effects. For example, the inhibitory effects of local anesthetics on cell receptors and neutrophil functions (see below) are greatly enhanced if the cells are incubated in the local anesthetics for hours rather than minutes [28]. Bupivacaine inhibits the signaling of thromboxane A_2 receptors by 10% after a 1-hour incubation and blocks the same receptors by 75% after 24 hours' incubation. Similarly, superoxide production in neutrophils primed with platelet-activating factor is essentially unaffected by a 10- to 30-minute incubation in low concentrations of bupivacaine, but these same concentrations depress neutrophil function by more than 60% after 6 hours' incubation. The mechanism behind this increased sensitivity after prolonged incubation rests in a time-dependent block by local anesthetics of Gq proteins at the cell membrane [29]. The clinical implication of these laboratory findings is that toxic actions that might be trivial when the compounds are administered for several hours may become greatly exaggerated and relevant when drugs are administered for a longer duration.

Second, compounds from novel drug classes may be used in concentrations or methods previously not administered clinically. For example, antidepressants, such as amitriptyline, have a structural similarity to local anesthetics and extremely long-lasting Na channel-blocking effects and thus provide prolonged skin anesthesia after cutaneous injection [30]. However, the concentrations required for these actions are orders of magnitude greater than when it is administered orally for indications such as depression or chronic pain. Hence, it is quite possible that these drugs may have effects not noticed previously. Recent animal and human studies [31] indicate that amitriptyline and related compounds administered at high concentrations may be associated with neuronal damage, and as a result, the compound has become a less likely candidate for local injection. We will return to this issue later.

Third, and maybe most importantly, we will be providing prolonged regional anesthesia to unmonitored patients in the home. If complications occur at home, no immediate expert help will be available. Even for the family physician, the complications from such highly specialized techniques might provide a serious challenge. Because of the setting where these approaches will be used, the requirement for demonstrated safety is greatly increased.

All of these factors interact, and it is imperative therefore that we define clearly the burden of proof required before a local anesthetic or new technique can be used in clinical practice. Therefore, it seems reasonable that the standards should exceed those used for approving drugs used in the highly monitored clinical setting. Whether this viewpoint is taken in reality is not so clear. Frequently, it seems to be assumed too easily that novel drugs with Na channel-blocking activity will have side effects similar to those of classic local anesthetics. Such is not necessarily the case. For example, antidepressants, when applied in the concentrations used when the compounds are injected for local anesthesia, have been shown to be lethal to neutrophils, whereas classic local anesthetics at such concentrations do not affect neutrophil viability [32]. The clinical impact of this finding has not yet been investigated, but one wonders what the effect on infection rates might be when neutrophils around a fresh surgical wound are eliminated by injecting a long acting local anesthetic.

Beneficial actions

Classic local anesthetics are likely to have a number of potentially beneficial effects that may not be necessarily shared by novel compounds. Although local anesthetics are used for their Na channel blockade, NNCA may also play an important role in clinical practice. However, the novel compounds may not only lack the NNCA effects of classic local anesthetics but may have NNCA that these local anesthetics lack.

One of the beneficial actions of local anesthetics that may not be shared by novel compounds is their inflammatory modulating action. This effect has been demonstrated in a number of clinical and animal studies [33]. This action most likely results in part from a subtle modulation of neutrophil function. Neutrophils, when activated by certain agonists, generate superoxide, which effectively kills invading bacteria. In addition to being activated, neutrophils can also be "primed." This refers to a process in which exposure to certain agonists does not itself induce superoxide release but greatly enhances superoxide production when the cells are subsequently activated [34]. It is as if a degree of "hypersensitization" is induced in the cell. Although priming might be quite useful in the setting of massive bacterial contamination, it is likely to be primarily detrimental in the surgical setting, where bacteria are essentially absent, and the increased superoxide formation only results in more host tissue damage. Indeed, priming has been shown to be a pathogenic factor in disease states such as acute respiratory distress syndrome. Local anesthetics selectively inhibit priming without affecting activation. This allows the neutrophil to function normally but prevents the hypersensitization that may lead to tissue damage. This effect is not Na channel-dependent (and in fact occurs at concentrations much lower than those required for Na channel blockade) and instead seems to be mediated by local anesthetic interactions with G protein signaling [35]. In addition, the effect is profoundly time-dependent, as mentioned above [28].

Numerous studies have demonstrated the clinical relevance of the inflammatory modulating activities of local anesthetics. In fact, it is suggested that some of beneficial effects of epidurally administered local anesthetic are caused by the anti-inflammatory action of local anesthetics absorbed into the blood stream [36]. This can be demonstrated by mimicking these effects by intravenous administration of low doses of local anesthetics. Cooke et al [37] have shown that the antithrombotic action (which is in essence an anti-inflammatory action) of epidural anesthesia can be mimicked by using intravenous lidocaine; the rate of deep venous thrombosis in patients undergoing hip replacement was reduced from 78% in the control group to 14% in the lidocaine-treated group. Groudine et al [38] studied the duration of postoperative ileus, which is essentially a response to the sterile inflammation induced by bowel manipulation, in patients undergoing prostatectomy. Those patients who received lidocaine intraoperatively and for 1 hour in the postanesthesia care unit had a 1-day earlier return of bowel function and were discharged from the hospital 1 day earlier than the control group (Fig. 1). These patients also had significantly less pain throughout their hospital course. This is in accordance with several other studies reporting decreased secondary hyperalgesia during local anesthetic infusion in experimental pain models [39]. In all these studies, local anesthetics were infused to the concentrations attained in blood during epidural anesthesia. Together, they

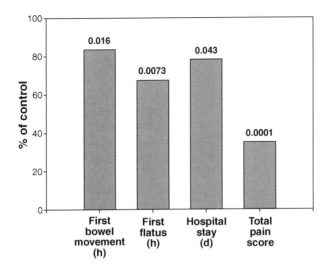

Fig. 1. Effect of intraoperative intravenous lidocaine infusion on bowel function, hospital stay, and pain after prostatectomy. Probability (*P*) values compared with placebo control are indicated above the bars. (*Data from* Groudine SB, Fisher HA, Kaufman RP Jr, et al. Intravenous lidocaine speeds the return of bowel function, decreases postoperative pain, and shortens hospital stay in patients undergoing radical retropubic prostatectomy. Anesth Analg 1998;86:235–9.)

indicate that at least part of the antithrombotic and analgesic actions of epidural anesthesia, as well as the beneficial effect on bowel function, are likely to result from anti-inflammatory action of absorbed local anesthetic rather than from the blockade of nerve transmission near the spinal cord. These actions are not mediated by Na channels and are therefore not necessarily mimicked by other compounds, even if they show similar Na channel-blocking activity.

Other actions of local anesthetics (eg, neuroprotective properties) are less established but are also possibly caused by NNCA. Local anesthetics in low concentrations significantly reduce cerebral infarct size after transient focal ischemia in rats [40,41] and have been shown to decrease the incidence of neuropsychologic dysfunction after cardiac surgery [42]. Local anesthetics are also effective in preventing the development of chronic pain after mastectomy [43].

The essential point is that novel compounds may not share these effects. For example, low concentrations (such as would be present in the blood during intravenous infusion) of antidepressants have been shown not to interfere with priming of neutrophils [32]. If priming inhibition is indeed a major part of the inflammatory modulating action of local anesthetics, it is conceivable that antidepressants may not provide the beneficial effects of local anesthetics on bowel function, coagulation, and even pain. Therefore, they should not be considered equivalent to existing local anesthetics unless these issues have been carefully investigated.

Summary

Our patients and surgical colleagues will be at our doorstep, asking us to provide intense, effective postoperative analgesia for long duration in patients undergoing major procedures in the ambulatory setting. It should be clear from the discussion above that we certainly do not presently have available a complement of local anesthetics and administration techniques required to serve us adequately in this task. Our current compounds may be satisfactory when they are applied in innovative ways (and catheter techniques are the main approach here), but in addition we will need new, much longer-acting local anesthetics than those available currently. It should also be clear that many safety issues will have to be addressed before we can confidently send patients home who have been treated with novel drugs and techniques (Table 1). Based on the comments above, we propose the following research plan.

Develop long-acting local anesthetics and delivery techniques. Without them, we will not be able to provide adequate care to our day surgery patients in the future. Test potential candidate compounds and techniques carefully for safety, both after short-term and long-term administration. We should be careful not to limit ourselves to side effects already known from our present compounds but look for unanticipated toxic actions. Determine the NNCA of the novel compounds. This may be particularly difficult, because even the NNCA of the presently available local anesthetics are largely unknown. Determine which beneficial and detrimental effects result from these NNCA. On this basis, make the decision about which compounds are suitable for further development as clinical, long-lasting local anesthetics. Finally, it is conceivable that drugs can be developed in which NNCA and Na channel blocking are separated (eg, a compound that inhibits neutrophil priming but does not block Na channels). Such compounds (which by definition would no longer be local anesthetics) might prove highly useful perioperative therapeutics in their own right.

Table 1
The road to long-lasting local anesthesia

	Advantages	Disadvantages
Catheter techniques	Flexibility	Technical complexity; potential for nerve damage
Encapsulated local anesthetics	Ease of application	No preparations currently clinically available; potential toxicity (with inadvertent fast release)
Novel long-lasting compounds	Ease of application; potential new beneficial non-Na channel-dependent effects	Potential toxicity; loss of beneficial non-Na channel-dependent effects; potential detrimental non-Na channel-dependent effects

References

[1] Butterworth JFt, Strichartz GR. Molecular mechanisms of local anesthesia: a review. Anesthesiology 1990;72:711-34.

[2] Graf BM. The cardiotoxicity of local anesthetics: the place of ropivacaine. Curr Top Med Chem 2001;1:207-14.

[3] Johnson ME. Potential neurotoxicity of spinal anesthesia with lidocaine. Mayo Clin Proc 2000; 75:921-32.

[4] Zink W, Seif C, Bohl JR, et al. The acute myotoxic effects of bupivacaine and ropivacaine after continuous peripheral nerve blockades. Anesth Analg 2003;97:1173-9.

[5] Nielsen KC, Steele SM. Outcome after regional anesthesia in the ambulatory setting-is it really worth it? Best Pract Res Clin Anaesthesiol 2002;16:145-57.

[6] Grant SA. The holy grail: long-acting local anaesthetics and liposomes. Best Pract Res Clin Anaesthesiol 2002;16:345-52.

[7] Enneking FK, Ilfeld BM. Major surgery in the ambulatory environment: continuous catheters and home infusions. Best Pract Res Clin Anaesthesiol 2002;16:285-94.

[8] Hollmann M, Durieux M, Graf B. Novel local anaesthetics and novel indications for local anaesthetics. Curr Opin Anaesthesiol 2001;14:741-9.

[9] Sharpe M, Easthope SE, Keating GM, et al. Polyethylene glycol-liposomal doxorubicin: a review of its use in the management of solid and haematological malignancies and AIDS-related Kaposi's sarcoma. Drugs 2002;62:2089-126.

[10] Hengge UR, Esser S, Rudel HP, et al. Long-term chemotherapy of HIV-associated Kaposi's sarcoma with liposomal doxorubicin. Eur J Cancer 2001;37:878-83.

[11] Arndt D, Zeisig R, Bechtel D, et al. Liposomal bleomycin: increased therapeutic activity and decreased pulmonary toxicity in mice. Drug Deliv 2001;8:1-7.

[12] Handzel O, Landau Z, Halperin D. Liposomal amphotericin B treatment for rhinocerebral mucormycosis: how much is enough? Rhinology 2003;41:184-6.

[13] Maesaki S. Drug delivery system of anti-fungal and parasitic agents. Curr Pharm Des 2002; 8:433-40.

[14] Lafont ND, Legros FJ, Boogaerts JG. Use of liposome-associated bupivacaine in a cancer pain syndrome. Anaesthesia 1996;51:578-9.

[15] Boogaerts JG, Lafont ND, Declercq AG, et al. Epidural administration of liposome-associated bupivacaine for the management of postsurgical pain: a first study. J Clin Anesth 1994;6:315-20.

[16] Grant GJ, Barenholz Y, Bolotin EM, et al. A novel liposomal bupivacaine formulation to produce ultralong-acting analgesia. Anesthesiology 2004;101:133-7.

[17] Boogaerts J, Lafont N, Donnay M, et al. Motor blockade and absence of local nerve toxicity induced by liposomal bupivacaine injected into the brachial plexus of rabbits. Acta Anaesthesiol Belg 1995;46:19-24.

[18] Hall SM, Gregson NA. The in vivo and ultrastructural effects of injection of lysophosphatidyl choline into myelinated peripheral nerve fibres of the adult mouse. J Cell Sci 1971;9:769-89.

[19] Malinovsky JM, Benhamou D, Alafandy M, et al. Neurotoxicological assessment after intra-cisternal injection of liposomal bupivacaine in rabbits. Anesth Analg 1997;85:1331-6.

[20] Kohane DS, Smith SE, Louis DN, et al. Prolonged duration local anesthesia from tetrodotoxin-enhanced local anesthetic microspheres. Pain 2003;104:415-21.

[21] Drager C, Benziger D, Gao F, et al. Prolonged intercostal nerve blockade in sheep using controlled-release of bupivacaine and dexamethasone from polymer microspheres. Anesthesiology 1998;89:969-79.

[22] Pedersen JL, Lilleso J, Hammer NA, et al. Bupivacaine in microcapsules prolongs analgesia after subcutaneous infiltration in humans: a dose-finding study. Anesthesiology 2004;99:912-8.

[23] Freiberg S, Xhu XX. Polymer microspheres for controlled drug release. Int J Pharm 2004; 282:1-18.

[24] Curley J, Castillo J, Hotz J, et al. Prolonged regional nerve blockade: injectable biodegradable bupivacaine/polyester microspheres. Anesthesiology 1996;84:1401-10.

[25] Capdevila X, Barthelet Y, Biboulet P, et al. Effects of perioperative analgesic technique on the surgical outcome and duration of rehabilitation after major knee surgery. Anesthesiology 1999;91:8–15.

[26] Salinas FV, Neal JM, Sueda LA, et al. Prospective comparison of continuous femoral nerve block with nonstimulating catheter placement versus stimulating catheter-guided perineural placement in volunteers. Reg Anesth Pain Med 2004;29:212–20.

[27] De Jong R. Local anesthetics. Saint Louis: Mosby-Year Book; 1994.

[28] Hollmann MW, Herroeder S, Kurz KS, et al. Time-dependent inhibition of G protein-coupled receptor signaling by local anesthetics. Anesthesiology 2004;100:852–60.

[29] Hollmann MW, McIntire WE, Garrison JC, et al. Inhibition of mammalian Gq protein function by local anesthetics. Anesthesiology 2002;97:1451–7.

[30] Khan MA, Gerner P, Kuo Wang G. Amitriptyline for prolonged cutaneous analgesia in the rat. Anesthesiology 2002;96:109–16.

[31] Gerner P, Mujtaba M, Khan M, et al. N-phenylethyl amitriptyline in rat sciatic nerve blockade. Anesthesiology 2002;96:1435–42.

[32] Strumper D, Durieux ME, Hollmann MW, et al. Effects of antidepressants on function and viability of human neutrophils. Anesthesiology 2003;98:1356–62.

[33] Hollmann MW, Durieux ME. Local anesthetics and the inflammatory response: a new therapeutic indication? Anesthesiology 2000;93:858–75.

[34] Condliffe AM, Kitchen E, Chilvers ER. Neutrophil priming: pathophysiological consequences and underlying mechanisms. Clin Sci 1998;94:461–71.

[35] Hollmann MW, Wieczorek KS, Berger A, et al. Local anesthetic inhibition of G protein-coupled receptor signaling by interference with Galpha (q) protein function. Mol Pharmacol 2001; 59:294–301.

[36] Hollmann M, Struemper D, Durieux M. The poor man's epidural: systemic local anesthetics for improving postoperative outcomes. Med Hypotheses 2004;63:386–9.

[37] Cooke ED, Bowcock SA, Lloyd MJ, et al. Intravenous lignocaine in prevention of deep venous thrombosis after elective hip surgery. Lancet 1977;2(8042):797–9.

[38] Groudine SB, Fisher HA, Kaufman Jr RP, et al. Intravenous lidocaine speeds the return of bowel function, decreases postoperative pain, and shortens hospital stay in patients undergoing radical retropubic prostatectomy. Anesth Analg 1998;86:235–9.

[39] Kawamata M, Takahashi T, Kozuka Y, et al. Experimental incision-induced pain in human skin: effects of systemic lidocaine on flare formation and hyperalgesia. Pain 2002;100:77–89.

[40] Lei B, Cottrell JE, Kass IS. Neuroprotective effect of low-dose lidocaine in a rat model of transient focal cerebral ischemia. Anesthesiology 2001;95:445–51.

[41] Lei B, Popp S, Capuano-Waters C, et al. Effects of delayed administration of low-dose lidocaine on transient focal cerebral ischemia in rats. Anesthesiology 2002;97:1534–40.

[42] Mitchell SJ, Pellett O, Gorman DF. Cerebral protection by lidocaine during cardiac operations. Ann Thorac Surg 1999;67:1117–24.

[43] Fassoulaki A, Sarantopoulos C, Melemeni A, et al. EMLA reduces acute and chronic pain after breast surgery for cancer. Reg Anesth Pain Med 2000;25:350–5.

ELSEVIER
SAUNDERS

Anesthesiology Clin N Am
23 (2005) 85–107

ANESTHESIOLOGY
CLINICS OF
NORTH AMERICA

Role of Analgesic Adjuncts in Postoperative Pain Management

Ashraf S. Habib, MBBCh, MSc, FRCA, Tong J. Gan, MB, FRCA*

Department of Anesthesiology, Duke University Medical Center, Box 3094, Durham, NC 27710, USA

Opioids remain the mainstay for postoperative analgesia, especially following major surgery. Pain, however, is a multi-factorial phenomenon that cannot be controlled adequately with simple monotherapy with opioids alone [1]. Furthermore, opioid use is associated with dose-related adverse effects such as respiratory depression, nausea, vomiting, urinary retention, itching, and sedation. Opioids also reduce gastrointestinal (GI) motility, which may contribute to postoperative ileus [2,3]. Their ability to control pain on movement also is limited, which may delay early mobilization and aggressive postoperative rehabilitation [4].

To improve pain relief, and reduce the incidence and severity of adverse effects, a multi-modal approach to postoperative analgesia should be used. This involves using different classes of analgesics, incorporating adjunct analgesics, and using different sites for administration of the analgesics [5]. The caudal administration of analgesic adjuncts in children is covered elsewhere in this issue. This article covers analgesic adjuncts, including N-methyl-D-aspartate (NMDA) receptor antagonists, α_2 agonists, anticonvulsants, opioid antagonists, neostigmine, and corticosteroids.

N-methyl-D-aspartate receptor antagonists

The NMDA receptor is an excitatory amino acid receptor that has been implicated in the modulation of prolonged pain states. Nociceptive stimuli induce

* Corresponding author.
E-mail address: gan00001@mc.duke.edu (T.J. Gan).

0889-8537/05/$ – see front matter © 2005 Elsevier Inc. All rights reserved.
doi:10.1016/j.atc.2004.11.007   *anesthesiology.theclinics.com*

the release of various substances, including excitatory amino acids, which activate the NMDA receptors and result in their hyperexcitability [6,7]. This creates a state of wind-up that leads to hyperactivity of the nociceptive system and increases the magnitude and duration of neurogenic responses to pain, even after the initial peripheral input is stopped [8]. The activation of the NMDA receptor by a painful stimulus increases intracellular calcium currents that amplify neuronal firing. This results in an increase in the intensity of the primary painful stimulus and a secondary pain perception. NMDA receptor antagonists block the receptors' gated calcium current and the evolving wind-up [9]. These agents are not antinociceptive on their own; their beneficial antinociceptive effects are secondary to their ability to inhibit central sensitization [10].

Ketamine

Ketamine is an intravenous (IV) anesthetic with analgesic properties in subanesthetic doses, secondary to its action on the NMDA receptor. Several trials are investigating the use of low-dose ketamine for managing postoperative pain. S (+)- ketamine is produced as a preservative-free solution. The S (+)- enantiomer was shown to be clinically superior to the racemic mixture of ketamine with regard to anesthetic potency, the extent of analgesia and amnesia, the incidence of adverse effects, and the psychotic reactions and agitation [11–13]. A review article [14] and two recent meta-analyses have reviewed the use of ketamine as a preemptive analgesic [15] and as an adjunct to opioid analgesia [16]. A detailed review of the literature about ketamine is beyond the scope of this article. The following section presents some of the conclusions reported by these articles.

The role of ketamine in preventive analgesia
In their meta-analysis, McCartney et al [15] reported that 24 studies examined the role of ketamine in preventive analgesia. The authors defined preventive analgesia as that which affects pain and/or analgesic consumption only beyond five half lives of ketamine administration. Of the 24 included studies, a positive pre-emptive or preventive analgesic effect was demonstrated in 14 studies (58%). Of those, ketamine was administered intravenously in nine studies, epidurally or intrathecally in four studies, and subcutaneously in one study. The doses used ranged from 0.15 to 1 mg/kg; the success of the preventive analgesic effect did not depend on the dose administered. Adverse effects, including psychomimetic effects, were evaluated in 20 of those studies. Only one study reported psychomimetic effects related to epidural ketamine dosed at 20 mg [17].

The role of ketamine as an adjunct to opioids
As part of patient-controlled analgesia.   The effect of adding ketamine to morphine for postoperative patient-controlled analgesia (PCA), compared with using morphine alone was investigated in six trials involving 330 patients. Only one trial in patients undergoing lumbar microdiscectomy [18] showed a beneficial effect of adding ketamine. There were no analgesic effects of ketamine in the

other five studies in patients undergoing abdominal surgery [19–23]. Adverse effects including vivid dreams, hallucinations, dysphoria, and disorientation were increased in ketamine-treated patients in two studies. Analysis of the pooled data from all six trials did not, however, reveal any significant differences in central nervous system (CNS) adverse effects between patients treated with ketamine plus morphine compared with those receiving morphine alone [16].

As a continuous intravenous infusion. Continuous IV infusion of ketamine in the perioperative period was investigated in 11 trials [24–34]. In seven of these trials, the ketamine infusion was used in addition to IV opioids, and in the remaining four, in combination with epidural opioids. The doses used were 0.6 mg/kg per hour to 20 mg per hour. Four studies reported significantly improved analgesia with the infusion of ketamine [25,26,28,30]. Pooled analysis of the mean visual analog scale (VAS) (0 to 100 mm) at rest from six studies reported a beneficial effect of the ketamine infusion with a weighted mean difference (WMD) for VAS of -8.2 mm (95% confidence interval [CI], -1.51, -0.14) (Fig. 1). CNS adverse effects were not increased significantly with IV ketamine infusion. There was a trend toward less postoperative nausea and vomiting (PONV) in patients receiving ketamine (P = 0.06) [16]. Two of 4 studies where IV ketamine infusion was given in combination with epidural opioids reported significant reductions in VAS and postoperative opioid consumption [32,34]. The dose of ketamine used was 0.5 mg/kg per hour. CNS adverse effects were not increased significantly in the ketamine-treated patients [16].

As a single intravenous bolus. A single IV bolus of 0.05 to 1 mg/kg of ketamine given in the perioperative period in conjunction with IV opioids was

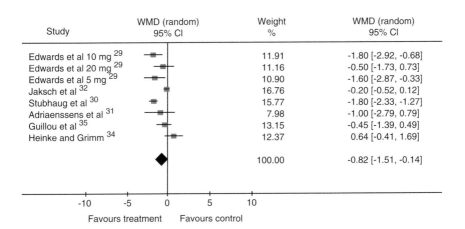

Fig. 1. Intravenous ketamine infusion with IV opioids (visual analog scale at rest). *Abbreviations:* WMD, weighted mean difference; CI, confidence interval. (*From* Subramaniam K, Subramaniam B, Steinbrook RA. Ketamine as adjuvant analgesic to opioids: a quantitative and qualitative systematic review. Anesth Analg 2004;99:489; with permission.)

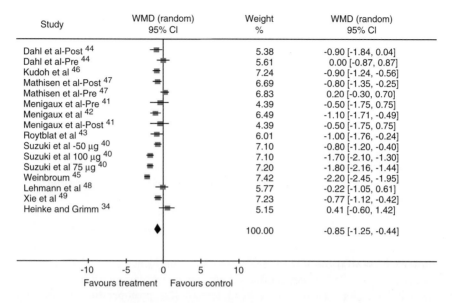

Study	WMD (random) 95% CI	Weight %	WMD (random) 95% CI
Dahl et al-Post [44]		5.38	-0.90 [-1.84, 0.04]
Dahl et al-Pre [44]		5.61	0.00 [-0.87, 0.87]
Kudoh et al [46]		7.24	-0.90 [-1.24, -0.56]
Mathisen et al-Post [47]		6.69	-0.80 [-1.35, -0.25]
Mathisen et al-Pre [47]		6.83	0.20 [-0.30, 0.70]
Menigaux et al-Pre [41]		4.39	-0.50 [-1.75, 0.75]
Menigaux et al [42]		6.49	-1.10 [-1.71, -0.49]
Menigaux et al-Post [41]		4.39	-0.50 [-1.75, 0.75]
Roytblat et al [43]		6.01	-1.00 [-1.76, -0.24]
Suzuki et al -50 µg [40]		7.10	-0.80 [-1.20, -0.40]
Suzuki et al 100 µg [40]		7.10	-1.70 [-2.10, -1.30]
Suzuki et al 75 µg [40]		7.20	-1.80 [-2.16, -1.44]
Weinbroum [45]		7.42	-2.20 [-2.45, -1.95]
Lehmann et al [48]		5.77	-0.22 [-1.05, 0.61]
Xie et al [49]		7.23	-0.77 [-1.12, -0.42]
Heinke and Grimm [34]		5.15	0.41 [-0.60, 1.42]
		100.00	-0.85 [-1.25, -0.44]

-10   -5   0   5   10
Favours treatment   Favours control

Fig. 2. Intravenous ketamine single bolus with IV opioids (visual analog scale at rest). *Abbreviations:* WMD, weighted mean difference; CI, confidence interval. (*From* Subramaniam K, Subramaniam B, Steinbrook RA. Ketamine as adjuvant analgesic to opioids: a quantitative and qualitative systematic review. Anesth Analg 2004;99:490; with permission.)

investigated in 11 clinical trials [29,35–44]. A beneficial analgesic effect was reported in seven studies. Pooling of the VAS scores of all studied revealed a WMD of -8.5 mm (95% CI, -1.25, -0.44) in favor of ketamine administration for VAS at rest (Fig. 2), and a WMD of -6.2 mm (95% CI, -0.83, -0.41) in favor of ketamine for VAS on movement. There was no difference in CNS adverse effects, and a trend toward less PONV in ketamine-treated patients compared with control patients [16].

Epidural ketamine. Epidural administration of ketamine (bolus 0.5 to 1 mg/kg or infusion 0.5 mg per hour to 0.25 mg/kg per hour) was investigated in eight trials in patients undergoing major intrathoracic and abdominal surgery [31, 44–50]. A useful analgesic effect was reported in five studies [44–46,49,50] with a WMD of -7.1 mm (95% CI, -1.01, -0.40) for mean VAS at rest in favor of ketamine-treated patients (Fig. 3). There was no difference in CNS adverse effects or PONV between ketamine-treated and control patients [16].

Dextromethorphan

Dextromethorphan is a weak, noncompetitive NMDA antagonist that has been used as an antitussive agent. It has been shown to inhibit development of cutaneous secondary hyperalgesia in people after peripheral burn injury [10]

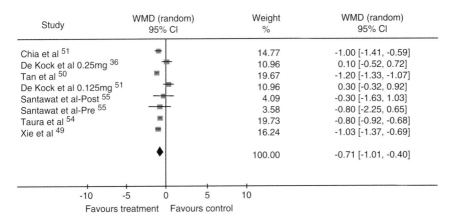

Study	WMD (random) 95% CI	Weight %	WMD (random) 95% CI
Chia et al [51]		14.77	-1.00 [-1.41, -0.59]
De Kock et al 0.25mg [36]		10.96	0.10 [-0.52, 0.72]
Tan et al [50]		19.67	-1.20 [-1.33, -1.07]
De Kock et al 0.125mg [51]		10.96	0.30 [-0.32, 0.92]
Santawat et al-Post [55]		4.09	-0.30 [-1.63, 1.03]
Santawat et al-Pre [55]		3.58	-0.80 [-2.25, 0.65]
Taura et al [54]		19.73	-0.80 [-0.92, -0.68]
Xie et al [49]		16.24	-1.03 [-1.37, -0.69]
		100.00	-0.71 [-1.01, -0.40]

-10   -5   0   5   10

Favours treatment   Favours control

Fig. 3. Epidural ketamine with epidural opioids (visual analog scale at rest). *Abbreviations:* WMD, weighted mean difference; CI, confidence interval. (*From* Subramaniam K, Subramaniam B, Steinbrook RA. Ketamine as adjuvant analgesic to opioids: a quantitative and qualitative systematic review. Anesth Analg 2004;99:491; with permission.)

and to reduce temporal summation of pain [51]. Several studies investigated the effect of the perioperative administration of dextromethorphan on acute postoperative pain. A recent meta-analysis reported that 8 out of 12 included studies demonstrated a useful pre-emptive and preventive analgesic effect of the perioperative administration of oral, intramuscular (IM), and IV dextromethorphan. The doses used ranged from 0.5 to 5 mg/kg and did not appear to be associated with the success of the intervention. Opiate-related adverse effects were similar between patients who received dextromethorphan and control patients [15]. Postoperative administration of IM dextromethorphan at a dose of 40 mg [52,53] and oral dextromethorphan (200 mg every 8 hours) [54] also were associated with a significant reduction in postoperative opioid consumption.

Magnesium

Magnesium acts as a noncompetitive antagonist of the NMDA glutamate receptors. Although some studies reported a useful analgesic effect from the perioperative administration of magnesium sulfate ($MgSO_4$) [55–58], others did not support these findings [59,60]. A recent meta-analysis [15] examined the preventive analgesic effect of Mg, as defined by its effects on pain or analgesic consumption only beyond five half-lives of $MgSO_4$ administration. The authors reported that none of the four included studies demonstrated a preventive analgesic effect. Two studies, however, reported a direct analgesic effect [57,58]. The intrathecal addition of 50 mg $MgSO_4$ to fentanyl 25 μg as part of a combined spinal epidural technique for labor analgesia resulted in a significant prolongation in the median duration of analgesia from 60 minutes in patients receiving spinal fentanyl alone to 75 minutes in those receiving added $MgSO_4$ [61].

Amantadine

Although amantadine is used primarily for the treatment of Parkinson's disease and as an antiviral drug, evidence shows that amantadine is a noncompetitive NMDA receptor antagonist. Although a single preoperative IV dose of 200 mg amantadine did not enhance postoperative analgesia [62], the regular administration of 200 mg of oral amantadine starting the evening before surgery and for 48 hours postoperatively, resulted in 32% reduction in morphine consumption after radical prostatectomy [63].

In summary, the available data suggest that ketamine has a useful analgesic effect with no increase in adverse effects when given as an IV bolus, as a continuous IV infusion, and with epidural administration. The addition of ketamine to PCA morphine did not confer any benefit. Although the use of dextromethorphan proved to have a useful preventive analgesic effect, the use of magnesium did not prove to be useful. More data are required regarding the use of amantadine as an adjunct analgesic.

α_2 agonists

α_2 agonists have been administered pre- and intraoperatively to provide sedative, anxiolytic, and analgesic effects. α_2 receptors are located in the presynaptic area of the sympathetic and CNS. α_2 receptors at the spinal cord level are thought to be responsible for the analgesic properties of α_2-adrenegic agonists, which inhibit the release of substance P. The sedative effect is secondary to action on the locus ceruleus [64]. Clonidine is a selective partial agonist for α_2 adrenoceptors with a ratio of approximately 220:1 (α_2: α_1). Dexmedetomidine is super selective for the α_2 receptors with an α_2: α_1 binding ratio of 1620:1. Its half-life is shorter (2 hours) compared with clonidine (9 to 12 hours) [65].

Systemic clonidine

The results of studies investigating the usefulness of oral clonidine on enhancing postoperative analgesia have been mixed. In children, premedication with oral clonidine dosed at 4 µg/kg reduced postoperative pain scores and analgesic consumption following minor surgery in one study [66], but had no analgesic effect following adenotonsillectomy in another study [67]. In adults, although clonidine dosed at 5 µg/kg enhanced the quality of postoperative analgesia by intrathecal and epidural morphine [68,69], the use of 3 µg/kg of oral clonidine did not produce a useful analgesic effect in patients receiving intrathecal morphine [70]. The preoperative administration 4 µg/kg of oral clonidine to women undergoing cesarean section under regional anesthesia reduced pain scores and PCA morphine consumption without compromising the condition of the newborn [71]. A 37% reduction in PCA morphine consumption and a reduction in the incidence of PONV also were reported following premedication with 5 μg/kg of oral clonidine in patients undergoing knee surgery [72]. The combination of 3 to 5 μg/kg of oral clonidine with 0.2 mg every 24 hours of transdermal clonidine was effective in reducing postoperative PCA morphine consumption in one study [73], but it failed to produce a similar effect in a more recent study [74]. Several studies also have demonstrated a morphine-sparing effect from the administration of 2 to 8 μg/kg of IV clonidine [75–78]. Hypotension, bradycardia, and sedation occurred with the higher doses of clonidine. In a dose-finding study, Marinangeli et al [79] found that the optimum analgesic dose of clonidine in the postoperative period was 3 μg/kg bolus followed by an infusion of 0.3 μg/kg per hour. The addition of clonidine to the PCA morphine also resulted in a significant reduction in morphine consumption and a reduction in the incidence of PONV compared with morphine PCA alone [80].

Neuraxial clonidine

There is evidence of a spinal action for clonidine [81,82]. Clonidine 150 μg, injected intrathecally after cesarean section or minor orthopedic surgery produced analgesia for 4 to 6 hours [83,84]. It also enhances and prolongs the effect of intrathecal local anesthetics [85]. Clonidine is approximately twice as potent given epidurally compared with intravenously [77]. Epidural clonidine alone at a dose of 3μg/kg was not better than placebo in one study after thoracic surgery [86]. In orthopedic and rectal surgery, a lower dose (2 μg/kg) of epidural clonidine was found to be more efficacious than placebo [87]. Armand et al [88] attempted to perform a meta-analysis of the studies investigating the use of extradural clonidine for postoperative analgesia. The main adverse effects reported were hypotension, bradycardia, and sedation. The tremendous variability in study design did not allow the authors to perform the meta-analysis. They reported that the efficacy of clonidine in combination with other drugs (local anesthetics or opioids) was almost always superior to that of each drug alone.

Peripheral nerve blocks

Clonidine, in doses of 0.5 μg/kg or greater, enhances and prolongs the effect of local anesthetics used for brachial plexus block [89–91], peribulbar [92,93] and retrobulbar [94] blocks, and IV regional anesthesia [95,96]. The intra-articular administration of clonidine dosed at 150 μg enhanced postoperative analgesia in patients undergoing knee arthroscopy [97–99]. Hemodynamic effects, namely bradycardia and hypotension, increase with doses of 1.5 μg/kg or more.

Dexmedetomidine

Dexmedetomidine has anesthetic and opioid-sparing effects [100–102]. It has a negligible respiratory depressant effect [103] and does not potentiate opioid-induced respiratory depression [104]. The IM administration of dexmedetomidine at a dose of 2.5 μg/kg 1 hour before anesthesia, led to a reduction in the

Table 1
Studies of the use of gabapentin in the perioperative period

Study	Type of surgery	Regimen (n patients) [duration of the study]	Pain scores versus control	Analgesic consumption versus control	Side effects
Dirks [115]	Mastectomy	Gabapentin 1200 mg 1h preop (31); placebo (34) [4 hours]	Reduced VAS on movement at 2 h (p < 0.0001) and 4 h (p = 0.018)	Reduced morphine consumption (p < 0.0001)	No difference
Fassoulaki [117]	Cancer breast surgery	Gabapentin 1200 mg/d for 10 days (22, 3) mexilitene 600 mg/d for 10 days (21) Placebo for 10 d (34) [3 months]	VAS rest and movement reduced by both drugs on day 3; VAS movement reduced by gabapentin between days 2 and 5	50% reduced codeine and paracetamol use from days 2 to 10	No difference
Turan [121]	Spinal surgery	Gabapentin 1200 mg 1 h preoperatively (25) Placebo 1 h preoperatively (25) [24 hours]	Reduced VAS at 1, 2, and 4 h	Reduced morphine consumption (p < 0.000)	Vomiting and urinary retention lower in gabapentin group (p < 0.05)
Dierking [116]	Abdominal hysterectomy	Gabapentin 1200 mg 1 h preoperatively followed by 600 mg at 6, 8, and 24 h after first dose (39) placebo 1 h preoperatively followed by placebo at 6, 8, and 24 h after first dose (32) [24 hours]	No difference	32% reduced morphine consumption (p < 0.001)	No difference

Study	Surgery	Intervention	Pain outcome	Analgesic consumption	Side effects
Turan [122]	Abdominal hysterectomy	Gabapentin 1200 mg 1 h preoperatively (25); placebo 1 h preoperatively (25) [24 hours]	Reduced VAS up to 20 h	Reduced tramadol consumption ($p < 0.000$)	No difference
Pandey [118]	Laparoscopic cholecystectomy	Gabapentin 300 mg 2 h preoperatively (153); Tramadol 100 mg 2 h preoperatively (153); placebo 2 h preoperatively (153) [24 hours]	Reduced VAS compared with tramadol (except at 0 to 6 h) and placebo	Reduced fentanyl consumption ($p < 0.05$)	Sedation and PONV higher in the gabapentin group
Rorarius [120]	Vaginal hysterectomy	Gabapentin 1200 mg 2.5 h preoperatively (38); oxazepam 15 mg 2.5 h preoperatively (37) [20 hours]	Trend towards reduced VAS in the first 2 h	40% reduced fentanyl consumption ($p < 0.005$)	Trend towards less PONV in the gabapentin group
Turan [119]	ENT surgery under MAC	Gabapentin 1200 mg 1 h preoperatively (25); placebo 1 h preoperatively (25) [24 hours]	VRS reduced postoperatively ($p < 0.001$) and at 45 and 60 min intraoperatively ($p < 0.05$)	Reduced intraoperative fentanyl use ($p < 0.05$), and postoperative diclofenac use ($p < 0.001$); prolonged time to first rescue analgesia ($p < 0.001$)	More dizziness in the gabapentin (24%) versus the placebo group (4%, $p < 0.05$)

Abbreviations: ENT, ear, nose, and throat; MAC, monitored anesthesia care.

intraoperative need for fentanyl by 60% and a reduction in the requirement for postoperative analgesics [104]. In women undergoing laparoscopic tubal ligation, morphine was required in 33% of women given 0.4 μg/kg of dexmedetomidine in the recovery room, compared with 83% of patients receiving diclofenac. Sedation and bradycardia, however, were associated with dexmedetomidine use [105]. In patients undergoing major surgery, the administration of dexmedetomidine (1 μg/kg loading dose followed by an infusion of 0.4 μg/kg per hour for 4 hours) reduced the early postoperative need for morphine by 66% compared with patients who received morphine sulfate at a dose of 0.08 mg/kg 30 minutes before the end of surgery [106]. The addition of 0.5 μg/kg of dexmedetomidine to lidocaine for IV regional anesthesia prolonged the duration of the block, and reduced tourniquet pain and analgesic supplementation for tourniquet pain [107].

In summary, the use of low doses of clonidine proved to be a useful adjunct analgesic when given neuraxially, and in combination with peripheral nerve blocks. Higher doses are associated with adverse effects and should be avoided. Data about the systemic administration of clonidine would support the usefulness of low-dose IV administration. More data are required regarding the use of dexmedetomidine as an analgesic adjunct.

Anticonvulsants

Gabapentin is a γ-aminobutyric acid (GABA) analog that was developed clinically as an anticonvulsant in the late 1980s [108]. It has been found to be effective for treating neuropathic pain [109], diabetic neuropathy [110], postherpetic neuralgia [111], and reflex sympathetic dystrophy [112]. Gabapentin also had a synergistic analgesic effect with morphine in animals [113], healthy volunteers [114], and patients with neuropathic cancer pain [115].

Despite its structural similarity to GABA, gabapentin does not act by means of mechanisms related to GABA [116]. Though the exact mechanism of action of gabapentin is not understood fully, there are several proposed explanations of its antihyperalgesic effects. These include an action at the $\alpha_2\delta_1$ subunits of voltage-dependent Ca^{2+} channels [117], which are up-regulated in the dorsal root ganglia and spinal cord after peripheral injury [118], suppression of glutaminergic transmission in the spinal cord [119], and suppression of substance P neurotransmission [120]. Alternatively, gabapentin may inhibit central sensitization through an action on voltage-dependent Ca^{2+} channels, resulting in a direct postsynaptic inhibition of Ca^{2+} influx or a presynaptic inhibition of Ca^{2+} influx that decreases excitatory amino acid neurotransmission [121].

Several recent studies reported a useful analgesic effect from the perioperative administration of gabapentin [122–129]. These studies are summarized in Table 1. Dizziness and somnolence have been reported to be the most common adverse effects of gabapentin in studies of chronic pain. With the exception of one study in patients receiving general anesthesia [125], and one study in patients receiving monitored anesthesia care [126], all the trials investigating the analgesic effect of gabapentin in the perioperative period reported no significant differences in adverse effects between patients who received gabapentin or placebo. Whether these adverse effects are masked by the effects of general anesthesia and post-operative opioids or if the short-term administration of gabapentin is devoid of sedative adverse effects remains unclear.

Pregabalin, another analog of GABA, also was found to have significant analgesic properties when given in a dose of 300 mg orally following third molar extraction. This dose of pregabalin was more effective than ibuprofen, placebo, and a 50 mg dose of pregabalin, but was associated with a higher incidence of dizziness and somnolence compared with the other three groups [130].

In summary, the available data support the use of gabapentin as an analgesic adjunct in the perioperative period.

Opioid antagonists

Preclinical in vivo and in vitro studies demonstrated that direct competitive antagonism of Gs-coupled excitatory opioid receptor functions by the administration of extremely low doses of clinically available opioid antagonists, markedly enhances the opioid's analgesic potency and simultaneously attenuates opioid tolerance and dependence [131–133]. These excitatory opioid receptors contribute to adverse effects and are involved in the tolerance and hyperalgesia often observed with opioid therapy [131,134,135]. It is also possible that block-ade of presynaptic opioid receptors responsible for auto-inhibition may cause exaggerated release of endogenous opioids [131]. The bimodal opioid modula-tion of the action potential of sensory neurons is illustrated in Fig. 4.

Several clinical studies investigated the possible enhancement of opioid anal-gesia by the concomitant administration of very low doses of opioid antagonists. In patients undergoing total abdominal hysterectomy, Gan et al reported that low-dose naloxone (0.25 µg/kg per hour) significantly reduced the PCA cumulative morphine consumption during the first 24 hours postoperatively. The incidence of PONV and pruritus also were significantly reduced in patients receiving low-dose naloxone. Patients receiving a higher dose of naloxone (1 µg/kg per hour) experienced a reduction in PONV and pruritus but consumed similar amounts of morphine compared with patients in the placebo group [134]. Joshi et al per-formed another study on 120 women undergoing lower abdominal surgery. At the end of surgery, patients were randomized to receive saline or 15 µg or 25 µg of nalmefene intravenously. The overall 24-hour pain scores were significantly lower in patients receiving nalmefene. The total consumption of morphine was however similar in the three groups. The need for antiemetic and antipruritic medications was significantly lower in patients receiving nalmefene [135]. These results were not reproduced in three subsequent studies in which naloxone was mixed with the PCA morphine in a dose of 6 µg/mL [136], 0.6µg/mL [137], and 26.6 µg/mL [138]. It is possible that the intermittent administration of naloxone

BIMODAL OPIOID MODULATION OF THE ACTION POTENTIAL OF SENSORY NEURONS

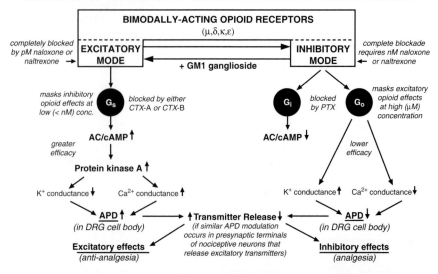

Fig. 4. Acute bimodal opioid modulation of the action potential of nociceptive dorsal root ganglion (DRG) neurons appears to be mediated by activation of GM1-regulated, interconvertible opioid receptors that can occur in a Gi/Go-coupled inhibitory mode (right) or in a Gs-coupled excitatory mode (left). The linkages of these Gi/Go sharply contrast with the Gs-coupled receptors to K and Ca conductances, which control action potential duration and transmitter release in presynaptic terminals of sensory neurons involved in opioid analgesic systems. Selective blockade of excitatory opioid effects in DRG by cotreatment with Pm naloxone or naltrexone attenuates the antianalgesic effects of morphine and other bimodally-acting opioid agonists and thereby enhances the analgesic efficacy of these opioid agonists. *Abbreviations:* AC, adenyl cyclase; Camp, cyclic AMP; CTX, cholera toxin; PTX, pertussis toxin. (*From* Crain SM, Shen KF. Antagonists of excitatory opioid receptor functions enhance morphine's analgesic potency and attenuate opioid tolerance/dependence liability. Pain 2000; 84:121–31; with permission.)

might have induced hyperalgesia at the excitatory opioid receptor that had become sensitized by opioid exposure [139].

These conflicting results suggest that further research is required in this area using naloxone infusions or longer-acting opioid antagonists.

Neostigmine

Intrathecal administration

Animal and human volunteer studies demonstrated the safety and analgesic efficacy of the intrathecal administration of neostigmine. Intrathecal neostigmine causes analgesia by inhibiting the breakdown of acetylcholine in the dorsal horn [140,141] and spinal meninges [142]. Acetylcholine may cause analgesia through direct action on spinal cholinergic muscarinic receptors M_1 and M_3 [143] and nicotinic receptors subtypes [144] and indirectly through stimulation of release of nitric oxide in the spinal cord [145]. The analgesia resulting from the combination of systemic opioid and intrathecal neostigmine is synergistic in animals [146] and additive in human volunteers [147]. A synergistic interaction also has been reported between nonsteroidal anti-inflammatory drugs (NSAIDs) and spinal neostigmine in mice [148].

Studies in human volunteers demonstrated no analgesia from doses less than 100 μg of intrathecal neostigmine [149]. Therefore, this dose was used in the initial studies evaluating the use of this drug for postoperative analgesia. Intrathecal doses ranging from 25 to 100 μg produced analgesia for several surgical procedures [150–159]. Despite this useful analgesic effect, significant adverse effects occurred, including a high incidence of intraoperative and postoperative nausea and vomiting, bradycardia, sweating, agitation, and distress. Dose–response studies reported that the analgesic effect of intrathecal neostigmine was dose-independent, but the adverse effects were dose-dependent [147,160,161]. Therefore, more recent studies have evaluated even smaller doses of intrathecal neostigmine. Doses as low as 1 to 5 μg still produced some analgesia without any adverse effects [162,163].

Epidural administration

Epidural administration of neostigmine has been suggested to produce analgesia without nausea in patients with chronic pain [164]. Doses of 1 to 10 μg/kg of epidural neostigmine had a useful analgesic effect in patients undergoing knee surgery [165,166], abdominal hysterectomy [167], abdominal surgery [17], and cesarean section [168]. Although there was no increase in the incidence of PONV in these studies, the use of neostigmine resulted in mild sedation in one study [168].

Intra-articular neostigmine

In vitro studies have shown that peripheral cholinergic-mediated antinociception at peripheral nerve endings is caused by a hyperpolarization of the neurons and by modulation of the nitric oxide pathways [169,170]. The intra-articular administration of neostigmine dosed at 500 μg resulted in improved postoperative analgesia, which lasted longer than that produced by morphine dosed at 2 mg, with no increase in adverse effects [97,171,172].

Neostigmine added to local anesthetics for brachial plexus block

The addition of 500 μg of neostigmine to mepivacaine or lidocaine for axillary brachial plexus bock (BPB) did not confer any advantages in two studies [173,174] but significantly increased the incidence of GI adverse effects (nausea, flatulence, difficulty in controlling anal sphincter) in one study [173]. Two other studies reported a delayed analgesic effect of 500 μg of neostigmine added to mepivacaine and bupivacaine for axillary BPB, with a reduction in pain scores and analgesic consumption starting 12 hours to 24 hours postoperatively, and no increase in adverse effects [175,176].

Neostigmine added to intravenous regional anesthesia

In one study, the addition of 0.5 mg of neostigmine to 3 mg/kg of prilocaine for IV regional anesthesia (IVRA) resulted in a quicker onset, prolonged duration, and improved quality of the block, and prolonged time to first rescue analgesic, compared with IVRA with prilocaine alone [177]. There results were not reproduced in a subsequent study in which 1 mg of neostigmine was added to 3 mg/kg of lidocaine for IVRA [178].

In summary, the intrathecal administration of neostigmine is associated with a high incidence of adverse effects and is not recommended. The epidural route seems to be promising, but more data are needed before this route of administration is recommended. Although the intra-articular administration of neostigmine is useful, more data are required regarding the addition of neostigmine to BPB or IVRA.

Corticosteroids

Corticosteroids inhibit the phospholipase enzyme and therefore block both the cyclo-oxygenase and the lipo-oxygenase pathways in the inflammatory chain reaction. They may be effective therefore in reducing pain by interfering with prostaglandins synthesis. Their anti-inflammatory and analgesic effects are well documented after oral surgery [179–181]. Betamethasone in a dose of 9 mg effectively alleviates postoperative pain and swelling after dental surgery [179]. A single dose of 12 mg betamethasone given intramuscularly before ambulatory surgery also reduced postoperative pain and nausea [182]. Analgesic effects also have been reported after general surgery [183], orthopedic surgery [184], and back surgery [185,186]. Other studies, however, did not confirm these findings [187–190]. Results of the studies investigating the impact of dexamethasone on postoperative pain following pediatric adenotonsillectomy have been conflicting [188,189,191–193]. A 27% reduction in postoperative emesis and an earlier tolerance of a soft or regular diet, however, have been reported in a meta-analysis of dexamethasone use with tonsillectomy [194].

In summary, although the use of steroids has a proven analgesic effect following oral surgery, the available data regarding their usefulness following other types of surgery are conflicting.

Summary

Many studies have investigated the use of analgesic adjuncts with the aim of reducing opioid consumption and opioid-related adverse effects. Most have shown beneficial effects, and some of these modalities have been adopted in clinical practice. The optimal use of these adjuncts, however, requires a better understanding of the dose–response relationships when combined with opioids to maximize the analgesic efficacy with minimal adverse effects from the combinations.

References

[1] Siddall PJ, Cousins MJ. Pain mechanisms and management: an update. Clin Exp Pharmacol Physiol 1995;22:679–88.

[2] Cali RL, Meade PG, Swanson MS, et al. Effect of morphine and incision length on bowel function after colectomy. Dis Colon Rectum 2000;43:163–8.

[3] Thorn SE, Wattwil M, Naslund I. Postoperative epidural morphine, but not epidural bupivacaine, delays gastric emptying on the first day after cholecystectomy. Reg Anesth 1992;17:91–4.

[4] Lynch EP, Lazor MA, Gellis JE, et al. Patient experience of pain after elective noncardiac surgery. Anesth Analg 1997;85:117–23.

[5] Kehlet H. Multi-modal approach to control postoperative pathophysiology and rehabilitation. Br J Anaesth 1997;78:606–17.

[6] Aanonsen LM, Wilcox GL. Nociceptive action of excitatory amino acids in the mouse: effects of spinally administered opioids, phencyclidine and sigma agonists. J Pharmacol Exp Ther 1987;243:9–19.

[7] Battaglia G, Rustioni A. Coexistence of glutamate and substance P in dorsal root ganglion neurons of the rat and monkey. J Comp Neurol 1988;277:302–12.

[8] Dickenson AH. Spinal cord pharmacology of pain. Br J Anaesth 1995;75:193–200.

[9] Mendell LM. Physiological properties of unmyelinated fiber projection to the spinal cord. Exp Neurol 1966;16:316–32.

[10] Ilkjaer S, Dirks J, Brennum J, et al. Effect of systemic N-methyl-D-aspartate receptor antagonist (dextromethorphan) on primary and secondary hyperalgesia in humans. Br J Anaesth 1997;79:600–5.

[11] White PF, Schuttler J, Shafer A, et al. Comparative pharmacology of the ketamine isomers. Studies in volunteers. Br J Anaesth 1985;57:197–203.

[12] Adams HA, Thiel A, Jung A, et al. Studies using S-(+)-ketamine on probands. Endocrine and circulatory reactions, recovery and dream experiences. Anaesthesist 1992;41:588–96.

[13] Calvey TN. Isomerism and anaesthetic drugs. Acta Anaesthesiol Scand Suppl 1995;106: 83–90.

[14] Schmid RL, Sandler AN, Katz J. Use and efficacy of low-dose ketamine in the management of acute postoperative pain: a review of current techniques and outcomes. Pain 1999;82: 111–25.

[15] McCartney CJ, Sinha A, Katz J. A qualitative systematic review of the role of N-methyl-D-aspartate receptor antagonists in preventive analgesia. Anesth Analg 2004;98:1385–400.

[16] Subramaniam K, Subramaniam B, Steinbrook RA. Ketamine as adjuvant analgesic to opioids: a quantitative and qualitative systematic review. Anesth Analg 2004;99:482–95.

[17] Kirdemir P, Ozkocak I, Demir T, et al. Comparison of postoperative analgesic effects of pre-emptively used epidural ketamine and neostigmine. J Clin Anesth 2000;12:543–8.

[18] Javery KB, Ussery TW, Steger HG, et al. Comparison of morphine and morphine with ketamine for postoperative analgesia. Can J Anaesth 1996;43:212–5.

[19] Reeves M, Lindholm DE, Myles PS, et al. Adding ketamine to morphine for patient-controlled analgesia after major abdominal surgery: a double-blinded, randomized controlled trial. Anesth Analg 2001;93:116–20.

[20] Murdoch CJ, Crooks BA, Miller CD. Effect of the addition of ketamine to morphine in patient-controlled analgesia. Anaesthesia 2002;57:484−8.

[21] Unlugenc H, Ozalevli M, Guler T, et al. Postoperative pain management with intravenous patient-controlled morphine: comparison of the effect of adding magnesium or ketamine. Eur J Anaesthesiol 2003;20:416−21.

[22] Burstal R, Danjoux G, Hayes C, et al. PCA ketamine and morphine after abdominal hysterectomy. Anaesth Intensive Care 2001;29:246−51.

[23] Hercock T, Gilham MJ, Sleigh J, et al. The addition of ketamine to patient-controlled morphine analgesia does not improve quality of analgesia after total abdominal hysterectomy. Acute Pain 1999;2:68−72.

[24] Edwards ND, Fletcher A, Cole JR, et al. Combined infusions of morphine and ketamine for postoperative pain in elderly patients. Anaesthesia 1993;48:124−7.

[25] Stubhaug A, Breivik H, Eide PK, et al. Mapping of punctuate hyperalgesia around a surgical incision demonstrates that ketamine is a powerful suppressor of central sensitization to pain following surgery. Acta Anaesthesiol Scand 1997;41:1124−32.

[26] Adriaenssens G, Vermeyen KM, Hoffmann VL, et al. Postoperative analgesia with IV patient-controlled morphine: effect of adding ketamine. Br J Anaesth 1999;83:393−6.

[27] Jaksch W, Lang S, Reichhalter R, et al. Perioperative small-dose S(+)-ketamine has no incremental beneficial effects on postoperative pain when standard-practice opioid infusions are used. Anesth Analg 2002;94:981−6.

[28] Guignard B, Coste C, Costes H, et al. Supplementing desflurane-remifentanil anesthesia with small-dose ketamine reduces perioperative opioid analgesic requirements. Anesth Analg 2002;95:103−8.

[29] Heinke W, Grimm D. Pre-emptive effects caused by coanalgesia with ketamine in gynecological laparotomies? Anaesthesiol Reanim 1999;24:60−4.

[30] Guillou N, Tanguy M, Seguin P, et al. The effects of small-dose ketamine on morphine consumption in surgical intensive care unit patients after major abdominal surgery. Anesth Analg 2003;97:843−7.

[31] De Kock M, Lavand'homme P, Waterloos H. Balanced analgesia in the perioperative period: is there a place for ketamine? Pain 2001;92:373−80.

[32] Aida S, Yamakura T, Baba H, et al. Pre-emptive analgesia by intravenous low-dose ketamine and epidural morphine in gastrectomy: a randomized double-blind study. Anesthesiology 2000;92:1624−30.

[33] Ilkjaer S, Nikolajsen L, Hansen TM, et al. Effect of IV ketamine in combination with epidural bupivacaine or epidural morphine on postoperative pain and wound tenderness after renal surgery. Br J Anaesth 1998;81:707−12.

[34] Kararmaz A, Kaya S, Karaman H, et al. Intraoperative intravenous ketamine in combination with epidural analgesia: postoperative analgesia after renal surgery. Anesth Analg 2003;97:1092−6.

[35] Suzuki M, Tsueda K, Lansing PS, et al. Small-dose ketamine enhances morphine-induced analgesia after outpatient surgery. Anesth Analg 1999;89:98−103.

[36] Menigaux C, Fletcher D, Dupont X, et al. The benefits of intraoperative small-dose ketamine on postoperative pain after anterior cruciate ligament repair. Anesth Analg 2000;90:129−35.

[37] Menigaux C, Guignard B, Fletcher D, et al. Intraoperative small-dose ketamine enhances analgesia after outpatient knee arthroscopy. Anesth Analg 2001;93:606−12.

[38] Roytblat L, Korotkoruchko A, Katz J, et al. Postoperative pain: the effect of low-dose ketamine in addition to general anesthesia. Anesth Analg 1993;77:1161−5.

[39] Dahl V, Ernoe PE, Steen T, et al. Does ketamine have pre-emptive effects in women undergoing abdominal hysterectomy procedures? Anesth Analg 2000;90:1419−22.

[40] Weinbroum AA. A single small dose of postoperative ketamine provides rapid and sustained improvement in morphine analgesia in the presence of morphine-resistant pain. Anesth Analg 2003;96:789−95.

[41] Kudoh A, Takahira Y, Katagai H, et al. Small-dose ketamine improves the postoperative state of depressed patients. Anesth Analg 2002;95:114−8.

[42] Mathisen LC, Aasbo V, Raeder J. Lack of pre-emptive analgesic effect of (R)-ketamine in laparoscopic cholecystectomy. Acta Anaesthesiol Scand 1999;43:220–4.

[43] Lehmann KA, Klaschik M. Lack of pre-emptive analgesic effect of low-dose ketamine in postoperative patients. A prospective, randomised double-blind study. Schmerz 2001;15:248–53.

[44] Xie H, Wang X, Liu G, Wang G. Analgesic effects and pharmacokinetics of a low dose of ketamine preoperatively administered epidurally or intravenously. Clin J Pain 2003;19:317–22.

[45] Tan PH, Kuo MC, Kao PF, et al. Patient-controlled epidural analgesia with morphine or morphine plus ketamine for post-operative pain relief. Eur J Anaesthesiol 1999;16:820–5.

[46] Chia YY, Liu K, Liu YC, et al. Adding ketamine in a multimodal patient-controlled epidural regimen reduces postoperative pain and analgesic consumption. Anesth Analg 1998;86:1245–9.

[47] Subramaniam B, Subramaniam K, Pawar DK, et al. Preoperative epidural ketamine in combination with morphine does not have a clinically relevant intra- and postoperative opioid-sparing effect. Anesth Analg 2001;93:1321–6.

[48] Subramaniam K, Subramaniam B, Pawar DK, et al. Evaluation of the safety and efficacy of epidural ketamine combined with morphine for postoperative analgesia after major upper abdominal surgery. J Clin Anesth 2001;13:339–44.

[49] Taura P, Fuster J, Blasi A, et al. Postoperative pain relief after hepatic resection in cirrhotic patients: the efficacy of a single small dose of ketamine plus morphine epidurally. Anesth Analg 2003;96:475–80.

[50] Santawat U, Pongraweewan O, Lertakayamanee J, et al. Can ketamine potentiate the analgesic effect of epidural morphine, preincisional or postincisional administration? J Med Assoc Thai 2002;85(Suppl 3):S1024–30.

[51] Price DD, Mao J, Frenk H, Mayer DJ. The N-methyl-D-aspartate receptor antagonist dextromethorphan selectively reduces temporal summation of second pain in man. Pain 1994;59:165–74.

[52] Chang FL, Wu CT, Yeh CC, et al. Postoperative intramuscular dextromethorphan injection provides postoperative pain relief and decreases opioid requirement after hemorrhoidectomy. Acta Anaesthesiol Sin 1999;37:179–83.

[53] Wu CT, Yu JC, Yeh CC, et al. Postoperative intramuscular dextromethorphan injection provides pain relief and decreases opioid requirement after modified radical mastectomy. Int J Surg Investig 2000;2:145–9.

[54] Wadhwa A, Clarke D, Goodchild CS, et al. Large-dose oral dextromethorphan as an adjunct to patient-controlled analgesia with morphine after knee surgery. Anesth Analg 2001;92:448–54.

[55] Koinig H, Wallner T, Marhofer P, et al. Magnesium sulfate reduces intra- and postoperative analgesic requirements. Anesth Analg 1998;87:206–10.

[56] Levaux C, Bonhomme V, Dewandre PY, et al. Effect of intra-operative magnesium sulphate on pain relief and patient comfort after major lumbar orthopaedic surgery. Anaesthesia 2003;58:131–5.

[57] Tramer MR, Schneider J, Marti RA, et al. Role of magnesium sulfate in postoperative analgesia. Anesthesiology 1996;84:340–7.

[58] Wilder-Smith CH, Knopfli R, Wilder-Smith OH. Perioperative magnesium infusion and postoperative pain. Acta Anaesthesiol Scand 1997;41:1023–7.

[59] Ko SH, Lim HR, Kim DC, et al. Magnesium sulfate does not reduce postoperative analgesic requirements. Anesthesiology 2001;95:640–6.

[60] Zarauza R, Saez-Fernandez AN, Iribarren MJ, et al. A comparative study with oral nifedipine, intravenous nimodipine, and magnesium sulfate in postoperative analgesia. Anesth Analg 2000;91:938–43.

[61] Buvanendran A, McCarthy RJ, Kroin JS, et al. Intrathecal magnesium prolongs fentanyl analgesia: a prospective, randomized, controlled trial. Anesth Analg 2002;95:661–6.

[62] Gottschalk A, Schroeder F, Ufer M, et al. Amantadine, a N-methyl-D-aspartate receptor antagonist, does not enhance postoperative analgesia in women undergoing abdominal hysterectomy. Anesth Analg 2001;93:192–6.

[63] Snijdelaar DG, Koren G, Katz J. Effects of perioperative oral amantadine on postoperative pain and morphine consumption in patients after radical prostatectomy: results of a preliminary study. Anesthesiology 2004;100:134–41.

[64] Maze M, Tranquilli W. Alpha-2 adrenoceptor agonists: defining the role in clinical anesthesia. Anesthesiology 1991;74:581–605.

[65] Dyck JB, Maze M, Haack C, et al. The pharmacokinetics and hemodynamic effects of intravenous and intramuscular dexmedetomidine hydrochloride in adult human volunteers. Anesthesiology 1993;78:813–20.

[66] Mikawa K, Nishina K, Maekawa N, et al. Oral clonidine premedication reduces postoperative pain in children. Anesth Analg 1996;82:225–30.

[67] Reimer EJ, Dunn GS, Montgomery CJ, et al. The effectiveness of clonidine as an analgesic in paediatric adenotonsillectomy. Can J Anaesth 1998;45:1162–7.

[68] Goyagi T, Nishikawa T. Oral clonidine premedication enhances the quality of postoperative analgesia by intrathecal morphine. Anesth Analg 1996;82:1192–6.

[69] Goyagi T, Tanaka M, Nishikawa T. Oral clonidine premedication enhances postoperative analgesia by epidural morphine. Anesth Analg 1999;89:1487–91.

[70] Mayson KV, Gofton EA, Chambers KG. Premedication with low dose oral clonidine does not enhance postoperative analgesia of intrathecal morphine. Can J Anaesth 2000;47:752–7.

[71] Yanagidate F, Hamaya Y, Dohi S. Clonidine premedication reduces maternal requirement for intravenous morphine after cesarean delivery without affecting newborn's outcome. Reg Anesth Pain Med 2001;26:461–7.

[72] Park J, Forrest J, Kolesar R, et al. Oral clonidine reduces postoperative PCA morphine requirements. Can J Anaesth 1996;43:900–6.

[73] Segal IS, Jarvis DJ, Duncan SR, et al. Clinical efficacy of oral-transdermal clonidine combinations during the perioperative period. Anesthesiology 1991;74:220–5.

[74] Owen MD, Fibuch EE, McQuillan R, et al. Postoperative analgesia using a low-dose, oral-transdermal clonidine combination: lack of clinical efficacy. J Clin Anesth 1997;9:8–14.

[75] De Kock MF, Pichon G, Scholtes JL. Intraoperative clonidine enhances postoperative morphine patient-controlled analgesia. Can J Anaesth 1992;39:537–44.

[76] Bernard JM, Hommeril JL, Passuti N, Pinaud M. Postoperative analgesia by intravenous clonidine. Anesthesiology 1991;75:577–82.

[77] Bernard JM, Kick O, Bonnet F. Comparison of intravenous and epidural clonidine for postoperative patient-controlled analgesia. Anesth Analg 1995;81:706–12.

[78] Lyons B, Casey W, Doherty P, et al. Pain relief with low-dose intravenous clonidine in a child with severe burns. Intensive Care Med 1996;22:249–51.

[79] Marinangeli F, Ciccozzi A, Donatelli F, et al. Clonidine for treatment of postoperative pain: a dose-finding study. Eur J Pain 2002;6:35–42.

[80] Jeffs SA, Hall JE, Morris S. Comparison of morphine alone with morphine plus clonidine for postoperative patient-controlled analgesia. Br J Anaesth 2002;89:424–7.

[81] Eisenach J, Detweiler D, Hood D. Hemodynamic and analgesic actions of epidurally administered clonidine. Anesthesiology 1993;78:277–87.

[82] Eisenach JC, Hood DD, Tuttle R, et al. Computer-controlled epidural infusion to targeted cerebrospinal fluid concentrations in humans. Clonidine. Anesthesiology 1995;83:33–47.

[83] Bonnet F, Boico O, Rostaing S, et al. Clonidine-induced analgesia in postoperative patients: epidural versus intramuscular administration. Anesthesiology 1990;72:423–7.

[84] Filos KS, Goudas LC, Patroni O, et al. Intrathecal clonidine as a sole analgesic for pain relief after cesarean section. Anesthesiology 1992;77:267–74.

[85] Bonnet F, Brun-Buisson V, Saada M, et al. Dose-related prolongation of hyperbaric tetracaine spinal anesthesia by clonidine in humans. Anesth Analg 1989;68:619–22.

[86] Gordh Jr T. Epidural clonidine for treatment of postoperative pain after thoracotomy. A double-blind placebo-controlled study. Acta Anaesthesiol Scand 1988;32:702–9.

[87] Bonnet F, Boico O, Rostaing S, et al. Postoperative analgesia with extradural clonidine. Br J Anaesth 1989;63:465–9.

[88] Armand S, Langlade A, Boutros A, et al. Meta-analysis of the efficacy of extradural clonidine to relieve postoperative pain: an impossible task. Br J Anaesth 1998;81:126–34.

[89] Casati A, Magistris L, Beccaria P, et al. Improving postoperative analgesia after axillary brachial plexus anesthesia with 0.75% ropivacaine. A double-blind evaluation of adding clonidine. Minerva Anestesiol 2001;67:407–12.

[90] Iskandar H, Guillaume E, Dixmerias F, et al. The enhancement of sensory blockade by clonidine selectively added to mepivacaine after midhumeral block. Anesth Analg 2001; 93:771–5.

[91] Erlacher W, Schuschnig C, Koinig H, et al. Clonidine as adjuvant for mepivacaine, ropivacaine and bupivacaine in axillary, perivascular brachial plexus block. Can J Anaesth 2001;48:522–5.

[92] Barioni MF, Lauretti GR, Lauretti-Fo A, et al. Clonidine as coadjuvant in eye surgery: comparison of peribulbar versus oral administration. J Clin Anesth 2002;14:140–5.

[93] Connelly NR, Camerlenghi G, Bilodeau M, et al. Use of clonidine as a component of the peribulbar block in patients undergoing cataract surgery. Reg Anesth Pain Med 1999;24:426–9.

[94] Madan R, Bharti N, Shende D, et al. A dose–response study of clonidine with local anesthetic mixture for peribulbar block: a comparison of three doses. Anesth Analg 2001;93:1593–7.

[95] Samkaoui MA, Bouaggad A, al Harrar R, et al. Addition of clonidine to 0.5% lidocaine for intravenous locoregional anesthesia. Ann Fr Anesth Reanim 2001;20:255–9.

[96] Gorgias NK, Maidatsi PG, Kyriakidis AM, et al. Clonidine versus ketamine to prevent tourniquet pain during intravenous regional anesthesia with lidocaine. Reg Anesth Pain Med 2001;26:512–7.

[97] Gentili M, Enel D, Szymskiewicz O, et al. Postoperative analgesia by intraarticular clonidine and neostigmine in patients undergoing knee arthroscopy. Reg Anesth Pain Med 2001;26: 342–7.

[98] Joshi W, Reuben SS, Kilaru PR, et al. Postoperative analgesia for outpatient arthroscopic knee surgery with intra-articular clonidine and/or morphine. Anesth Analg 2000;90:1102–6.

[99] Reuben SS, Connelly NR. Postoperative analgesia for outpatient arthroscopic knee surgery with intra-articular clonidine. Anesth Analg 1999;88:729–33.

[100] Aantaa R, Jaakola ML, Kallio A, et al. Reduction of the minimum alveolar concentration of isoflurane by dexmedetomidine. Anesthesiology 1997;86:1055–60.

[101] Aantaa R, Jaakola ML, Kallio A, et al. A comparison of dexmedetomidine, and alpha 2-adrenoceptor agonist, and midazolam as IM premedication for minor gynaecological surgery. Br J Anaesth 1991;67:402–9.

[102] Aantaa R, Kanto J, Scheinin M, et al. Dexmedetomidine, an alpha 2-adrenoceptor agonist, reduces anesthetic requirements for patients undergoing minor gynecologic surgery. Anesthesiology 1990;73:230–5.

[103] Belleville JP, Ward DS, Bloor BC, et al. Effects of intravenous dexmedetomidine in humans. I. Sedation, ventilation, and metabolic rate. Anesthesiology 1992;77:1125–33.

[104] Scheinin H, Jaakola ML, Sjovall S, et al. Intramuscular dexmedetomidine as premedication for general anesthesia. A comparative multi-center study. Anesthesiology 1993;78:1065–75.

[105] Aho MS, Erkola OA, Scheinin H, et al. Effect of intravenously administered dexmedetomidine on pain after laparoscopic tubal ligation. Anesth Analg 1991;73:112–8.

[106] Arain SR, Ruehlow RM, Uhrich TD, et al. The efficacy of dexmedetomidine versus morphine for postoperative analgesia after major inpatient surgery. Anesth Analg 2004;98:153–8.

[107] Memis D, Turan A, Karamanlioglu B, et al. Adding dexmedetomidine to lidocaine for intravenous regional anesthesia. Anesth Analg 2004;98:835–40.

[108] Gilron I. Is gabapentin a broad-spectrum analgesic? Anesthesiology 2002;97:537–9.

[109] Rosner H, Rubin L, Kestenbaum A. Gabapentin adjunctive therapy in neuropathic pain states. Clin J Pain 1996;12:56–8.

[110] Backonja M, Beydoun A, Edwards KR, et al. Gabapentin for the symptomatic treatment of painful neuropathy in patients with diabetes mellitus: a randomized controlled trial. JAMA 1998;280:1831–6.

[111] Rowbotham M, Harden N, Stacey B, et al. Gabapentin for the treatment of postherpetic neuralgia: a randomized controlled trial. JAMA 1998;280:1837–42.

[112] Mellick GA, Mellick LB. Reflex sympathetic dystrophy treated with gabapentin. Arch Phys Med Rehabil 1997;78:98–105.

[113] Shimoyama M, Shimoyama N, Inturrisi CE, et al. Gabapentin enhances the antinociceptive effects of spinal morphine in the rat tail-flick test. Pain 1997;72:375–82.

[114] Eckhardt K, Ammon S, Hofmann U, et al. Gabapentin enhances the analgesic effect of morphine in healthy volunteers. Anesth Analg 2000;91:185–91.

[115] Caraceni A, Zecca E, Martini C, et al. Gabapentin as an adjuvant to opioid analgesia for neuropathic cancer pain. J Pain Symptom Manage 1999;17:441–5.

[116] Field MJ, Holloman EF, McCleary S, et al. Evaluation of gabapentin and S-(+)-3-isobutylgaba in a rat model of postoperative pain. J Pharmacol Exp Ther 1997;282:1242–6.

[117] Gee NS, Brown JP, Dissanayake VU, et al. The novel anticonvulsant drug, gabapentin (Neurontin), binds to the alpha2delta subunit of a calcium channel. J Biol Chem 1996;271: 5768–76.

[118] Luo ZD, Chaplan SR, Higuera ES, et al. Upregulation of dorsal root ganglion (alpha)2(delta) calcium channel subunit and its correlation with allodynia in spinal nerve-injured rats. J Neurosci 2001;21:1868–75.

[119] Maneuf YP, McKnight AT. Block by gabapentin of the facilitation of glutamate release from rat trigeminal nucleus following activation of protein kinase C or adenylyl cyclase. Br J Pharmacol 2001;134:237–40.

[120] Fehrenbacher JC, Taylor CP, Vasko MR. Pregabalin and gabapentin reduce release of substance P and CGRP from rat spinal tissues only after inflammation or activation of protein kinase C. Pain 2003;105:133–41.

[121] Hurley RW, Chatterjea D, Rose Feng M, et al. Gabapentin and pregabalin can inter-act synergistically with naproxen to produce antihyperalgesia. Anesthesiology 2002;97: 1263–73.

[122] Dirks J, Fredensborg BB, Christensen D, et al. A randomized study of the effects of single-dose gabapentin versus placebo on postoperative pain and morphine consumption after mastectomy. Anesthesiology 2002;97:560–4.

[123] Dierking G, Duedahl TH, Rasmussen ML, et al. Effects of gabapentin on postoperative morphine consumption and pain after abdominal hysterectomy: a randomized, double-blind trial. Acta Anaesthesiol Scand 2004;48:322–7.

[124] Fassoulaki A, Patris K, Sarantopoulos C, et al. The analgesic effect of gabapentin and mexiletine after breast surgery for cancer. Anesth Analg 2002;95:985–91.

[125] Pandey CK, Priye S, Singh S, et al. Pre-emptive use of gabapentin significantly decreases postoperative pain and rescue analgesic requirements in laparoscopic cholecystectomy. [L'usage preventif de gabapentine diminue significativement la douleur postoperatoire et les besoins d'analgesique de secours lors d'une cholecystectomie laparoscopique]. Can J Anesth 2004;51:358–63.

[126] Turan A, Memis D, Karamanlioglu B, et al. The analgesic effects of gabapentin in monitored anesthesia care for ear-nose-throat surgery. Anesth Analg 2004;99:375–8.

[127] Rorarius MGF, Mennander S, Suominen P, et al. Gabapentin for the prevention of postopera-tive pain after vaginal hysterectomy. Pain 2004;110:175–81.

[128] Turan A, Karamanlioglu B, Memis D, et al. Analgesic effects of gabapentin after spinal surgery. Anesthesiology 2004;100:935–8.

[129] Turan A, Karamanlioglu B, Memis D, et al. The analgesic effects of gabapentin after total abdominal hysterectomy. Anesth Analg 2004;98:1370–3.

[130] Hill CM, Balkenohl M, Thomas DW, et al. Pregabalin in patients with postoperative dental pain. Eur J Pain 2001;5:119–24.

[131] Crain SM, Shen KF. Antagonists of excitatory opioid receptor functions enhance mor-phine's analgesic potency and attenuate opioid tolerance/dependence liability. Pain 2000;84:121–31.

[132] Crain SM, Shen KF. Modulation of opioid analgesia, tolerance and dependence by Gs-

coupled, GM1 ganglioside-regulated opioid receptor functions. Trends Pharmacol Sci 1998; 19:358–65.

[133] Shen KF, Crain SM. Ultra-low doses of naltrexone or etorphine increase morphine's antinociceptive potency and attenuate tolerance/dependence in mice. Brain Res 1997; 757:176–90.

[134] Gan TJ, Ginsberg B, Glass PS, et al. Opioid-sparing effects of a low-dose infusion of naloxone in patient-administered morphine sulfate. Anesthesiology 1997;87:1075–81.

[135] Joshi JP, Duffy L, Chehade J, et al. Effects of prophylactic nalmefene on the incidence of morphine-related side effects in patients receiving intravenous patient-controlled analgesia. Anesthesiology 1999;90:1007–11.

[136] Cepeda MS, Africano JM, Manrique AM, et al. The combination of low dose of naloxone and morphine in PCA does not decrease opioid requirements in the postoperative period. Pain 2002;96:73–9.

[137] Cepeda MS, Alvarez H, Morales O, et al. Addition of ultra-low dose naloxone to postoperative morphine PCA: unchanged analgesia and opioid requirement but decreased incidence of opioid side effects. Pain 2004;107:41–6.

[138] Sartain JB, Barry JJ, Richardson CA, et al. Effect of combining naloxone and morphine for intravenous patient-controlled analgesia. Anesthesiology 2003;99:148–51.

[139] Mehlisch DR. The combination of low dose of naloxone and morphine in patient-controlled (PCA) does not decrease opioid requirements in the postoperative period. Pain 2003;101: 209–11.

[140] Yaksh TL, Grafe MR, Malkmus S, et al. Studies on the safety of chronically administered intrathecal neostigmine methylsulfate in rats and dogs. Anesthesiology 1995;82:412–27.

[141] Abram SE, Winne RP. Intrathecal acetyl cholinesterase inhibitors produce analgesia that is synergistic with morphine and clonidine in rats. Anesth Analg 1995;81:501–7.

[142] Ummenhofer WC, Brown SM, Bernards CM. Acetylcholinesterase and butyrylcholinesterase are expressed in the spinal meninges of monkeys and pigs. Anesthesiology 1998;88: 1259–65.

[143] Naguib M, Yaksh TL. Characterization of muscarinic receptor subtypes that mediate antinociception in the rat spinal cord. Anesth Analg 1997;85:847–53.

[144] Chiari A, Tobin JR, Pan HL, et al. Sex differences in cholinergic analgesia I: a supplemental nicotinic mechanism in normal females. Anesthesiology 1999;91:1447–54.

[145] Xu Z, Tong C, Eisenach JC. Acetylcholine stimulates the release of nitric oxide from rat spinal cord. Anesthesiology 1996;85:107–11.

[146] Eisenach JC, Gebhart GF. Intrathecal amitriptyline. Antinociceptive interactions with intravenous morphine and intrathecal clonidine, neostigmine, and carbamylcholine in rats. Anesthesiology 1995;83:1036–45.

[147] Krukowski JA, Hood DD, Eisenach JC, et al. Intrathecal neostigmine for postcesarean section analgesia: dose response. Anesth Analg 1997;84:1269–75.

[148] Miranda HF, Sierralta F, Pinardi G. Neostigmine interactions with non steroidal anti-inflammatory drugs. Br J Pharmacol 2002;135:1591–7.

[149] Hood DD, Eisenach JC, Tuttle R. Phase I safety assessment of intrathecal neostigmine methylsulfate in humans. Anesthesiology 1995;82:331–43.

[150] Lauretti GR, Reis MP, Prado WA, et al. Dose–response study of intrathecal morphine versus intrathecal neostigmine, their combination, or placebo for postoperative analgesia in patients undergoing anterior and posterior vaginoplasty. Anesth Analg 1996;82:1182–7.

[151] Lauretti GR, Reis MP. Postoperative analgesia and antiemetic efficacy after subarachnoid neostigmine in orthopedic surgery. Reg Anesth 1997;22:337–42.

[152] Klamt JG, Slullitel A, Garcia IV, et al. Postoperative analgesic effect of intrathecal neostigmine and its influence on spinal anaesthesia. Anaesthesia 1997;52:547–51.

[153] Lauretti GR, Mattos AL, Gomes JM, et al. Postoperative analgesia and antiemetic efficacy after intrathecal neostigmine in patients undergoing abdominal hysterectomy during spinal anesthesia. Reg Anesth 1997;22:527–33.

[154] Pan PM, Huang CT, Wei TT, et al. Enhancement of analgesic effect of intrathecal neostigmine and clonidine on bupivacaine spinal anesthesia. Reg Anesth Pain Med 1998;23:49–56.

[155] Lauretti GR, Azevedo VM. Intravenous ketamine or fentanyl prolongs postoperative analgesia after intrathecal neostigmine. Anesth Analg 1996;83:766–70.

[156] Tan PH, Chia YY, Lo Y, et al. Intrathecal bupivacaine with morphine or neostigmine for postoperative analgesia after total knee replacement surgery. Can J Anaesth 2001;48:551–6.

[157] Chung CJ, Kim JS, Park HS, et al. The efficacy of intrathecal neostigmine, intrathecal morphine, and their combination for postcesarean section analgesia. Anesth Analg 1998; 87:341–6.

[158] Klamt JG, Garcia LV, Prado WA. Analgesic and adverse effects of a low dose of intrathecally administered hyperbaric neostigmine alone or combined with morphine in patients submitted to spinal anaesthesia: pilot studies. Anaesthesia 1999;54:27–31.

[159] Lauretti GR, Mattos AL, Reis MP, et al. Combined intrathecal fentanyl and neostigmine: therapy for postoperative abdominal hysterectomy pain relief. J Clin Anesth 1998;10:291–6.

[160] Lauretti GR, Mattos AL, Reis MP, et al. Intrathecal neostigmine for postoperative analgesia after orthopedic surgery. J Clin Anesth 1997;9:473–7.

[161] Lauretti GR, Hood DD, Eisenach JC, et al. A multi-center study of intrathecal neostigmine for analgesia following vaginal hysterectomy. Anesthesiology 1998;89:913–8.

[162] Almeida RA, Lauretti GR, Mattos AL. Antinociceptive effect of low-dose intrathecal neostigmine combined with intrathecal morphine following gynecologic surgery. Anesthesiology 2003;98:495–8.

[163] Lauretti GR, Oliveira AP, Juliao MC, et al. Transdermal nitroglycerine enhances spinal neostigmine postoperative analgesia following gynecological surgery. Anesthesiology 2000; 93:943–6.

[164] Lauretti GR, Gomes JM, Reis MP, et al. Low doses of epidural ketamine or neostigmine, but not midazolam, improve morphine analgesia in epidural terminal cancer pain therapy. J Clin Anesth 1999;11:663–8.

[165] Lauretti GR, de Oliveira R, Reis MP, et al. Study of three different doses of epidural neostigmine coadministered with lidocaine for postoperative analgesia. Anesthesiology 1999;90:1534–8.

[166] Omais M, Lauretti GR, Paccola CA. Epidural morphine and neostigmine for postoperative analgesia after orthopedic surgery. Anesth Analg 2002;95:1698–701.

[167] Nakayama M, Ichinose H, Nakabayashi K, et al. Analgesic effect of epidural neostigmine after abdominal hysterectomy. J Clin Anesth 2001;13:86–9.

[168] Kaya FN, Sahin S, Owen MD, et al. Epidural neostigmine produces analgesia but also sedation in women after cesarean delivery. Anesthesiology 2004;100:381–5.

[169] Urban L, Willetts J, Murase K, et al. Cholinergic effects on spinal dorsal horn neurons in vitro: an intracellular study. Brain Res 1989;500:12–20.

[170] Iwamoto ET, Marion L. Pharmacologic evidence that spinal muscarinic analgesia is mediated by an L-arginine/nitric oxide/cyclic GMP cascade in rats. J Pharmacol Exp Ther 1994;271: 601–8.

[171] Yang LC, Chen LM, Wang CJ, Buerkle H. Postoperative analgesia by intra-articular neostigmine in patients undergoing knee arthroscopy. Anesthesiology 1998;88:334–9.

[172] Lauretti GR, de Oliveira R, Perez MV, et al. Postoperative analgesia by intraarticular and epidural neostigmine following knee surgery. J Clin Anesth 2000;12:444–8.

[173] Bouaziz H, Paqueron X, Bur ML, et al. No enhancement of sensory and motor blockade by neostigmine added to mepivacaine axillary plexus block. Anesthesiology 1999;91:78–83.

[174] Van Elstraete AC, Pastureau F, Lebrun T, et al. Neostigmine added to lidocaine axillary plexus block for postoperative analgesia. Eur J Anaesthesiol 2001;18:257–60.

[175] Bone HG, Van Aken H, Booke M, et al. Enhancement of axillary brachial plexus block anesthesia by coadministration of neostigmine. Reg Anesth Pain Med 1999;24:405–10.

[176] Bouderka MA, Al-Harrar R, Bouaggad A, Harti A. Neostigmine added to bupivacaine in axillary plexus block: which benefit? Ann Fr Anesth Reanim 2003;22:510–3.

[177] Turan A, Karamanlyoglu B, Memis D, et al. Intravenous regional anesthesia using prilocaine and neostigmine. Anesth Analg 2002;95:1419–22.

[178] McCartney CJ, Brill S, Rawson R, et al. No anesthetic or analgesic benefit of neostigmine 1 mg added to intravenous regional anesthesia with lidocaine 0.5% for hand surgery. Reg Anesth Pain Med 2003;28:414–7.

[179] Skjelbred P, Lokken P. Postoperative pain and inflammatory reaction reduced by injection of a corticosteroid. A controlled trial in bilateral oral surgery. Eur J Clin Pharmacol 1982;21:391–6.

[180] Olstad OA, Skjelbred P. Comparison of the analgesic effect of a corticosteroid and paracetamol in patients with pain after oral surgery. Br J Clin Pharmacol 1986;22:437–42.

[181] Baxendale BR, Vater M, Lavery KM. Dexamethasone reduces pain and swelling following extraction of third molar teeth. Anaesthesia 1993;48:961–4.

[182] Aasboe V, Raeder JC, Groegaard B. Betamethasone reduces postoperative pain and nausea after ambulatory surgery. Anesth Analg 1998;87:319–23.

[183] Schulze S, Sommer P, Bigler D, et al. Effect of combined prednisolone, epidural analgesia, and indomethacin on the systemic response after colonic surgery. Arch Surg 1992;127:325–31.

[184] Vargas 3rd JH, Ross DG. Corticosteroids and anterior cruciate ligament repair. Am J Sports Med 1989;17:532–4.

[185] Glasser RS, Knego RS, Delashaw JB, et al. The perioperative use of corticosteroids and bupivacaine in the management of lumbar disc disease. J Neurosurg 1993;78:383–7.

[186] Watters III WC, Temple AP, Granberry M. The use of dexamethasone in primary lumbar disc surgery. A prospective, randomized, double-blind study. Spine 1989;14:440–2.

[187] Highgenboten CL, Jackson AW, Meske NB. Arthroscopy of the knee. Ten-day pain profiles and corticosteroids. Am J Sports Med 1993;21:503–6.

[188] Catlin FI, Grimes WJ. The effect of steroid therapy on recovery from tonsillectomy in children. Arch Otolaryngol Head Neck Surg 1991;117:649–52.

[189] Ohlms LA, Wilder RT, Weston B. Use of intraoperative corticosteroids in pediatric tonsillectomy. Arch Otolaryngol Head Neck Surg 1995;121:737–42.

[190] Lavyne MH, Bilsky MH. Epidural steroids, postoperative morbidity, and recovery in patients undergoing microsurgical lumbar discectomy. J Neurosurg 1992;77:90–5.

[191] April MM, Callan ND, Nowak DM, et al. The effect of intravenous dexamethasone in pediatric adenotonsillectomy. Arch Otolaryngol Head Neck Surg 1996;122:117–20.

[192] Tom LW, Templeton JJ, Thompson ME, et al. Dexamethasone in adenotonsillectomy. Int J Pediatr Otorhinolaryngol 1996;37:115–20.

[193] Giannoni C, White S, Enneking FK. Does dexamethasone with pre-emptive analgesia improve pediatric tonsillectomy pain? Otolaryngol Head Neck Surg 2002;126:307–15.

[194] Goldman AC, Govindaraj S, Rosenfeld RM. A meta-analysis of dexamethasone use with tonsillectomy. Otolaryngol Head Neck Surg 2000;123:682–6.

ELSEVIER
SAUNDERS

Anesthesiology Clin N Am
23 (2005) 109–123

ANESTHESIOLOGY
CLINICS OF
NORTH AMERICA

Intravenous Patient-Controlled Analgesia: One Size Does Not Fit All

Pamela E. Macintyre, BMedSc, MBBS, FANZCA, MHA, FFPMANZCA

Department of Anaesthesia, Acute Pain Service, Hyperbaric and Pain Medicine,
Royal Adelaide Hospital and University of Adelaide, Adelaide, South Australia, 5000 Australia

Patient-controlled analgesia (PCA) was introduced as a technique that would allow patients to self-administer small doses of intravenous (IV) opioids at frequent intervals and as needed. It was hoped that the flexibility of this technique would allow the amount of opioid delivered to better match interpatient variations in dose requirements and enable the patient to better cover episodes of incident pain. It was anticipated that PCA would lead to significant improvements in analgesic efficacy compared with the more traditional methods used in the management of acute pain, such as intermittent intramuscular (IM) opioid injections. Although to an extent this has proven to be the case, the benefits have not been as great as expected.

Efficacy of IV-PCA compared with conventional opioid analgesia

The first meta-analysis that compared IV-PCA with conventional IM opioid analgesia was performed by Ballantyne et al [1] and included randomized controlled trials published up until 1991. They concluded that patients reported higher satisfaction with IV-PCA and that pain relief was better (although the mean additional benefit was only 5.6 on a pain score scale of 0 to 100), with no difference in side effects or opioid consumption. A later meta-analysis by Walder

E-mail address: pamela.macintyre@adelaide.edu.au

et al [2], in 2001, included randomized controlled trials published up until 2000. Again, patients preferred IV-PCA, and there were no differences in the amount of opioid used or opioid-related adverse effects. There was also some evidence that the incidence of pulmonary complications after surgery was decreased. Analgesia was better when all pain outcomes (pain intensity, pain relief, and requirement for rescue analgesia) were combined, but there was no difference in pain scores. That is, as with the first meta-analysis, analgesia with IV-PCA was only a little better than conventional methods of pain relief.

Given the continuing popularity of IV-PCA, these results are probably a little unexpected. These results could indicate that there is truly no great difference between IV-PCA and conventional methods of opioid analgesia or that conventional opioid analgesia is more effective under study conditions when greater attention is paid to the technique by investigators and staff alike—the "Hawthorne effect" [3]; or they may mean that the way in which PCA was used did not adequately allow for interpatient variations. Walder et al [2] noted from the studies included in their analysis that there was a large variability in pain intensity scores in both groups and therefore there was "still room for improvement" with both IV-PCA and the traditional methods of opioid analgesia. They also commented that the enormous variability in programmed PCA parameters (bolus doses, lockout intervals, and maximum permitted cumulative doses) used in the studies suggested continued uncertainty about the ideal PCA program. Certainly, in many if not most of the studies, PCA program parameters were fixed, which could significantly limit the flexibility of the technique.

Less rigorous evidence from information obtained through audit data and formal studies suggests that IV-PCA may be appreciably more effective in the clinical setting than intermittent IM opioid analgesia. Dolin et al [4] reviewed all publications (randomized controlled trials, cohort studies, case control studies, and audit reports) up until 1999 that concerned the management of postoperative pain. They looked at the percentage of patients who experienced moderate to severe pain and severe pain associated with "as needed" IM opioid analgesia, IV-PCA, and epidural analgesia during the first 24 hours after surgery. The mean (95% confidence interval [CI]) percentage of patients with moderate to severe pain was 67.2% (58.1%–76.2%) for IM analgesia, 35.8% (31.4%–40.2%) for IV-PCA, and 20.9% (17.8%–24.0%) for epidural analgesia. The results for severe pain were 29.1% (18.8%–39.4%), 10.4% (8.0%–12.8%), and 7.8% (6.1%–9.5%), respectively. Again, although IV-PCA resulted in better pain relief than as-needed IM opioids, there was considerable room for improvement with all techniques.

In 1999, in a review of patient-controlled analgesia (PCA), Etches [5] remarked that PCA was not "a set and forget" or a "one size fits all" therapy. That is, the success of PCA may depend on how well it is used. He suggested that the effective and safe use of PCA requires frequent patient assessment, adjustment to PCA orders as needed, and knowledgeable nursing staff [5]. It may be that IV-PCA could be more effective and possibly safer if individual PCA prescriptions, including the programmed parameters, the opioid chosen, the use of adjuvant drugs, and the treatment of opioid-related adverse effects, were adjusted more frequently and if relevant patient factors, including patient selection and education, were addressed. To do this, the following need to be considered:

- Which opioid, if any, might be best to use with IV-PCA and which adjuvant drugs might be useful when added to the IV-PCA opioid or given separately but concurrently with IV-PCA.
- The evidence, if any, behind commonly prescribed IV-PCA program parameters and how these parameters might be adjusted to better suit individual patients.
- Patient factors, including psychological aspects and education, that might affect the efficacy of IV-PCA.
- Whether adjustments need to be made to IV-PCA in specific patient groups, for example, for patients who are opioid-tolerant, or morbidly obese, or who have obstructive sleep apnea, and the elderly.

Choice of IV-PCA opioid

On a population basis, there are no major differences between the various opioids prescribed for IV-PCA. Morphine and other commonly used opioids such as fentanyl [6], hydromorphone [7], meperidine [6,8,9], oxycodone [10], and tramadol [11–13] provide equally effective analgesia and have a similar incidence of side effects, although more patients may report pruritus with morphine [6]. The choice of opioid may be more important when there is a need to consider the possible effects of opioid metabolites. In patients with renal impairment, the use of a drug with no active metabolites, such as fentanyl, might be preferred [14].

Problems resulting from the use of meperidine and the accumulation of its active metabolite, normeperidine, may occur even in the absence of renal impairment. The accumulation of normeperidine occurs after prolonged use or high doses of meperidine and can result in a spectrum of side effects ranging from anxiety and agitation to myoclonic jerks and grand mal seizures, all of which may occur within 24 hours of starting therapy [15]. Meperidine is no more effective than morphine [16] or hydromorphone [17] in the treatment of renal colic, and both meperidine and morphine have similar effects on the sphincter of Oddi and the biliary [18]. Because meperidine has no advantage over other opioids, its use is discouraged [18].

Therefore, for most patients, no one opioid is preferable for initial use with IV-PCA. However, on an individual basis, some opioids may be better in some patients, and if a patient is experiencing intolerable side effects that are unresponsive or incompletely responsive to treatment, an alternative opioid may improve the effectiveness of IV-PCA.

In a randomized double-blind three-way cross-over study, Woodhouse et al [19] administered morphine, meperidine, and fentanyl in a random sequence to each of 82 postsurgical patients. Although overall patient responses were similar for all three drugs (consistent with the studies cited above), there was considerable variability in individual patient responses. Some patients were able to tolerate all three opioids, some were intolerant to all, and others appeared to be sensitive only to one or two opioids.

Opioid-related side effects

Any of the opioid-related side effects can occur during IV-PCA therapy, but the side effect that causes most concern is respiratory depression. The overall incidence ranges from 0.1% to 0.8%; however, incidences of 1.1% to 3.9% have been recorded when a concurrent background infusion is used [20]. Comparisons of PCA with more conventional opioid analgesic techniques are difficult because there is a paucity of data relating to the latter methods. The incidence of respiratory depression with conventional methods of opioid administration is approximately in the range of 0.2% to 0.9% [20].

The occurrence of side effects may also have an impact on the effectiveness of analgesia with IV-PCA. When asked to rate potential postoperative outcomes from most undesirable to least undesirable, patients ranked vomiting the most undesirable followed by gagging on an endotracheal tube, incisional pain, and nausea [21]. Similarly, patients seen before and after surgery gave comparable "importance" scores to pain control and the combination of type and severity of side effects [22]. The side effects that were least preferred were vomiting, nightmares, hallucinations, and nausea. It is not surprising therefore that when given the choice, many patients will balance the positive effect of an analgesic technique (effective pain relief) against the negative outcomes (opioid-related side effects) and limit their analgesic use in an attempt reduce the severity of a troublesome side effect [23]. More effective management of side effects, especially postoperative nausea and vomiting (see below), may encourage patients to attempt better pain relief using IV-PCA.

Adjuvant drugs and IV-PCA

In the attempt to improve analgesia or minimize side effects, a variety adjuvant drugs have been added to the IV-PCA regimens, administered either separately or added to the opioid syringe or reservoir.

Adjuvants administered separately

Nonsteroidal anti-inflammatory drugs
The addition of nonsteroidal anti-inflammatory drugs to opioid analgesic regimens is known to improve the quality of pain relief and reduce the amount of opioid required; however such opioid sparing does not always reduce the incidence of opioid-related side effects [24]. Studies of the use of selective cyclooxygenase-2 (COX-2) inhibitors suggest that the same is also true. Valdecoxib used for up to 48 hours after total knee arthroplasty [25] and

parecoxib given to patients undergoing total knee arthroplasty [26] or hysterectomy [27] improved pain relief and reduced PCA morphine consumption but had no effect on the incidence of opioid-related side effects. However, in another study [28], parecoxib in doses of 40 mg but not 20 mg given to patients undergoing total knee arthroplasty reduced morphine consumption, improved analgesia, and resulted in a reduction in the incidence of postoperative vomiting.

Acetaminophen

Intravenously [29], rectally [30], and orally [31] administered acetaminophen given as an adjunct to IV-PCA morphine may lead to opioid sparing and better pain relief, although this is not inevitable [32]; but again, there is no difference in opioid-related adverse effects.

Ketamine

Similarly, the use of ketamine as an adjunct to IV opioids, including IV-PCA, reduces the amount of opioid needed but no consistent decrease in opioid-related adverse effects has been demonstrated [33].

Adjuvants added to the IV-PCA solution

The routine addition of adjuvant drugs to the IV-PCA opioid solution means that all patients receive the adjuvant whether or not they need it; even if they require it, some patients may receive inadequate doses, whereas others receive inappropriately high doses. Therefore, the routine addition of adjunctive drugs to IV-PCA opioid is not recommended. However, if the addition of an adjuvant drug is contemplated, the cost-benefit and risk-benefit should be considered for each patient [20].

Antiemetics

The efficacy of antiemetics added to IV-PCA opioid solutions and the incidence of their adverse effects were systematically reviewed by Tramèr et al [34]. The antiemetic most commonly used in the studies was droperidol, for which the number needed to treat was 2.7 for nausea and 3.1 for vomiting. The risk of nausea or vomiting in control patients was 43% and 55%, respectively. The authors concluded that 100 patients would need to be treated with droperidol in this manner for 30 patients who would otherwise have had emetic symptoms to avoid these side effects. They also reported that there was no evidence of dose-responsiveness with droperidol but that the absolute risk of adverse effects increased when cumulative doses of more than 4 mg/d were used. Tramèr et al [34] suggest that mixing droperidol with morphine "may be the most effective and sensible approach to reducing morphine PCA related nausea and vomiting." However, it does mean than some patients will be exposed to the risk of adverse effects from a drug that they do not need.

A later study by Culebras et al [35] comparing the effects of adding 0.5, 1.5, and 5 mg of droperidol to 100 mg of PCA morphine found that droperidol did show dose-responsiveness. Although the 0.5 mg dose had no significant antiemetic effect, the 1.5 mg dose was effective against nausea but not vomiting, and the 5 mg dose significantly reduced both nausea and vomiting. However, the largest dose was associated with unacceptable sedation.

The second most reported group of antiemetics added to IV-PCA opioids analyzed by Tramèr et al [34] was 5-hydroxytryptamine$_3$ receptor antagonists (ondansetron and tropisetron). The number needed to treat to prevent vomiting was approximately 5, but these agents had no effect on nausea. Promethazine "showed promising results," but patient numbers were small [34]. The use of any drug that may cause patient sedation and increase the risk of respiratory depression, especially promethazine, must be carefully considered in light of the proven effectiveness of other antiemetics.

Other drugs

A number of other drugs have also been added to IV-PCA opioid solutions in an attempt to improve analgesia or minimize side effects. The addition of ketamine [33], lidocaine [36], or naloxone does not improve pain relief [37–39], but naloxone used in very low doses may decrease the incidence of nausea and pruritus [39]. Clonidine added to IV-PCA morphine resulted in significantly better pain relief for the first 12 hours only and less nausea and vomiting compared with morphine administered alone [40].

Program parameters for IV-PCA

Postoperative IV-PCA requirements vary at least 10-fold between patients, with doses decreasing as patient age increases [41]. The parameters programmed into PCA devices should therefore allow for this wide interpatient variability. However, in many clinical and research settings, the parameters used (which are often fixed) would not permit this range of opioid doses to be delivered. In general, standard orders are for standard patients; the effectiveness of IV-PCA may be increased when such orders are adjusted to suit individual patient needs.

Bolus dose

There are few studies that have investigated the optimal IV-PCA bolus dose (one which provides good pain relief with minimal side effects). Owen et al [42] compared 0.5-, 1-, and 2-mg bolus doses of morphine and found that most patients who were prescribed 0.5 mg were unable to achieve adequate analgesia, whereas those who received a 2-mg bolus had a high incidence of respiratory depression. They concluded that the best size for a morphine IV-PCA bolus dose was 1 mg. Similarly, Camu et al [43] found that the risk of respiratory depression was higher in patients who were prescribed 60-μg bolus doses of fentanyl compared with those who received 20- or 40-μg doses (all doses were given as a

10-minute infusion, which is not the usual clinical practice) and concluded that the optimal bolus dose (given as an infusion) for fentanyl was 40 μg.

Rigid adherence to an "optimal" dose may, however, not lead to the best pain relief for all patients. Initial orders for bolus doses should take into account factors such as a history of previous opioid use (discussed elsewhere in this issue) and patient age [41], and these doses should then be adjusted according to patient pain reports or the onset of any side effects. Initial IV-PCA bolus doses that are commonly used (for opioid-naive patients) are morphine, 1 to 2 mg; hydromorphone, 0.2 to 0.4 mg; fentanyl, 20 to 40 μg; and diamorphine, 0.5 to 1 mg.

Lockout interval

The lockout interval is used to limit the frequency of demands made by the patient within a certain time. In some institutions, the lockout interval is decreased when patients report inadequate analgesia. However, decreasing the lockout interval is unlikely to improve pain relief because patients may not increase their demand rate enough to compensate for inadequate or smaller bolus doses, even though the length of the lockout interval would allow more doses [42]. In the study by Owen et al [42] it was noted that even patients complaining of poor pain relief averaged only four demands per hour. It may be that patients will not sustain a high demand rate to try and achieve better analgesia, even though they understand the concept and use of IV-PCA. If a patient is uncomfortable and already receiving an average of three or more bolus doses per hour, it may be reasonable to consider an increase in the size of the bolus dose [20].

Lockout periods between 5 and 10 minutes are commonly prescribed in clinical practice, but Ginsberg et al [44] were unable to find any differences in pain relief, side effects, or anxiety with lockout intervals of 7 or 11 minutes for morphine and 5 or 8 minutes for fentanyl. Importantly, if a patient is uncomfortable and already receiving an average of three or more bolus doses per hour, it may be more effective to increase the size of the bolus dose rather than decrease the lockout interval [20].

Concurrent background (continuous) infusions

When it was first introduced, it was anticipated that the use of a background infusion with IV-PCA, in addition to bolus doses on demand, would improve patient comfort and sleep. However, this has not been the case; instead, studies report no benefit to pain relief or sleep and no decrease in the number of demands made but a marked increase in the risk of respiratory depression [42,45–51]. This has led to the general recommendation that background infusions should not be used with IV-PCA. However, a better recommendation could be that the relative safety of background infusions is increased if a patient's opioid requirements are already known and the rate of infusion is based on those requirements [5,20]. There may be times when background infusions may improve the effectiveness of IV-PCA, for example, in patients who are opioid-tolerant (discussed elsewhere in this issue) or in opioid-naive patients with high opioid requirements or who complain of waking in severe pain at night [20].

Dose limits

If IV-PCA is to be used effectively, a wide range of opioid doses will be required. There is, however, no reliable way of knowing how much opioid a patient will need for analgesia, far less how much will result in respiratory depression. Although the limits to the amount of opioid that can be delivered over a certain period (commonly 1 or 4 hours) can be programmed into most PCA machines, there is no good evidence of any benefit that can be attributed to these limits [20].

Patient factors

A number of patient factors, including psychological characteristics and patient education, may also affect IV-PCA use and need to be taken into account if efficacy is to be maximized.

Psychological characteristics

The subjective experience of pain depends on a number of factors, including patients' psychological characteristics. These characteristics may affect how well patients use PCA and therefore their pain relief. Anxiety seems to be the most important psychological factor affecting PCA use, and high levels of preoperative anxiety are associated with an increase in the number of demands made by the patient (often during the lockout interval), a higher level of dissatisfaction with PCA, and increased postoperative pain [52–57]. There is also a relationship between preoperative depression and pain intensity, morphine requirements, PCA demands, and the degree of dissatisfaction [53]. However there appears to be no association between the locus of control and postoperative pain intensity, satisfaction with PCA, or PCA dose-demand ratio [57].

Patient education

The evidence concerning the benefits of patient education on PCA effectiveness is mixed. It is known that patient may have concerns about some aspects of IV-PCA, and if these concerns led to reduced PCA use, efficacy would be affected. Chumbley et al [23] surveyed 200 patients who used PCA and reported that approximately 20% were worried that they might become addicted and that 20% and 30%, respectively, felt that the machine could give them too much drug or that they could self-administer too much opioid.

However, in a later study from the same group [58], it was noted that, although patients given preoperative education about IV-PCA were better informed, less confused about the technique, and more rapidly became familiar with its use, pain relief was not improved, and there were no effects on their concerns about addiction and safety or knowledge of side effects. The lack of effect of patient education on pain scores and opioid consumption has also been reported by Lam et al [59] and Griffen et al [60].

Specific patient groups

Opioid-tolerant patients

Patients with a history of opioid consumption (whether legally prescribed or illegally obtained) before admission to hospital may require higher than average opioid doses if adequate analgesia is to be obtained. This means that significant deviations from "standard" IV-PCA prescriptions are often needed.

Rapp et al [61] reported that the average postoperative 24-hour IV-PCA requirements of opioid-tolerant patients (patients with cancer pain, chronic noncancer pain, and those with an opioid addiction) were three times the average requirements of matched opioid-naive controls and that the opioid-tolerant patients had higher pain scores and fewer emetic and pruritic symptoms. Surprisingly, this group also had higher sedation scores than would normally be expected for tolerance to this side effect. Although these patients were much more likely to be given concurrent anxiolytics, the authors state that this did not correlate with increased sedation. It may be that if opioid doses are rapidly increased to levels that are significantly in excess of preadmission basal doses, oversedation (a better clinical indicator of early respiratory depression than a decrease in respiratory rate; see discussion below) can result (for more detail on acute pain management in opioid-tolerant patients see elsewhere in this issue).

Morbidly obese patients and patients with obstructive sleep apnea

Epidemiologic studies show that the prevalence of obstructive sleep apnea (OSA) in the adult population is high. Up to 20% of adults have at least mild OSA, and 7% have moderate to severe OSA. It is more common in males than females (a ratio of 8 to 1), and approximately 75% of those who could benefit from treatment remain undiagnosed [62].

Although IV-PCA has therefore probably been used in many patients with undiagnosed OSA, there have been case reports of complications after its use in patients with OSA. VanDercar et al [63] reported a case of severe postoperative respiratory depression in a patient who weighed 136 kg (~300 lb) and, despite a history suggestive of OSA, was not diagnosed with OSA until after the incident. The patient was found unconscious 10.5 hours after starting IV-PCA; his $PaCO_2$ was 94 mm Hg, and his PaO_2 was 44 mm Hg. Excessive self-administration of morphine was deemed to be a contributing factor. However, the PCA machine was programmed to deliver a bolus dose of 1.5 mg and a background infusion of 2 mg/h. There is no mention of any assessment of his level of sedation, nor is there a reference to any oxygen administration.

It is known that the use of a background infusion with IV-PCA increases the risk of respiratory depression (see discussion above). It is also known that a decrease in respiratory rate is an unreliable indicator of the presence or absence of opioid-induced respiratory depression and that the best early clinical indicator of respiratory depression is increasing sedation [20,64–66]. The addition of the background infusion and the lack of sedation scoring may increase the risk of respiratory depression even without the presence of OSA. Finally, it has been shown that oxygen therapy can reduce the likelihood of significant hypoxemia in patients with OSA even if it does not prevent disruption of sleep pattern or symptoms such as daytime somnolence [67,68]. Because patients with OSA are more at risk for hypoxemia after surgery or if given opioids, and despite concerns about reducing respiratory drive during the apneic periods [69], the use of supplemental oxygen would seem appropriate.

Lofsky [69] gives another example case, from a composite of claims cases reported, in which a patient with OSA (diagnosed retrospectively from his history) was prescribed IV-PCA with a background infusion for postoperative analgesia. One hour after "his last normal vital signs," the patient was "found in respiratory arrest." Similarly, respiratory depression occurring in two other patients with OSA was noticed only when one patient "was found to be unrousable" with a PCO_2 of 94 mm Hg [70], and the other "was heavily sedated and hypercapnic" [71]. Severe opioid-induced respiratory depression caused by IV-PCA is unlikely to occur suddenly (unless there are additional adverse events such as a programming error or machine malfunction leading to the delivery of a large dose of the opioid), and patients will become progressively rather than suddenly sedated. If sedation is noted at an earlier stage, the opioid can be withheld and restarted at a lower dose when the patient is more awake.

The importance of sedation as an early indicator of respiratory depression is highlighted in another case report [72] in which morphine, 4 mg IM, was given to a patient with OSA. Over the following 2 hours, the patient was noted to be "sleepy" and then "unresponsive." An order was given to continue monitoring "vital signs," and no additional oxygen was given; the patient was found in cardiac arrest 30 minutes later.

Morbid obesity is common in patients with OSA [62], but the use of PCA in morbidly obese patients is probably no less safe than other opioid analgesic techniques in these patients [73–75]. There is no evidence that morbidly obese patients require smaller or larger IV-PCA bolus doses. However, in view of the risks associated with opioids and OSA, smaller initial bolus doses have been suggested [5,20].

Elderly patients

For IV-PCA to be used effectively and safely, patients need to have reasonably normal cognitive function. Patients who have preadmission evidence of cognitive impairment may not be suitable candidates for IV-PCA. Delirium (confusion) is a common form of acute cognitive impairment in the elderly, especially during acute illnesses and in the postoperative setting [76]. Should this develop in a patient already using IV-PCA, alternative forms of analgesia will usually need to be organized.

Apart from old age, some of the risk factors associated with the development of delirium in previously cognitively intact patients include infection, pre-existing depression, hypoxemia, anemia, certain drugs (eg, anticholinergic drugs, psychoactive drugs, benzodiazepines, opioids, and some antiemetics), and drug withdrawal (eg, alcohol and benzodiazepines) [76,77].

Patient-controlled analgesia has been shown to be an effective method of pain relief in the elderly [78–81]. In a comparison with IM morphine, IV-PCA resulted in better pain relief, less confusion, and fewer severe pulmonary complications [80]. Similarly, pain scores were lower in elderly patients using IV-PCA compared with intermittent subcutaneous injections of morphine [82]. The risk of respiratory depression with IV-PCA use appears to be higher in the elderly patient [70], and it has therefore been suggested that a lower PCA bolus dose should be used [5,41,82].

Summary

Patient-controlled analgesia was introduced as a technique that would allow greater flexibility in opioid delivery both between and within patients for the management of acute pain. However, any improvements in pain relief compared with conventional methods of pain relief appear to be small. In both clinical and research settings, relatively inflexible PCA prescriptions are often used. These may reduce the chance of good pain relief in some patients and lead to increased risk in others. On the basis that "one size does not fit all," it is possible that the efficacy and safety of IV-PCA could be improved if such orders are adjusted to suit individual patient needs.

References

[1] Ballantyne JC, Carr DB, Chalmers TC, et al. Postoperative patient-controlled analgesia: meta-analyses of initial randomized control trials. J Clin Anesth 1993;5:182–93.

[2] Walder B, Schafer M, Henzi H, et al. Efficacy and safety of patient-controlled opioid analgesia for acute postoperative pain. Acta Anaesthesiol Scand 2001;45:795–804.

[3] Watson TJ. Sociology, work and industry. London: Routledge & Kegan Paul Ltd.; 1987.

[4] Dolin SJ, Cashman JN, Bland JM. Effectiveness of acute postoperative pain management: evidence from published data. Br J Anaesth 2002;89:409–23.

[5] Etches RC. Patient-controlled analgesia. Surg Clin North Am 1999;79:297–312.

[6] Woodhouse A, Hobbes AF, Mather LE, et al. A comparison of morphine, pethidine and fentanyl in the postsurgical patient-controlled analgesia environment. Pain 1996;64:115–21.

[7] Rapp SE, Egan KJ, Ross BK, et al. A multidimensional comparison of morphine and hydromorphone patient-controlled analgesia. Anesth Analg 1996;82:1043–8.

[8] Stanley G, Appadu B, Mead M, et al. Dose requirements, efficacy and side effects of morphine and pethidine delivered by patient-controlled analgesia after gynaecological surgery. Br J Anaesth 1996;76:484–6.

[9] Sinatra RS, Lodge K, Sibert K, et al. A comparison of morphine, meperidine and oxymorphone as utilized in patient-controlled analgesia following cesarean delivery. Anesthesiology 1989;70:585–90.

[10] Silvasti M, Rosenberg P, Seppala T, et al. Comparison of analgesic efficacy of oxycodone and morphine in postoperative intravenous patient-controlled analgesia. Acta Anaesthesiol Scand 1998;42:576–80.

[11] Pang WW, Mok MS, Lin CH, et al. Comparison of patient-controlled analgesia (PCA) with tramadol or morphine. Can J Anaesth 1999;46:1030–5.

[12] Silvasti M, Tarkkila P, Tuominen M, et al. Efficacy and side effects of tramadol versus oxycodone for patient-controlled analgesia after maxillofacial surgery. Eur J Anaesthesiol 1999;16:834–9.

[13] Stamer UM, Maier C, Grond S, et al. Tramadol in the management of postoperative pain: a double blind placebo and active drug controlled study. Eur J Anaesthesiol 1997;14:646–54.

[14] Mather LE, Woodhouse A. Pharmacokinetics of opioids in the context of patient controlled analgesia. Pain Reviews 1997;4:20–32.

[15] Simopoulos TT, Smith HS, Peeters-Asdourian C, et al. Use of meperidine in patient-controlled analgesia and the development of a normeperidine toxic reaction. Arch Surg 2002 Jan;137:84–8.

[16] O'Connor A, Schug SA, Cardwell HJ. A comparison of the efficacy and safety of morphine and pethidine as analgesia for suspected renal colic in the emergency setting. J Accid Emerg Med 2000;17:261–4.

[17] Jasani NB, O'Conner RE, Bouzoukis JK. Comparison of hydromorphone and meperidine for ureteral colic. Acad Emerg Med 1994;1:539–43.

[18] Latta KS, Ginsberg B, Barkin RL. Meperidine: a critical review. Am J Ther 2002;9:53–68.

[19] Woodhouse A, Ward ME, Mather LE. Intra subject variability in postoperative patient-controlled analgesia (PCA): is the patient equally satisfied with morphine, pethidine and fentanyl? Pain 1999;80:545–53.

[20] Macintyre PE. Safety and efficacy of patient-controlled analgesia. Br J Anaesth 2001;87:36–46.

[21] Macario M, Weinger M, Carney S, et al. Which clinical anesthesia outcomes are important to avoid: the perspective of patients. Anesth Analg 1999;89:652–8.

[22] Gan TJ, Lubarsky DA, Flood EM, et al. Patient preferences for acute pain treatment. Br J Anaesth 2004;92:681–8.

[23] Chumbley GM, Hall GM, Salmon P. Patient-controlled analgesia: an assessment by 200 patients. Anaesthesia 1998;53:216–21.

[24] Royal College of Anaesthetists. Guidelines for the use of non-steroidal anti-inflammatory drugs in the perioperative period. Oxford (UK): Royal College of Anaesthetists (London, UK); 1998.

[25] Reynolds LW, Hoo RK, Brill RJ, et al. The COX-s specific inhibitor, valdecoxib, is an effective opioid-sparing analgesia in patients undergoing total knee arthroplasty. J Pain Symptom Manage 2003;25:133–41.

[26] Hubbard RC, Naumann TM, Traylor L, et al. Parecoxib sodium has opioid-sparing effects in patients undergoing total knee arthroplasty under spinal anaesthesia. Br J Anaesth 2003; 90:166–72.

[27] Ng A, Smith G, Davidson AC. Analgesic effects of parecoxib following total abdominal hysterectomy. Br J Anaesth 2003;90:746–9.

[28] Malan TP, Marsh G, Hakki S, et al. Parecoxib sodium, a parenteral cyclooxygenase 2 selective inhibitor, improves morphine analgesia and is opioid sparing following total hip arthroplasty. Anesthesiology 2003;98:950–6.

[29] Hernandez-Palazon J, Tortosa JA, Martinez-Lage JF, et al. Intravenous administration of propacetamol reduced morphine consumption after spinal surgery. Anesth Analg 2001;92: 1473–6.

[30] Cobby TF, Crighton IM, Kyriakides K, et al. Rectal paracetamol has a significant morphine-sparing effect after hysterectomy. Br J Anaesth 2000;85:658–9.

[31] Schug SA, Sidebotham DA, McGuinnety M, et al. Acetaminophen as an adjunct to morphine by patient-controlled analgesia in the management of acute postoperative pain. Anesth Analg 1998;87:368–72.

[32] Lahtinen P, Kokki H, Hendolin H, et al. Propacetamol as adjunctive treatment for postoperative pain after cardiac surgery. Anesth Analg 2002;95:813–9.

[33] Subramaniam K, Subramaniam B, Steinbrook RA. Ketamine as adjuvant analgesic to opioids: a quantitative and qualitative systematic review. Anesth Analg 2004;99:482–95.

[34] Tramèr MR, Walder B. Efficacy and adverse effects of prophylactic antiemetics during patient-controlled analgesia therapy: a quantitative systematic. Anesth Analg 1999;88:1354–61.

[35] Culebras X, Corpataux JB, Gaggero G, et al. The antiemetic effect of droperidol added to morphine patient-controlled analgesia: a randomized, controlled, multicenter dose-finding study. Anesth Analg 2003;97:816–21.

[36] Cepeda MS, Delgado M, Ponce M, et al. Equivalent outcomes during postoperative patient-controlled intravenous analgesia with lidocaine plus morphine versus morphine alone. Anesth Analg 1996;83:102–6.

[37] Sartain JB, Barry JJ, Richardson CA, et al. Effect of combining naloxone and morphine for intravenous patient-controlled analgesia. Anesthesiology 2003;99:148–51.

[38] Cepeda MS, Africano JM, Manrique AM, et al. The combination of low dose of naloxone and morphine in PCA does not decrease opioid requirements in the postoperative period. Pain 2002;96:73–9.

[39] Cepeda MS, Alvarez H, Morales O, et al. Addition of ultra low dose naloxone to postoperative morphine PCA: unchanged analgesia and opioid requirements but decreased incidence of opioid side effects. Pain 2004;107:41–6.

[40] Jeffs SA, Hall JE, Morris S. Comparison of morphine alone with morphine plus clonidine for postoperative patient-controlled analgesia. Br J Anaesth 2002;89:424–7.

[41] Macintyre PE, Jarvis DA. Age is the best predictor of postoperative morphine requirements. Pain 1996;64:357–64.

[42] Owen H, Plummer JL, Armstrong I, et al. Variables of patient-controlled analgesia: bolus size. Anaesthesia 1989;44:7–10.

[43] Camu F, Van Aken H, Bovill JG. Postoperative analgesic effects of three demand-dose sizes of fentanyl administered by patient-controlled analgesia. Anesth Analg 1998;87:890–5.

[44] Ginsberg B, Gil KM, Muir M, et al. The influence of lockout intervals and drug selection on patient-controlled analgesia following gynecological surgery. Pain 1995;62:95–100.

[45] Parker RK, Holtmann B, White PF. Effects of a nighttime opioid infusion with PCA therapy on patient comfort and analgesic requirements after abdominal hysterectomy. Anesthesiology 1992;76:362–7.

[46] Parker RK, Holtmann B, White PF. Patient-controlled analgesia. Does a concurrent opioid infusion improve pain management after surgery? JAMA 1991;266:1947–52.

[47] Dal D, Kanbak M, Caglar M, et al. A background infusion of morphine does not enhance postoperative analgesia after cardiac surgery. Can J Anaesth 2003;50:476–9.

[48] Fleming BM, Coombs DW. A survey of complications documented in a quality-control analysis of patient-controlled analgesia in the postoperative patient. J Pain Symptom Manage 1992;7:463–9.

[49] Notcutt WG, Morgan RJ. Introducing patient-controlled analgesia for postoperative pain control into a district general hospital. Anaesthesia 1990;45:401–6.

[50] Schug SA, Torrie JJ. Safety assessment of postoperative pain management by an acute pain service. Pain 1993;55:387–91.

[51] Sidebotham D, Dijkhuizen MR, Schug SA. The safety and utilization of patient-controlled analgesia. J Pain Symptom Manage 1997;14:202–9.

[52] Gil KM, Ginsberg B, Muir M, et al. Patient-controlled analgesia in postoperative pain: the relation of psychological factors to pain and analgesic use. Clin J Pain 1990;6:137–42.

[53] Ozalp G, Sarioglu R, Tuncel G, et al. Preoperative emotional states in patients with breast cancer and postoperative pain. Acta Anaesthesiol Scand 2003;47:26–9.

[54] Jamieson RN, Taft K, O'Hara JP, et al. Psychosocial and pharmacological predictors of satisfaction with intravenous patient-controlled analgesia. Anesth Analg 1993;77:121–5.

[55] Perry F, Parker RK, White PF, et al. Role of psychological factors in postoperative pain control and recovery with patient-controlled analgesia. Clin J Pain 1994;10:57–63.

[56] Thomas V, Heath M, Rose D, et al. Psychological characteristics and the effectiveness of patient-controlled analgesia. Br J Anaesth 1995;74:271–6.

[57] Brandner B, Bromley L, Blagrove M. Influence of psychological factors in the use of patient controlled analgesia. Acute Pain 2002;4:53–6.

[58] Chumbley GM, Ward L, Hall GM, et al. Pre-operative information and patient-controlled analgesia: much ado about nothing. Anaesthesia 2004;59:354–8.

[59] Lam KK, Chan MTV, Chen PP, et al. Structured preoperative patient education for patient-controlled analgesia. J Clin Anesth 2001;13:465–9.

[60] Griffin MJ, Brennan L, McShane AJ. Preoperative education and outcome of patient-controlled analgesia. Can J Anaesth 1998;45:943–8.

[61] Rapp SE, Ready BL, Nessly ML. Acute pain management in patients with prior opioid consumption: a case-controlled retrospective review. Pain 1995;61:195–201.

[62] Young T, Skatrud J, Peppard PE. Risk factors for obstructive sleep apnoea in adults. JAMA 2004;291:2013–6.

[63] VanDercar DH, Martinez AP, De Lisser EA. Sleep apnea syndromes: a potential contraindication for patient-controlled analgesia. Anesthesiology 1991;74(3):623–4.

[64] Ready LB, Oden R, Chadwick HS, et al. Development of an anesthesiology-based postoperative pain management service. Anesthesiology 1988;68:100–6.

[65] Leith S, Wheatley RG, Jackson IJB, et al. Extradural infusion analgesia for postoperative pain relief. Br J Anaesth 1994;73:552–8.

[66] Chaney MA. Side effects of intrathecal and epidural opioids. Can J Anaesth 1995;42:891–903.

[67] Phillips BA, Schmitt FA, Berry DT, et al. Treatment of obstructive sleep apnea: a preliminary report comparing nasal CPAC to nasal oxygen in patients with mild OSA. Chest 1990;98:325–30.

[68] Landsberg R, Freidman M, Ascher-Landsberg J. Treatment of hypoxemia in obstructive sleep apnea. Am J Rhinol 2001;15:311–3.

[69] Lofsky A. Sleep apnea and narcotic postoperative pain medication: morbidity and mortality risk. Anesthesia Patient Safety Foundation Newsletter 2002;17:24.

[70] Etches RC. Respiratory depression associated patient-controlled analgesia: a review of eight cases. Can J Anaesth 1994;41:125–32.

[71] Parikh SN, Stuchin SA, Maca C, et al. Sleep apnea syndrome in patients undergoing total joint arthroplasty. J Arthroplasty 2002;17(5):635–42.

[72] Cullen DJ. Obstructive sleep apnea and postoperative analgesia–a potentially dangerous combination. J Clin Anesth 2001;13:83–5.

[73] Kyzer S, Ramadan E, Gersch M, et al. Patient-controlled analgesia following vertical gastroplasty: a comparison with intramuscular narcotics. Obes Surg 1995;5:18–21.

[74] Choi YK, Brolin RE, Bertil KJ, et al. Efficacy and safety of patient-controlled analgesia for morbidly obese patients following gastric bypass surgery. Obes Surg 2000;10:154–9.

[75] Charghi R, Backman S, Christou N, et al. Patient controlled IV analgesia is an acceptable management strategy in morbidly obese patients undergoing gastric bypass surgery: a retrospective comparison with epidural analgesia. Can J Anesth 2003;50:672–8.

[76] Beckker AY, Weeks EJ. Cognitive function after anaesthesia in the elderly. Best Pract Res Clin Anesthesiol 2003;17:259–72.

[77] Macintyre PE, Upton R, Ludbrook GL. Pain in the elderly. In: Rowbotham DJ, Macintyre PE, editors. Clinical pain management: acute pain. London: Arnold Publishers; 2003. p. 463–84.

[78] Gagliese L, Jackson M, Ritvo P, et al. Age is not an impediment to effective use of patient-controlled analgesia by surgical patients. Anesthesiology 2000;93:601–10.

[79] Mann C, Pouzeratte Y, Boccara G, et al. Comparison of intravenous or epidural patient-controlled analgesia in the elderly after major abdominal surgery. Anesthesiology 2000;92:433–41.

[80] Egbert AM, Parks LH, Short LM, et al. Randomised trial of postoperative patient-controlled analgesia v. intramuscular opioids in frail elderly men. Arch Intern Med 1990;150: 1897–903.
[81] Keita H, Geachan N, Dahmani S, et al. Comparison between patient-controlled analgesia and subcutaneous morphine in elderly patients after total hip replacement. Br J Anaesth 2002; 90:53–7.
[82] Lavand'Homme P, De Kock M. Practical guidelines on the postoperative use of patient-controlled analgesia in the elderly. Drugs Aging 1998;13:9–16.

ELSEVIER
SAUNDERS

Anesthesiology Clin N Am
23 (2005) 125–140

ANESTHESIOLOGY
CLINICS OF
NORTH AMERICA

Epidural Analgesia for Postoperative Pain

Jeffrey M. Richman, MD[a,b], Christopher L. Wu, MD[a,b,*]

[a]Department of Anesthesiology, The Johns Hopkins Hospital, Carnegie 280, 600 North Wolfe Street, Baltimore, MD 21287, USA
[b]Anesthesiology and Critical Care Medicine, The Johns Hopkins University, Carnegie 280, 600 North Wolfe Street, Baltimore, MD 21287, USA

Although we have significantly increased our knowledge of the neurobiology of nociception and have made improvements in analgesic techniques, postoperative pain continues to be undertreated [1,2]. Poorly controlled postoperative pain may result in both short- and long-term consequences, including a decrease in quality of life, an increase in postoperative cognitive dysfunction, and a higher incidence of chronic pain after surgery [3–5]. Recently published evidence-based guidelines highlight the deficiencies in our understanding of postoperative pain and the recovery process and provide a menu of analgesic choices categorized by surgical procedure; these guidelines may ultimately result in the development of reliable, comprehensive, and individualized analgesic plans for specific surgical procedures [6].

There is sufficient evidence to suggest that epidural analgesia offers superior postoperative analgesia compared with systemic opioids, including intravenous patient-controlled analgesia [7]. In addition to improved pain control, epidural anesthesia and analgesia can improve patient outcomes (including reduced major morbidity and possibly mortality) by attenuating detrimental perioperative physiology [8–11]. The use of epidural analgesia for the management of postoperative pain has evolved as a critical component of a multimodal approach to achieving the goal of adequate analgesia with improved outcomes. An evidence-based strategy for postoperative analgesia that uses both regional analgesia techniques in conjunction with other modalities tailored to each patient's needs may prove to offer the best outcomes for patients.

* Corresponding author. Department of Anesthesiology, The Johns Hopkins Hospital, Carnegie 280, 600 North Wolfe Street, Baltimore, MD 21287.
E-mail address: chwu@jhmi.edu (C.L. Wu).

0889-8537/05/$ – see front matter © 2005 Elsevier Inc. All rights reserved.
doi:10.1016/j.atc.2004.11.004
anesthesiology.theclinics.com

Benefits of epidural analgesia on patient outcomes

The overall efficacy of perioperative epidural analgesia on patient outcomes is controversial. There are many methodology issues that contribute to this controversy (especially considering the limitations of the various types of study designs examining this issue) [12–15]. One of the most problematic issues is that epidural analgesia is often considered a generic entity. It is a misnomer to refer to epidural anesthesia and analgesia as a homogeneous technique because many factors (eg, congruency of epidural catheter location and surgical incision, choice of analgesic and local anesthetic concentrations, adjunctive agent, infusion rates, and epidural placement technique [16]) contribute to the overall efficacy and effectiveness of this technique.

Morbidity and mortality

The effect of perioperative epidural anesthesia-analgesia on mortality is unclear. Several randomized controlled trials and database analyses found no reduction in mortality [10,17,18], whereas other investigators report reduced postoperative mortality with epidural anesthesia-analgesia [11,19,20]. Although the perioperative use of epidural anesthesia-analgesia does not appear to decrease certain morbidity (eg, cognitive dysfunction or immunosuppression), the physiologic benefits provided by epidural analgesia may result in decreased cardiovascular, pulmonary, gastrointestinal, and coagulation-related morbidity as well as improvements in patient-oriented outcomes [7,21–25].

Cardiovascular

Sympathetic nervous system activation (eg, neuroendocrine stress response or uncontrolled pain) may not only increase heart rate, contractility, and blood pressure, but it may also theoretically precipitate atherosclerotic plaque rupture through increases in stress-induced mechanical forces and precipitate coronary artery vasoconstriction [26]. Therefore, thoracic epidural analgesia using a local anesthetic-based solution may be beneficial in patients who are at high risk for myocardial ischemia and infarction because of the blockade of cardiac sympathetic outflow from the vasomotor center and cardiac sympathetic reflexes at the segmental level that attenuate increases in heart rate, blood pressure, inotropy, and myocardial oxygen consumption [21,27]. By diminishing sympathetic outflow, thoracic epidural analgesia may also improve coronary blood flow to subendocardial areas that are at risk for ischemia, which has been shown to reduce the anatomic extent of experimentally induced myocardial infarction and ischemia-induced malignant arrhythmias [21,27].

Despite the experimental evidence suggesting a physiologic benefit of thoracic epidural analgesia for patients at high risk for myocardial ischemia and infarction, randomized trials [28–32] evaluating these benefits have been equivocal. However, a recent meta-analysis has revealed that thoracic but not lumbar epidural analgesia significantly decreases the incidence of postoperative myocardial infarction, corroborating some of the experimental evidence demonstrating the physiologic benefits of thoracic epidural analgesia on cardiovascular outcomes [8].

Pulmonary

Thoracic epidural anesthesia-analgesia may improve postoperative pulmonary function in part by enhancing diaphragmatic function by attenuating reflex spinal inhibition of diaphragmatic activity [33] as well as by preserving hypoxic pulmonary vasoconstriction in poorly ventilated segments [21,34]. In addition, the superior pain relief provided by epidural analgesia may result in improved patient participation and compliance with rehabilitative physiotherapy [7]. Compared with epidural or systemic opioids, epidural local anesthetic solutions appear to result in a lower incidence of postoperative pulmonary complications [9,10,35]. Although no improvement has been clearly demonstrated in surrogate measures of pulmonary function (and there has been controversy over the definition of pulmonary complications in various studies), some data suggest that perioperative epidural anesthesia-analgesia leads to a decrease in atelectasis and respiratory complications [9] and a lower incidence of respiratory failure in high risk patients [10], and it facilitates early postoperative extubation in high-risk thoracic surgical patients [35].

Gastrointestinal

Postoperative gastrointestinal ileus is a common problem that results in patient discomfort and prolonged hospitalization, and it may contribute to other morbidity, including pulmonary complications, septic complications, and decreased wound healing [21,36]. The cause of postoperative ileus is multifactorial and includes systemic inflammatory response, somatic and visceral neural stimuli, and intravenous opioids [21,36]. A local anesthetic-based thoracic epidural may inhibit somatic and visceral nociceptive afferent fibers and attenuate spinal reflexes, contributing to gastrointestinal ileus and an increase in gut mucosal blood flow in the presence of decreased perfusion pressure, and it reduces ileus associated with bowel ischemia [21,37]. A systematic review of randomized trials reveals reduced gastrointestinal paralysis in patients undergoing abdominal surgery with local anesthetic-based epidural analgesia compared with systemic or epidural opioids [38–40]. Thoracic epidural analgesia also may provide earlier fulfillment of discharge criteria [41]. However, these benefits are not observed with lumbar epidural analgesia and the use of epidural opioids (either alone or in combination with local anesthetics), which may delay the return of gastrointestinal motility [14,21,41]. Of note, there is no evidence that epidural analgesia increases the risk of anastomotic leakage after abdominal surgery [42].

Coagulation

Attenuating the hypercoagulable state that occurs postoperatively may be important in decreasing postoperative mortality and morbidity [21]. The administration of local anesthetic-based epidural analgesia has been demonstrated to attenuate perioperative hypercoagulability by increasing peripheral blood flow, preserving fibrinolytic activity, attenuating increases in coagulation factors, and decreasing blood viscosity [43,44]. Randomized-controlled trials and meta-analyses [11,32,45–57] suggest that intraoperative epidural and spinal anesthesia (versus general anesthesia) decrease postoperative hypercoagulable-related adverse events such as vascular graft thrombosis, deep venous thrombosis, and pulmonary embolism. However, many early studies did not concurrently use systemic anticoagulant prophylaxis, which is now a standard practice. Thus, the true benefit of intraoperative neuraxial anesthesia in decreasing deep venous thrombosis and pulmonary embolism remains unclear.

Perioperative blood loss

Epidural anesthesia-analgesia may decrease perioperative blood loss in part through a decrease in arterial or venous blood pressure [48]. Although there are contradicting studies with regard to the effect of regional anesthesia on intraoperative blood loss, a meta-analysis of randomized trials [11] examining neuraxial versus general anesthesia revealed that neuraxial anesthesia decreased perioperative blood loss and the need for blood transfusion. Another recent meta-analysis [49] demonstrated a significant decrease in intraoperative blood loss with neuraxial anesthesia compared with general anesthesia or combined general and epidural anesthesia. It is possible that a decrease in transfusion requirements may decrease transfusion-related morbidity and mortality as well as costs.

Patient-oriented outcomes

Compared with systemic opioids, epidural analgesia provides superior postoperative pain control [7] and is associated with an improvement in patient-oriented outcomes such as patient satisfaction [25] and health-related quality of life [23,24]. Although there are no data measuring patient satisfaction as a primary endpoint, in a comparison of epidural analgesia and systemic opioids for postoperative pain control, a systematic review [25] suggests that the use of regional analgesic techniques compared with systemic opioids results in higher patient satisfaction. The assessment of health-related quality of life is a widely accepted outcome measurement and is adversely affected by an increase in postoperative pain [3]. Available data suggest that the use of epidural analgesia (versus systemic opioids) is associated with an improvement in health-related quality of life in the postoperative period [23,24]. Thus, postoperative epidural analgesia may improve patient-oriented outcomes, although there are many methodology issues in measuring these endpoints [25,50].

Factors affecting efficacy of epidural analgesia

Epidural catheter location

The location of epidural catheter placement affects the efficacy of epidural analgesia and influences patient outcomes. Insertion of the epidural catheter in a location congruent to the incisional dermatome provides equal or superior analgesia and improved postoperative outcome with reduced side effects [11,14,51]. The reduced side effects with thoracic epidural analgesia are probably caused by avoidance of the blockade of the sympathetic nerve fibers from T9–L1 [52,53]. For example, the thoracic rather than the lumbar placement of an epidural catheter for a patient undergoing upper abdominal surgery provides a segmental blockade of thoracic dermatomes corresponding to the incision and will likely reduce the total volume of the local anesthetic required, possibly decreasing side effects such as lower extremity motor weakness, urinary retention, and hypotension [52,54,55]. The higher side effects caused by catheter-incision incongruence (eg, placement of the lumbar epidural for upper abdominal surgery) may prompt a reduction in the infusion rate, resulting in inadequate pain relief or the early termination of epidural analgesia [56–59]. Thoracic epidural catheter placement for upper abdominal or thoracic procedures may improve coronary blood flow, decrease pulmonary complications, and reduce inhibitory gastrointestinal tone, allowing a faster return of bowel function [21,27,60]. Despite concerns that the placement of a thoracic epidural may involve greater risk because of potential spinal cord injury, the current evidence does not support any increased danger compared with lumbar epidural [61,62].

Choice of Analgesic Agent

The choice of analgesic agents infused through the epidural catheter play a significant role in the achievement of optimal analgesia. The primary choices for postoperative epidural analgesia are opioids alone, local anesthetics alone, and a combination of local anesthetics and opioids. In addition, adjuvant agents may be administered epidurally in an attempt to enhance postoperative analgesia.

Opioids

Epidural opioids confer several benefits compared with epidural local anesthetics, related primarily to the absence of sensory and motor blockade as well as the absence of sympathetic blockade. One of the most important factors in the choice of an opioid is its hydrophilicity (versus lipophilicity). Hydrophilic opioids, such as morphine and hydromorphone, have a slower onset but a longer duration of action and generally a higher incidence of side effects caused in part by a greater cephalad spread in the cerebrospinal fluid [63]. Hydrophilic opioids have an analgesic site of action that is primarily spinal and may be beneficial in situations in which the location of the epidural catheter is incongruent to the incision or side effects attributed to local anesthetics are excessive. It is important to recognize that lower opioid doses may be required for thoracic epidural and in elderly patients [63,64].

In contrast to hydrophilic opioids, lipophilic opioids (eg, fentanyl and sufentanil) provide a more rapid onset of analgesia and decreased side effects (eg, delayed respiratory depression), but they have a shorter duration of action [63]. The site of action of lipophilic opioids is unclear, although several randomized controlled trials suggest a systemic rather than a spinal effect [65,66]. Thus, there may be only a marginal advantage of epidurally administered lipophilic opioid compared with intravenous opioids [67,68]. Therefore, epidural lipophilic opioids are generally administered in conjunction with local anesthetics.

Local anesthetics

Only epidural local anesthetics have a significant ability to block afferent and efferent signals to and from the spinal cord, resulting in the suppression of the surgical stress response, which may decrease perioperative morbidity and mortality [21]. In addition, systemic absorption of local anesthetics may facilitate the return of gastrointestinal motility, diminish inflammation, and decrease blood viscosity [21,41,43]. However, the sole use of local anesthetics is less common than local anesthetic-opioid combinations because of the relatively high incidence of motor blockade and hypotension, and the use of lower concentrations may not provide adequate analgesia [68–70]. Nevertheless, epidural infusions of local anesthetic alone may be warranted in situations in which the side effects of opioids are troublesome to the patient.

Local anesthetic-opioid combinations

Epidural analgesia is most commonly provided using a combination of local anesthetic and an opioid (typically a lipophilic opioid). Compared with opioids or local anesthetic alone, a local anesthetic-opioid combination provides superior postoperative analgesia with lower local anesthetic doses [38,68,69]. It is not clear whether the analgesic effects of the combination of local anesthetic and opioids are additive or synergistic [69,71], but experimental studies [72] imply a synergistic effect.

Of the local anesthetics available for epidural use, bupivacaine, ropivacaine, and levobupivacaine are probably the most widely used in clinical settings because of their preferential sensory blockade with minimal motor blockade at low doses [73–75]. A higher concentration of bupivacaine (eg, 0.1%–0.125%) may typically be used for thoracic epidural analgesia although a lower concentration (eg, 0.0625%) is used for lumber epidural analgesia because of the higher incidence of motor blockade of the lower extremities with a lumbar epidural. Although the newer more expensive local anesthetics (eg, ropivacaine and levobupivacaine) may be relatively less cardiotoxic, this advantage may not be clinically important because relatively low doses of local anesthetics are used for postoperative epidural analgesia.

Hydrophilic opioids (eg, morphine, 0.05–0.1 mg/ml, or hydromorphone, 0.01–0.05 mg/ml) may be added to the local anesthetic; however, they are difficult to titrate compared with lipophilic opioids [76,77]. The concentration commonly used for fentanyl is 2 to 10 μg/ml and for sufentanil (used less frequently than fentanyl) is 0.5–1 μg/ml [68,76,77]. The optimal concentration and combination of opioids and local anesthetics and the infusion rate remain controversial and dependent on the type of surgery and the location of the epidural catheter as well as the patient's susceptibility to side effects. Clinically, however, the most commonly used combination is probably bupivacaine (0.05%–0.1%) with fentanyl (4–5 μg/ml). Infusions of local anesthetics alone are not as common as the bupivacaine-fentanyl combinations (for reasons discussed earlier), and infusions of hydrophilic opioids can be used for catheter-incision incongruent analgesia.

Analgesic adjuncts

A number of adjunctive agents have been examined for postoperative epidural analgesia, but none have been shown to confer significant benefits (eg, enhancing analgesia or minimizing side effects) and thus have not gained widespread acceptance. Epidural clonidine (5–20 μg/h) may improve analgesia, but its clinical application is limited by its dose-dependent side effects, particularly hypotension and sedation [78]. Epinephrine (2–5 μg/ml) may improve postoperative analgesia, but its use also remains controversial [79,80]. Finally, the use of N-methyl-D-aspartate antagonists, such as ketamine, may potentiate the analgesic effect of epidural opioids; however, its safety needs to be determined before it can be recommended for routine use [81–84].

Duration of epidural analgesia

The duration of postoperative epidural analgesia may influence the efficacy of analgesia and affect postoperative outcome. Because many of the adverse perioperative pathophysiologies begin intraoperatively and continue well into the postoperative period, the continuation of epidural analgesia from the intraoperative into the postoperative period will maximize the analgesic and physiologic benefits, which may translate into improved patient outcomes. Typically, to optimize these benefits, the epidural analgesic regimen is started in the intraoperative period and continued postoperatively. However, the optimal duration of epidural analgesia in the postoperative period to maximize physiologic and analgesic benefits is not clearly defined. Although there is no defined time frame, which would be needed to obtain these benefits, generally, epidural analgesia should be continued (as long as there are no contraindications [see subsequent sections on the risks of epidural analgesia]) for a period of 2 to 4 days after major surgery. For instance, epidural analgesia of less than 24 hours demonstrated no benefit of epidural analgesia with respect to return of gastrointestinal function, whereas studies [60,85–88] that continued epidural analgesia beyond 24 hours demonstrated an improvement. Postoperative thoracic epidural analgesia [8] but not intraoperative neuraxial anesthesia [11] reduced the incidence of postoperative myocardial infarction. However, because most postoperative myocardial infarctions occur during the first 2 to 3 postoperative days, it would be necessary to maintain the duration of epidural analgesia for at least 2 to 3 days [89].

Continuous infusion versus patient-controlled epidural analgesia

Patient-controlled epidural analgesia (PCEA) individualizes postoperative analgesic requirements and would theoretically confer several benefits such as greater patient satisfaction, superior analgesia, and lower drug use, which may minimize some medication-related side effects such as motor weakness [90]. Observational data from two series [54,91] of more than 1000 patients reveal that over 90% of the patients with PCEA had adequate analgesia and median pain scores of 1 (of a possible 10) at rest and 4 with activity. The use of a continuous or background infusion in addition to the demand is more common with PCEA and may provide superior analgesia than the use of a demand dose alone [92,93]. The incidence of side effects with PCEA are 1.8%–16.7% for pruritus, 3.8%–14.8% for nausea, 13.2% for sedation, 4.3%–6.8% for hypotension, 0.1%–2% for motor block, and 0.2%–0.3% for respiratory depression, which are comparable to that seen with continuous epidural infusions [54,1]. Although the benefits of PCEA versus continuous epidural infusions are not clearly defined at this point, if it is available, PCEA may be the preferable choice in most clinical situations because it allows the patient to individualize his or her analgesic regimen. Further research is needed to define the optimal settings for individual surgical procedures, although it does seem that a background infusion would be of benefit for PCEA.

Risks of epidural analgesia

Despite the numerous benefits of perioperative epidural analgesia, there are associated risks. Although most of the adverse events are minor and are related to the analgesic agents used in the epidural regimen (eg, hypotension and motor blockade from local anesthetics and nausea and pruritus from opioids), there are a few rare but potentially devastating complications.

Epidural hematoma

The incidence of epidural hematoma has been small, with 1:150,000 reported for epidural block; however, after the introduction of low molecular weight heparin (LMWH) in the United States, the incidence of epidural hematoma increased to as high as 1:6,600 for epidural anesthetics (1:3,100 for postoperative epidural analgesia) [94–98]. Interestingly, LMWH had been used in Europe without significant problems before this [99]. A series of consensus statements for the administration (insertion and removal) of neuraxial techniques in the presence of various anticoagulants, including oral anticoagulants (warfarin) [100], antiplatelet agents [101], fibrinolytics-thrombolytics [102], standard unfractionated heparin [103], and LMWH [98] have been published by the American Society of Regional Anesthesia [95]. In patients receiving anticoagulants in the presence of neuraxial techniques, clinicians should consider that the timing of the neuraxial needle or catheter insertion and removal should reflect the pharmacokinetic properties of the specific anticoagulant; that there should be frequent neurologic monitoring and that the concurrent use of multiple anticoagulants may increase the risk of epidural hematoma; that the analgesic regimen should be tailored to facilitate neurological monitoring; and that there should be a high degree of suspicion because early recognition followed by emergent operative decompression may significantly improve patient outcomes. Epidural hematoma may occur even in the absence of any risk factors [104].

Infection

Although there may be a relatively high incidence of superficial inflammation or cellulitis (4%–14%) and catheter colonization (20%–35%) with increasing duration of catheterization, these problems rarely result in serious long-term consequences [105–107]. Despite the use of solutions such as 10% povidine iodine, there may be a relatively high incidence of epidural needle and catheter contamination. Serious infections (eg, meningitis or spinal abscess) associated with postoperative epidural analgesia are rare ($\leq$1:10,000) [108–110]. These potentially devastating complications may increase (1:1000–1:2000) with a relatively long duration of catheterization or in immunocompromised patients (eg, conditions of malignancy) [68,111,112]. The use of an epidural analgesia for a typical postoperative course (2–4 days) is rarely associated with epidural abscess formation in patients without other significant risk factors [54,91]. The treatment of an epidural abscess requires the early recognition of associated symptoms (eg, back pain, erythema, leukocytosis, and progressive neurologic deficit), the administration of antibiotics, and possibly surgical decompression.

Other complications

Migration of the catheter out of the epidural space may result in an unintentional intrathecal or intravascular delivery of local anesthetic. Fortunately, the rate of intrathecal (0.15% [113,114]) and intravascular (0.07–0.18% [114,115]) migration of an epidural catheter is low. The local anesthetics used in the epidural solutions may cause rare complications including cardiotoxicity [116,117]. Another relatively uncommon complication is the development of pressure sores associated with postoperative epidural analgesia [118]. Of note, occasionally a complication is incorrectly attributed to the epidural catheter, and the clinician must also be cognizant of other possible causes [119]. Another common complication is the early discontinuation of the epidural catheter (typically 6%–25%), which exceeds the incidence of actual premature dislodgement (mean, 5.7%; 95% confidence interval: 4.0%–7.4%) [54,59,70,91,120–122]. This may be related to numerous factors including one-sided block, hypotension, and motor blockade, which may also play a significant role in the premature termination of epidural catheters.

Finally, common side effects can occur and are the result of the medications used in the epidural regimen. The prevention and treatment of pruritus include opioid antagonists (naloxone, ~2 μg/kg/h; naltrexone, 6–9 mg orally; nalbuphine up to 40 mg), proprofol (10 mg intravenously), and ondansetron (0.1 mg/kg intravenously) [123]. The use of opioid antagonists may also antagonize the analgesic effects of neuraxial opioids. Antihistamines probably are not effective because histamine release does not appear to be a significant mechanism for neuraxial-induced pruritus [123]. Intravenous ondansetron (4 mg), dexamethasone (5 mg), or droperidol (1.25 mg) have been used for prophylaxis for postoperative nausea and vomiting related to neuraxial opioids [124–126]. In addition, the opioid can be decreased or removed from the epidural regimen (if used as part of a local anesthetic-opioid combination) in an attempt to treat neuraxial-opioid-induced pruritus or nausea.

Summary

Epidural analgesia is an important analgesic option in the control of postoperative pain. The analgesic and physiologic benefits conferred by epidural analgesia may potentially result in an improvement in many outcomes including reduced morbidity (eg, coagulation, cardiovascular, pulmonary, and gastrointestinal) and improved patient-oriented endpoints, although there are several methodology issues that confound the findings. "Epidural analgesia" should not be used as a generic technique because multiple factors (eg, catheter-incision congruent analgesia, duration of use, and analgesic regimen) may influence the efficacy of this technique on patient outcomes, especially in the high-risk patient population. The use of postoperative epidural analgesia as part of a multimodal approach may result in early patient convalescence and improvement in outcomes. Despite the benefits of perioperative epidural analgesia, there are risks (some of which can be devastating) associated with use of epidural analgesia, and clinicians should weigh the risks and benefits of epidural analgesia for each patient on an individual basis.

References

[1] Wu CL, Berenholtz SM, Pronovost PJ, et al. Systematic review and analysis of postdischarge symptoms after outpatient surgery. Anesthesiology 2002;96:994–1003.
[2] Apfelbaum JL, Chen C, Mehta SS, et al. Postoperative pain experience: results from a national survey suggest postoperative pain continues to be undermanaged. Anesth Analg 2003;97: 534–40.

[3] Wu CL, Naqibuddin M, Rowlingson AJ, et al. The effect of pain on health-related quality of life in the immediate postoperative period. Anesth Analg 2003;97:1078–85.

[4] Lynch EP, Lazor MA, Gellis JE, et al. The impact of postoperative pain on the development of postoperative delirium. Anesth Analg 1998;86:781–5.

[5] Perkins FM, Kehlet H. Chronic pain as an outcome of surgery. A review of predictive factors. Anesthesiology 2000;93:1123–33.

[6] Rosenquist RW, Rosenberg J. Postoperative pain guidelines. Reg Anesth Pain Med 2003;28: 279–88.

[7] Block BM, Liu SS, Rowlingson AJ, et al. Efficacy of postoperative epidural analgesia: a meta-analysis. JAMA 2003;290:2455–63.

[8] Beattie WS, Badner NH, Choi P. Epidural analgesia reduces postoperative myocardial infarction: a meta-analysis. Anesth Analg 2001;93:853–8.

[9] Ballantyne JC, Carr DB, deFerranti S, et al. The comparative effects of postoperative analgesic therapies on pulmonary outcome: cumulative meta-analyses of randomized, controlled trials. Anesth Analg 1998;86:598–612.

[10] Rigg JR, Jamrozik K, Myles PS, et al. Epidural anaesthesia and analgesia and outcome of major surgery: a randomised trial. Lancet 2002;359:1276–82.

[11] Rodgers A, Walker N, Schug S, et al. Reduction of postoperative mortality and morbidity with epidural or spinal anaesthesia: results from overview of randomised trials. BMJ 2000; 321:1493.

[12] Liu SS. Bank robbers and outcomes research. Reg Anesth Pain Med 2003;28:262–4.

[13] Halpern S. Why meta-analysis? Reg Anesth Pain Med 2002;27:3–5.

[14] Wu CL, Fleisher LA. Outcomes research in regional anesthesia and analgesia. Anesth Analg 2000;91:1232–42.

[15] Silber JH. Medicare claims and anesthesia clinical research: a perfect match. Reg Anesth Pain Med 2003;28:259–61.

[16] Shenouda PE, Cunningham BJ. Assessing the superiority of saline versus air for use in the epidural loss of resistance technique: a literature review. Reg Anesth Pain Med 2003;28:48–53.

[17] Wu CL, Anderson GF, Herbert R, et al. Effect of postoperative epidural analgesia on morbidity and mortality after total hip replacement surgery in medicare patients. Reg Anesth Pain Med 2003;28.

[18] Norris EJ, Beattie C, Perler BA, et al. Double-masked randomized trial comparing alternate combinations of intraoperative anesthesia and postoperative analgesia in abdominal aortic surgery. Anesthesiology 2001;95:1054–67.

[19] Wu CL, Hurley RW, Anderson GF, et al. The effect of perioperative epidural analgesia on patient mortality and morbidity in the Medicare population. Reg Anesth Pain Med, in press.

[20] Park WY, Thompson JS, Lee KK. Effect of epidural anesthesia and analgesia on perioperative outcome: a randomized, controlled Veterans Affairs cooperative study. Ann Surg 2001; 234:560–9.

[21] Liu S, Carpenter RL, Neal JM. Epidural anesthesia and analgesia: their role in postoperative outcome. Anesthesiology 1995;82:1474–506.

[22] Correll DJ, Viscusi ER, Grunwald Z, et al. Epidural analgesia compared with intravenous morphine patient-controlled analgesia: postoperative outcome measures after mastectomy with immediate TRAM flap breast reconstruction. Reg Anesth Pain Med 2001;26:444–9.

[23] Carli F, Mayo N, Klubien K, et al. Epidural analgesia enhances functional exercise capacity and health-related quality of life after colonic surgery: results of a randomized trial. Anesthesiology 2002;97:540–9.

[24] Gottschalk A, Smith DS, Jobes DR, et al. Preemptive epidural analgesia and recovery from radical prostatectomy: a randomized controlled trial. JAMA 1998;279:1076–82.

[25] Wu CL, Naqibuddin M, Fleisher LA. Measurement of patient satisfaction as an outcome of regional anesthesia and analgesia: a systematic review. Reg Anesth Pain Med 2001;26: 196–208.

[26] Mollhoff T. Regional Anesthesia in patients at coronary risk for noncardiac and cardiac surgery. Curr Opinion Anesthesiol 2001;14:17–25.

[27] Veering BT, Cousins MJ. Cardiovascular and pulmonary effects of epidural anaesthesia. Anaesth Intensive Care 2000;28:620–35.

[28] Boylan JF, Katz J, Kavanagh BP, et al. Epidural bupivacaine-morphine analgesia versus patient-controlled analgesia following abdominal aortic surgery: analgesic, respiratory, and myocardial effects. Anesthesiology 1998;89:585–93.

[29] Bois S, Couture P, Boudreault D, et al. Epidural analgesia and intravenous patient-controlled analgesia result in similar rates of postoperative myocardial ischemia after aortic surgery. Anesth Analg 1997;85:1233–9.

[30] Bode Jr RH, Lewis KP, Zarich SW, et al. Cardiac outcome after peripheral vascular surgery: comparison of general and regional anesthesia. Anesthesiology 1996;84:3–13.

[31] Yeager MP, Glass DD, Neff RK, et al. Epidural anesthesia and analgesia in high-risk surgical patients. Anesthesiology 1987;66:729–36.

[32] Tuman KJ, McCarthy RJ, March RJ, et al. Effects of epidural anesthesia and analgesia on coagulation and outcome after major vascular surgery. Anesth Analg 1991;73:696–704.

[33] Warner DO, Warner MA, Ritman EL. Human chest wall function during epidural anesthesia. Anesthesiology 1996;85:761–73.

[34] Brimioulle S, Vachiery JL, Brichant JF, et al. Sympathetic modulation of hypoxic pulmonary vasoconstriction in intact dogs. Cardiovasc Res 1997;34:384–92.

[35] Liu SS, Block BM, Wu CL. Effects of perioperative central neuraxial analgesia on outcome after coronary artery bypass surgery: a meta-analysis. Anesthesiology 2004;101(SA Supl): 153–61.

[36] Kehlet H, Holte K. Review of postoperative ileus. Am J Surg 2001;182:3S–10S.

[37] Groudine SB, Fisher HA, Kaufman RP, et al. Intravenous lidocaine speeds the return of bowel function, decreases postoperative pain, and shortens hospital stay in patients undergoing radical retropubic prostatectomy. Anesth Analg 1998;86:235–9.

[38] Jorgensen H, Wetterslev J, Moiniche S, et al. Epidural local anaesthetics versus opioid-based analgesic regimens on postoperative gastrointestinal paralysis, PONV and pain after abdominal surgery. Cochrane Database Syst Rev 2000:CD001893.

[39] Cassady Jr JF, Lederhaas G, Cancel DD, et al. A randomized comparison of the effects of continuous thoracic epidural analgesia and intravenous patient-controlled analgesia after posterior spinal fusion in adolescents. Reg Anesth Pain Med 2000;25:246–53.

[40] Liu SS. Anesthesia and analgesia for colon surgery. Reg Anesth Pain Med 2004;29:52–7.

[41] Liu SS, Carpenter RL, Mackey DC, et al. Effects of perioperative analgesic technique on rate of recovery after colon surgery. Anesthesiology 1995;83:757–65.

[42] Holte K, Kehlet H. Epidural analgesia and risk of anastomotic leakage. Reg Anesth Pain Med 2001;26:111–7.

[43] Hollmann MW, Wieczorek KS, Smart M, et al. Epidural anesthesia prevents hypercoagulation in patients undergoing major orthopedic surgery. Reg Anesth Pain Med 2001;26:215–22.

[44] Rosenfeld BA. Benefits of regional anesthesia on thromboembolic complications following surgery. Reg Anesth 1996;21:9–12.

[45] Sorenson RM, Pace NL. Anesthetic techniques during surgical repair of femoral neck fractures: a meta-analysis. Anesthesiology 1992;77:1095–104.

[46] Christopherson R, Beattie C, Frank SM, et al, for the Perioperative Ischemia Randomized Anesthesia Trial Study Group. Perioperative morbidity in patients randomized to epidural or general anesthesia for lower extremity vascular surgery. Anesthesiology 1993;79:422–34.

[47] Rosenfeld BA, Beattie C, Christopherson R, et al, for the Perioperative Ischemia Randomized Anesthesia Trial Study Group. The effects of different anesthetic regimens on fibrinolysis and the development of postoperative arterial thrombosis. Anesthesiology 1993;79:435–43.

[48] Juelsgaard PLU, Larsen VT, Sorensen JV, Madsen F, et al. Hypotensive epidural anesthesia in total knee replacement without tournquet: reduced blood loss and transfusion. Reg Anesth Pain Med 2001;26:105–10.

[49] Maine DN, Richman JM, Rowlingson AJ, et al. Efficacy of neuraxial anesthesia on intraoperative blood loss: a meta-analysis [poster]. Presented at the 29th Annual American Society of Regional Anesthesia. Orlando, Florida, March 12, 2004.

[50] Wu CL, Richman JM. Postoperative pain and quality of recovery. Curr Opinion Anesthesiol 2004;17:455–60.

[51] Liu SS, Bernards CM. Exploring the epidural trail. Reg Anesth Pain Med 2002;27:122–4.

[52] Magnusdottir H, Kirno K, Ricksten SE, et al. High thoracic epidural anesthesia does not inhibit sympathetic nerve activity in the lower extremities. Anesthesiology 1999;91:1299–304.

[53] Basse L, Werner M, Kehlet H. Is urinary drainage necessary during continuous epidural analgesia after colonic resection? Reg Anesth Pain Med 2000;25:498–501.

[54] Liu SS, Allen HW, Olsson GL. Patient-controlled epidural analgesia with bupivacaine and fentanyl on hospital wards: prospective experience with 1,030 surgical patients. Anesthesiology 1998;88:688–95.

[55] Chisakuta AM, George KA, Hawthorne CT. Postoperative epidural infusion of a mixture of bupivacaine 0.2% with fentanyl for upper abdominal surgery: a comparison of thoracic and lumbar routes. Anaesthesia 1995;50:72–5.

[56] Broekema AA, Gielen MJ, Hennis PJ. Postoperative analgesia with continuous epidural sufentanil and bupivacaine: a prospective study in 614 patients. Anesth Analg 1996;82:754–9.

[57] Kahn L, Baxter FJ, Dauphin A, et al. A comparison of thoracic and lumbar epidural techniques for post-thoracoabdominal esophagectomy analgesia. Can J Anaesth 1999;46:415–22.

[58] Brodner G, Mertes N, Buerkle H, et al. Acute pain management: analysis, implications and consequences after prospective experience with 6349 surgical patients. Eur J Anaesthesiol 2000;17:566–75.

[59] Ready LB. Acute pain: lessons learned from 25,000 patients. Reg Anesth Pain Med 1999; 24:499–505.

[60] Hodgson PS. Thoracic epidural anaesthesia and analgesia for abdominal surgery: effects on gastrointestinal function and perfusion. Balliere's Clin Anaesthesiol 1999;13:9–22.

[61] Tanaka K, Watanabe R, Harada T, et al. Extensive application of epidural anesthesia and analgesia in a university hospital: incidence of complications related to technique. Reg Anesth 1993;18:34–8.

[62] Giebler RM, Scherer RU, Peters J. Incidence of neurologic complications related to thoracic epidural catheterization. Anesthesiology 1997;86:55–63.

[63] Grass JA. Epidural Analgesia. Problems in Anesthesia 1998;10:445.

[64] Mulroy MF. Epidural opioid delivery methods: bolus, continuous infusion, and patient-controlled epidural analgesia. Reg Anesth 1996;21:100–4.

[65] Sandler AN, Stringer D, Panos L, et al. A randomized, double-blind comparison of lumbar epidural and intravenous fentanyl infusions for postthoracotomy pain relief. Analgesic, pharmacokinetic, and respiratory effects. Anesthesiology 1992;77:626–34.

[66] Guinard JP, Mavrocordatos P, Chiolero R, et al. A randomized comparison of intravenous versus lumbar and thoracic epidural fentanyl for analgesia after thoracotomy. Anesthesiology 1992;77:1108–15.

[67] Salomaki TE, Laitinen JO, Nuutinen LS. A randomized double-blind comparison of epidural versus intravenous fentanyl infusion for analgesia after thoracotomy. Anesthesiology 1991;75:790–5.

[68] Wheatley RG, Schug SA, Watson D. Safety and efficacy of postoperative epidural analgesia. Br J Anaesth 2001;87:47–61.

[69] Kopacz DJ, Sharrock NE, Allen HW. A comparison of levobupivacaine 0.125%, fentanyl 4 microg/mL, or their combination for patient-controlled epidural analgesia after major orthopedic surgery. Anesth Analg 1999;89:1497–503.

[70] Scott DA, Beilby DS, McClymont C. Postoperative analgesia using epidural infusions of fentanyl with bupivacaine: a prospective analysis of 1,014 patients. Anesthesiology 1995;83: 727–37.

[71] Camann W, Abouleish A, Eisenach J, et al. Intrathecal sufentanil and epidural bupivacaine for labor analgesia: dose-response of individual agents and in combination. Reg Anesth Pain Med 1998;23:457–62.

[72] Kaneko M, Saito Y, Kirihara Y, et al. Synergistic antinociceptive interaction after epidural coadministration of morphine and lidocaine in rats. Anesthesiology 1994;80:137–50.

[73] Stevens RA, Bray JG, Artuso JD, et al. Differential epidural block. Reg Anesth 1992;17:22–5.

[74] White JL, Stevens RA, Beardsley D, et al. Differential epidural block: does the choice of local anesthetic matter? Reg Anesth 1994;19:335–8.

[75] Zaric D, Nydahl PA, Philipson L, et al. The effect of continuous lumbar epidural infusion of ropivacaine (0.1%, 0.2%, and 0.3%) and 0.25% bupivacaine on sensory and motor block in volunteers: a double-blind study. Reg Anesth 1996;21:14–25.

[76] de Leon-Casasola OA, Lema MJ. Postoperative epidural opioid analgesia: what are the choices? Anesth Analg 1996;83:867–75.

[77] Hamber EA, Viscomi CM. Intrathecal lipophilic opioids as adjuncts to surgical spinal anesthesia. Reg Anesth Pain Med 1999;24:255–63.

[78] Curatolo M, Schnider TW, Petersen-Felix S, et al. A direct search procedure to optimize combinations of epidural bupivacaine, fentanyl, and clonidine for postoperative analgesia. Anesthesiology 2000;92:325–37.

[79] Niemi G, Breivik H. Adrenaline markedly improves thoracic epidural analgesia produced by a low-dose infusion of bupivacaine, fentanyl and adrenaline after major surgery. A randomised, double-blind, cross-over study with and without adrenaline. Acta Anaesthesiol Scand 1998; 42:897–909.

[80] Sakaguchi Y, Sakura S, Shinzawa M, et al. Does adrenaline improve epidural bupivacaine and fentanyl analgesia after abdominal surgery? Anaesth Intensive Care 2000;28:522–6.

[81] Wong CS, Liaw WJ, Tung CS, et al. Ketamine potentiates analgesic effect of morphine in postoperative epidural pain control. Reg Anesth 1996;21:534–41.

[82] Yaksh TL. Epidural ketamine: a useful, mechanistically novel adjuvant for epidural morphine? Reg Anesth 1996;21:508–13.

[83] Hawksworth C, Serpell M. Intrathecal anesthesia with ketamine. Reg Anesth Pain Med 1998; 23:283–8.

[84] Hodgson PS, Neal JM, Pollock JE, et al. The neurotoxicity of drugs given intrathecally (spinal). Anesth Analg 1999;88:797–809.

[85] Wallin G, Cassuto J, Hogstrom S, et al. Failure of epidural anesthesia to prevent postoperative paralytic ileus. Anesthesiology 1986;65:292–7.

[86] Kanazi GE, Thompson JS, Boskovski NA. Effect of epidural analgesia on postoperative ileus after ileal pouch-anal anastomosis. Am Surg 1996;62:499–502.

[87] Hjortso NC, Neumann P, Frosig F, et al. A controlled study on the effect of epidural analgesia with local anaesthetics and morphine on morbidity after abdominal surgery. Acta Anaesthesiol Scand 1985;29:790–6.

[88] Neudecker J, Schwenk W, Junghans T, et al. Randomized controlled trial to examine the influence of thoracic epidural analgesia on postoperative ileus after laparoscopic sigmoid resection. Br J Surg 1999;86:1292–5.

[89] Badner NH, Knill RL, Brown JE, et al. Myocardial infarction after noncardiac surgery. Anesthesiology 1998;88:572–8.

[90] Assad SA, Wu CL. An update on patient-controlled epidural analgesia. Tech Reg Anes Pain Med 2003;7:127–32.

[91] Wigfull J, Welchew E. Survey of 1057 patients receiving postoperative patient-controlled epidural analgesia. Anaesthesia 2001;56:70–5.

[92] Komatsu H, Matsumoto S, Mitsuhata H. Comparison of patient-controlled epidural analgesia with and without night-time infusion following gastrectomy. Br J Anaesth 2001;87:633–5.

[93] Komatsu H, Matsumoto S, Mitsuhata H, et al. Comparison of patient-controlled epidural analgesia with and without background infusion after gastrectomy. Anesth Analg 1998;87: 907–10.

[94] Schroeder DR. Statistics: detecting a rare adverse drug reaction using spontaneous reports. Reg Anesth Pain Med 1998;23:183–9.

[95] Horlocker TT, Wedel DJ, Benzon H, et al. Regional anesthesia in the anticoagulated patient: defining the risks. Reg Anesth Pain Med 2004;29:1–12

[96] Landow L. Monitoring adverse drug events: the Food and Drug Administration MedWatch reporting system. Reg Anesth Pain Med 1998;23:190–3.

[97] Vandermeulen EP, Van Aken H, Vermylen J. Anticoagulants and spinal-epidural anesthesia. Anesth Analg 1994;79:1165–77.

[98] Horlocker TT, Wedel DJ. Neuraxial block and low-molecular-weight heparin: balancing perioperative analgesia and thromboprophylaxis. Reg Anesth Pain Med 1998;23:164–77.

[99] Tryba M. European practice guidelines: thromboembolism prophylaxis and regional anesthesia. Reg Anesth Pain Med 1998;23:178–82.

[100] Enneking FK, Benzon H. Oral anticoagulants and regional anesthesia: a perspective. Reg Anesth Pain Med 1998;23:140–5.

[101] Urmey WF, Rowlingson J. Do antiplatelet agents contribute to the development of perioperative spinal hematoma? Reg Anesth Pain Med 1998;23:146–51.

[102] Rosenquist RW, Brown DL. Neuraxial bleeding: fibrinolytics/thrombolytics. Reg Anesth Pain Med 1998;23:152–6.

[103] Liu SS, Mulroy MF. Neuraxial anesthesia and analgesia in the presence of standard heparin. Reg Anesth Pain Med 1998;23:157–63.

[104] Sidiropoulou T, Pompeo E, Bozzao A, et al. Epidural hematoma after thoracic epidural catheter removal in the absence of risk factors. Reg Anesth Pain Med 2003;28:531–4.

[105] Kost-Byerly S, Tobin JR, Greenberg RS, et al. Bacterial colonization and infection rate of continuous epidural catheters in children. Anesth Analg 1998;86:712–6.

[106] McNeely JK, Trentadue NC, Rusy LM, et al. Culture of bacteria from lumbar and caudal epidural catheters used for postoperative analgesia in children. Reg Anesth 1997;22:428–31.

[107] Simpson RS, Macintyre PE, Shaw D, et al. Epidural catheter tip cultures: results of a 4-year audit and implications for clinical practice. Reg Anesth Pain Med 2000;25:360–7.

[108] Horlocker TT, Wedel DJ. Neurologic complications of spinal and epidural anesthesia. Reg Anesth Pain Med 2000;25:83–98.

[109] Brookman CA, Rutledge ML. Epidural abscess: case report and literature review. Reg Anesth Pain Med 2000;25:428–31.

[110] Rathmell JP, Garahan MB, Alsofrom GF. Epidural abscess following epidural analgesia. Reg Anesth Pain Med 2000;25:79–82.

[111] Rygnestad T, Borchgrevink PC, Eide E. Postoperative epidural infusion of morphine and bupivacaine is safe on surgical wards. Organisation of the treatment, effects and side-effects in 2000 consecutive patients. Acta Anaesthesiol Scand 1997;41:868–76.

[112] Wang LP, Hauerberg J, Schmidt JF. Incidence of spinal epidural abscess after epidural analgesia: a national 1-year survey. Anesthesiology 1999;91:1928–36.

[113] Schug SA, Torrie JJ. Safety assessment of postoperative pain management by an acute pain service. Pain 1993;55:387–91.

[114] Ready LB, Loper KA, Nessly M, et al. Postoperative epidural morphine is safe on surgical wards. Anesthesiology 1991;75:452–6.

[115] Lema MJ. Monitoring epidural local anesthetic action during the postoperative period. Reg Anesth 1996;21:94–9.

[116] Mulroy MF. Systemic toxicity and cardiotoxicity from local anesthetics: incidence and preventive measures. Reg Anesth Pain Med 2002;27:556–61.

[117] Drasner K. Local anesthetic neurotoxicity: clinical injury and strategies that may minimize risk. Reg Anesth Pain Med 2002;27:576–80.

[118] Cherng CH, Wong CS. Pressure sore induced by epidural catheter in a patient recieving postoperative pain control. Reg Anesth Pain Med 2003;28:580.

[119] Crystal Z, Katz Y. Postoperative epidural analgesia and possible transient anterior spinal artery syndrome. Reg Anesth Pain Med 2001;26:274–7.

[120] Dolin SJ, Cashman JN, Bland JM. Effectiveness of acute postoperative pain management: I. Evidence from published data. Br J Anaesth 2002;89:409–23.

[121] de Leon-Casasola OA, Parker B, Lema MJ, et al. Postoperative epidural bupivacaine-morphine therapy: experience with 4,227 surgical cancer patients. Anesthesiology 1994;81:368–75.

[122] Burstal R, Wegener F, Hayes C, et al. Epidural analgesia: prospective audit of 1062 patients. Anaesth Intensive Care 1998;26:165–72.

[123] Szarvas S, Harmon D, Murphy D. Neuraxial opioid-induced pruritus: a review. J Clin Anesth 2003;15:234–9.

[124] Tzeng JI, Chu KS, Ho ST, et al. Prophylactic iv ondansetron reduces nausea, vomiting and pruritus following epidural morphine for postoperative pain control. Can J Anaesth 2003; 50:1023–6.

[125] Wang JJ, Ho ST, Wong CS, et al. Dexamethasone prophylaxis of nausea and vomiting after epidural morphine for post-Cesarean analgesia. Can J Anaesth 2001;48:185–90.

[126] Tzeng JI, Wang JJ, Ho ST, et al. Dexamethasone prophylaxis of nausea and vomiting after epidural morphine for post-Cesarean section analgesia: comparison of droperidol and saline. Br J Anaesth 2000;85:865–8.

ELSEVIER
SAUNDERS

Anesthesiology Clin N Am
23 (2005) 141–162

ANESTHESIOLOGY
CLINICS OF
NORTH AMERICA

Peripheral Nerve Blocks and Continuous Catheter Techniques

Holly Evans, MD, FRCP(C), Susan M. Steele, MD,
Karen C. Nielsen, MD, Marcy S. Tucker, MD, PhD,
Stephen M. Klein, MD*

Department of Anesthesiology, Duke University Medical Center, Box 3094, Durham, NC 27710, USA

The provision of extended analgesia after painful surgery continues to be a major challenge in health care. This challenge must also be met in a changing environment that emphasizes shorter hospital stays, cost-effective use of resources, and a continued shift toward outpatient surgery. The peripheral nerve block (PNB) is an analgesic modality with unique characteristics that meet this challenge and complement multimodal therapies. Newer continuous catheter techniques can also sustain the benefits of postoperative pain control while single injection blocks regress 10 to 18 hours after the injection of long-acting local anesthetic (LA). This article reviews and highlights the potential advantages of individual PNBs and summarizes the data related to the use of continuous PNBs for postoperative pain control.

Interscalene brachial plexus block

The interscalene block is performed at the level of C6 where the roots of the brachial plexus (C5 through T1) pass between the anterior and middle scalene muscles. This proximal brachial plexus block is ideal for postoperative analgesia for shoulder and upper arm surgery [1]. The superficial nature of the plexus at this

This work was supported by the Department of Anesthesiology, Duke University Medical Center, Durham, North Carolina.

* Corresponding author.
E-mail address: klein006@mc.duke.edu (S.M. Klein).

anesthesiology.theclinics.com

location, the easily identifiable landmarks, and high success rate of this block as well as the preponderance of shoulder surgery contribute to making this one of the most commonly performed regional anesthesia techniques [2,3].

The interscalene block is highly effective at managing the intense post-operative pain that results from shoulder surgery; consequently, many authors consider this the gold standard in shoulder analgesia. A number of studies have documented the superior pain relief provided by this block when compared with opioid analgesia for arthroscopic and open shoulder surgery. Greater than 50% reduction in the pain verbal analog scale (VAS) scores [4–6], delayed time until first analgesic use [5], and reduced total opioid requirements [4–7] result from this technique. An example of this approach was provided by Kinnard et al [6] in a comparison of bupivacaine interscalene block versus opioids for postoperative analgesia in patients who had general anesthesia (GA) for acromioplasty or rotator cuff repair. During the first 24 hours after surgery, the mean postoperative pain VAS score was 1.8 on 10 in the treatment group versus 5.2 in the control group, and the hydromorphone consumption was 0.1 and 2.5 mg per patient, respectively. Other investigators have compared interscalene block versus sub-acromial bursa block [8] or the intra-articular administration of LA [9] and have demonstrated similarly superior analgesic efficacy from this PNB. Postoperative oxycodone consumption after interscalene block was one fourth that after sub-acromial bursa block [8], and pain VAS scores were 2 to 5 times higher with intra-articular LA compared with interscalene block [9].

The decreased incidence of pain and use of postoperative opioids lead to further beneficial effects, including a reduced incidence of postoperative nausea and vomiting (PONV) by 65% to 81% [4,5], improved postoperative mood [6], and up to 2 hours more sleep on the night after surgery [6]. Additional results include a faster discharge of the ambulatory patient [5], reduced in-patient length of stay [7], and lower rates of unanticipated hospital admission [4,10,11]. In an attempt to further improve on these effects, adjuvants to LA such as clonidine [12–14], ketamine [15], and morphine [16] have been examined. Although some studies have demonstrated that clonidine prolongs the analgesic effects of short-acting LA, controversy exists as to whether this is systemically or periph-erally mediated.

In an effort to prolong the duration of postoperative analgesia, continuous interscalene nerve blocks have been investigated. Several authors have documented the safety and efficacy of this technique for painful procedures such as open rotator cuff repair and arthroplasty [17–26]. Two prospective studies by Borgeat et al [23,26] are representative. In both studies, patients had GA and an interscalene block for open shoulder procedures. The investigators compared postoperative analgesia with intravenous patient-controlled analgesia (IVPCA) versus patient-controlled interscalene block with ropivacaine [26] or bupivacaine [23]. Patient-controlled interscalene block with a basal infusion and patient-administered boluses was associated with a greater than 50% reduction in postoperative pain VAS scores from 12 to 48 hours, reduced PONV, and higher patient satisfaction.

Several interscalene catheter infusion strategies have been successfully implemented: continuous infusion alone [20,22], infusion with patient-administered boluses [22,23,25–27], and patient-controlled boluses alone [22]. Singelyn et al [22] compared these three modalities over a 48-hour period in patients who underwent open shoulder surgery. They found that the continuous infusion achieved excellent analgesia and minimal opioid consumption but was associated with the greatest use of LA. Infusion with patient-administered boluses provided excellent analgesia with intermediate consumption of LA. A regimen of patient-controlled boluses was associated with up to four times higher pain VAS scores and greater opioid consumption; however, this strategy did result in the lowest overall LA consumption.

Dilute bupivacaine [22,23,25], levobupivacaine [27], and ropivacaine [19,20,25–27] have all been used for postoperative infusions. Ropivacaine may offer advantages because it has a favorable safety profile and is associated with minimal motor block. This was quantified in a study by Borgeat et al [25]. After a 24-hour infusion of ropivacaine or bupivacaine, they found a reduction of 48% and 66%, respectively, in hand strength, compared with preoperative values. The most common challenges of the continuous technique include pain experienced during the transition from a dense surgical block to an analgesic block with dilute LA [24,28] and catheter-related problems such as dislodgement [19,23,24], kinking [22], and leaking [28].

Recent literature has focused on the use of continuous interscalene catheter infusions for outpatients [19,29–31]. This has enabled prompt hospital discharge with excellent pain control and few side effects after painful and complex procedures. In addition, this technique diminishes breakthrough pain that outpatients may experience after the resolution of a single-injection block [32]. The added benefits such as reduction in sleep disturbances and preservation of cognitive function are also observed [31]. Appropriate patient selection, education, and follow-up are crucial when prescribing outpatient infusions in an unmonitored environment.

Supraclavicular brachial plexus block

The supraclavicular block is performed at the level of the trunks of the brachial plexus. In this technique, LA is injected where the brachial plexus is most compact, leading to consistent, rapid-onset anesthesia distal to the shoulder [1,33]. Bedder et al [34] documented sensory block onset within 3.6 to 4.0 minutes using bupivacaine; this is faster than onset times reported with infraclavicular or axillary blocks. Up to 17 hours of analgesia result after a single injection of bupivacaine or ropivacaine [35,36], and some studies have shown further prolongation from the addition of clonidine, 150 μg [37], or buprenorphine, 300 μg [38,39]. Although the "plumb-bob" technique has historically been associated with a high incidence of pneumothorax, the safety and efficacy of the subclavian perivascular approach has been demonstrated by Franco and

Vieira [40]. They reported no pneumothoraces or neurologic deficits related to supraclavicular block insertion in a series of 1001 blocks performed by both residents and staff anesthesiologists. Despite these attractive features, few studies have investigated the postoperative analgesic efficacy of this block compared with placebo or IVPCA with opioids. Furthermore, although the authors have used continuous supraclavicular brachial plexus infusions of LA for post-operative analgesia with good success, the literature on this subject is sparse. The rapid onset of sensory block, broad upper extremity coverage, and long-lasting analgesia provided by this block make it invaluable for postoperative pain management after upper extremity procedures.

Infraclavicular brachial plexus block

The infraclavicular block targets the brachial plexus at the divisions and cords, where the plexus is in close proximity to the axillary artery and vein. This block is used for procedures of the elbow, forearm, wrist, and hand. Two large series of infraclavicular blocks [41,42] document efficient block performance in as little as 5 minutes, good analgesic efficacy, and a favorable safety profile with a very low incidence of pneumothoraces or postoperative neurologic deficits. In a prospective study of outpatients who underwent hand and wrist procedures, Hadzic et al [43] compared infraclavicular block versus GA and found lower pain VAS scores on arrival to the postanesthesia care unit (PACU) in the infraclavicular block group. Analgesia was required in the PACU by 48% of those in the GA group and by none of the patients in the infraclavicular block group. The use of the short-acting LA chloroprocaine led to similar pain VAS scores and opioid consumption in both groups at 24 and 48 hours; however, substitution with a long-acting LA could be used to prolong analgesia and improve on these results.

Several studies have reported the use of continuous infraclavicular brachial plexus nerve block catheters for postoperative pain management [44–46]. Ilfeld et al [44] compared 0.2% ropivacaine versus saline for ambulatory infraclavicular brachial plexus infusion and demonstrated greater than 50% decrease in pain VAS scores for the duration of the infusion, reduced opioid consumption, and fewer opioid-related side effects in the ropivacaine group. In addition, no pa-tients receiving the ropivacaine infusion reported difficulty sleeping, in con-trast to 60% of those in the saline group. Patient satisfaction was higher in the ropivacaine group, in which all patients were willing to repeat the same technique in the future, compared with 53% of those who received a saline infusion. A subsequent study that evaluated the effect of the addition of clonidine to the LA infusion [45] demonstrated a reduction in overall LA use but determined that this difference was not clinically significant. A comparison of infraclavicular infusion regimens produced results comparable with similar studies involving interscalene brachial plexus infusions. A regimen consisting of a basal infusion with patient-controlled boluses yielded the optimal analgesia of long duration compared with a basal infusion alone or patient-controlled boluses alone [46]. Compared with other upper extremity approaches, the only real advantage of this continuous brachial plexus block may relate to the ability to maintain a secure catheter insertion site.

Axillary brachial plexus block

This technique blocks the terminal branches of the brachial plexus as they surround the axillary artery. This is the most commonly performed PNB in the United States [2,3] likely because of its favorable safety profile [47], ease of performance, high patient acceptance [48], and broad applicability for hand, wrist, and forearm procedures [1]. Variations of the axillary block have been investigated for postoperative pain management for nearly 100 years; hence, the literature base is broad.

In the axilla, the terminal nerves of the brachial plexus are contained within a fascial sheath [49,50]. The presence of septae within the sheath [49,50] and the exclusion of the musculocutaneous, intercostobrachial, and medial antebrachial cutaneous nerves from the sheath at this level may affect the spread of LA as well as the consistency and extent of anesthesia achieved. These anatomical features contribute to the variability in success rates and onset times reported with single-stimulation techniques [51–53] and the improved results obtained with multiple-stimulation techniques [54,55]. The multiple-stimulation technique can also be used to provide selective incisional analgesia of long duration with the early return of partial sensorimotor function in areas outside the surgical field [56]. This is accomplished by blocking the nerves that supply the surgical field with long-acting LA and the remaining nerves with short-acting LA.

Further attempts to prolong postoperative analgesia and minimize motor block have focused on the addition of adjuvant solutions to the LA. The $\alpha 2$ agonist, clonidine, in a dosage range of 0.1 to 2 µg/kg, has been shown to double the duration of postoperative analgesia when added to short-acting LA [57,58]. Hypotension, bradycardia, and sedation, however, may limit the use of perineural clonidine in certain patient populations. There is also evidence that the perineural administration of tramadol [59,60], buprenorphine [61], fentanyl [62,63], and morphine [64] may prolong the duration of analgesia or reduce opioid requirements postoperatively. The controversy continues as to whether these additives act locally at the peripheral nerve or more systemically.

Two prospective studies have compared axillary block with short-acting LA versus GA in patients undergoing hand surgery [65,66]. The benefits attributed to the axillary block include greater than 50% reduction in pain VAS scores, from 30 to 120 min after surgery [66], lower in-hospital opioid requirements [65,66], and longer time until the first analgesic [66]. Additional postoperative advantages include a 75% reduction in the incidence of immediate PONV [65,66] as well as a more expedient discharge from both the PACU and the hospital [66]. However, when long-term benefits were investigated, there was no difference in pain, opioid consumption, adverse effects, or patient satisfaction on the first, seventh, or fourteenth postoperative day [66]. When an axillary block was compared with intravenous regional anesthesia for hand surgery [65], the intravenous regional anesthesia technique was associated with similar postoperative analgesia but a 30% reduction in intra- and postoperative costs, a shorter duration of recovery, and fewer PACU nursing interventions.

Axillary blocks have also been used for the creation of vascular access grafts for dialysis and for the reimplantation of traumatic amputations. The sympathectomy that occurs from this plexus block enhances distal blood flow and perfusion [67] and is of particular benefit for these procedures.

Continuous axillary brachial plexus infusions have further lengthened the duration of analgesia and sympathectomy after upper extremity procedures. A large descriptive series by Bergman et al [68] documented successful axillary catheter insertion in more than 90% of patients, with very few complications. Among 405 catheter insertions, there was one infection that resolved with antibiotic therapy and four new postoperative neurologic deficits. Two of these deficits were attributed to surgical technique, and only one of the four deficits was noted to have incomplete recovery. Given the location of catheter placement, the challenges of continuous axillary catheter management include maintaining a clean, sterile site and avoiding catheter dislodgement from this very mobile area.

In a study of patients undergoing hand microsurgery, a continuous basal infusion was compared with patient-controlled bolus administration of 0.25% bupivacaine [69]. Investigators found that both regimens produced low pain VAS scores and opioid requirements; however, lower plasma bupivacaine levels were measured with the bolus strategy despite similar hourly LA consumption in each group. In an early report on the use of ambulatory continuous axillary infusions for patients undergoing outpatient hand surgery, Rawal et al [70] described a regimen involving patient-controlled boluses of 0.125% bupivacaine or ropivacaine administered as often as once every hour. This technique achieved reductions in pain VAS scores after every bolus and a high rate of patient satisfaction.

Because the axillary block requires multiple injections to achieve complete distal upper extremity analgesia, prolonged performance and onset time may result, and efficacy similar to other approaches to the brachial plexus may not be achieved. Despite this, the ease of performance and low incidence of side effects associated with the axillary block have made it the most commonly performed PNB.

Lumbar plexus block

The ventral rami of the spinal nerve roots L1–4 combine to form the lumbar plexus within the substance of the psoas muscle. A number of methods of lumbar plexus block are described. Each provides reliable anesthesia of the three main terminal nerves of the lumbar plexus—the femoral, lateral femoral cutaneous, and the obturator nerves [71]; however, anesthesia of the more proximal plexus nerves (ilioinguinal, iliohypogastric, and genitofemoral nerves) is inconsistent.

The extent to which sensory analgesia is achieved makes lumbar plexus block suitable for knee and hip procedures. This block has been used safely and effectively for outpatient knee arthroscopy. Jankowski et al [72] compared a mepivacaine lumbar plexus block versus subarachnoid block (SAB) versus GA and found that the two regional anesthetics were associated with three times more frequent PACU bypass, lower pain VAS scores from 30 to 120 minutes after surgery, and 53% to 69% fewer patients requiring analgesics in the hospital before same-day discharge. Hadzic et al (Admir Hadzic, MD, PhD, personal communication, 2004) contrasted chloroprocaine lumbar plexus and sciatic nerve blocks versus GA and documented early postoperative benefits from the PNBs, including a reduced incidence and severity of PONV, sore throat and concentration difficulties, and a shorter time to both oral intake and discharge readiness by 1 hour. However, reflecting the low incidence of severe postoperative pain that occurs with this procedure and the use of short-acting LA in these studies, neither report demonstrated long-lasting benefit from the lumbar plexus block compared with GA.

Greater postoperative analgesic benefit is evident when a lumbar plexus block is used for invasive and more painful procedures such as anterior cruciate ligament (ACL) repair or total knee arthroplasty (TKA). In a study of patients undergoing arthroscopic ACL repair, Matheny et al [73] found 89% lower opioid requirements and a reduced incidence of opioid-related side effects in the group that received continuous lumbar plexus block versus those who had IVPCA. In an investigation of TKA patients by Luber et al [74], a subset of patients described an easier and more comfortable recovery with lumbar plexus and sciatic nerve blocks compared with previous experience with GA and IVPCA. Kaloul et al [75] compared continuous lumbar plexus block versus continuous femoral nerve block versus IVPCA in TKA patients and found that the PNB techniques reduced 48-hour morphine consumption by 48% to 50%. This benefit was most apparent in the first 12 hours after surgery but was less obvious after 12 to 24 hours when the surgical block resolved and less intense analgesia was provided with an infusion of dilute LA. Pain originating from the sciatic nerve contributions to the knee may also have been a factor. As expected, investigators found more frequent obturator nerve block in the lumbar plexus group than the femoral group; however, this failed to translate into any clinical advantage, again, possibly related to overriding discomfort from the territory of the unblocked sciatic nerve.

Several studies have described the use of a lumbar plexus block for hip fractures and total hip arthroplasty [76,77]. Overall results have been excellent. Hevia-Sanchez et al [78] evaluated patients having total hip arthroplasty under SAB and found that a lumbar plexus block provided low pain VAS scores and infrequent use of opioids in the postoperative period. Most impressively, no patients required morphine in the first 12 hours postoperatively, and only 15% of patients used morphine after 12 to 24 hours. When patients evaluated their experience on the first day after surgery, 90% described their pain as mild or moderate, and only 10% reported pain as intense. Two other groups [77,79] have investigated patients undergoing total hip arthroplasty, and both groups found that a lumbar plexus block reduced pain VAS scores and opioid use for 6 to 12 hours, respectively, after surgery, compared with the use of parenteral opioids alone.

Prolongation of analgesia after total hip arthroplasty can be achieved using a continuous lumbar plexus catheter [80]. Using this technique, Capdevila et al [81] documented low pain VAS scores for over 48 hours. In a study by Turker et al [82], the block was as successful as a lumbar epidural in providing analgesia, minimizing opioid use, and enhancing patient satisfaction. More importantly, patients who received the continuous lumbar plexus block experienced a reduction of more than 80% in the incidence of orthostatic hypotension, urinary retention, and PONV, as well as earlier ambulation than those who received the epidural.

Quantitative summaries regarding overall efficacy of lumbar plexus block for painful hip and knee procedures are difficult to make because the existing studies have numerous variations in methodology. Although the benefits of this technique are shown repeatedly, the extent and duration of analgesia vary depending on whether single-injection or continuous blocks are used and whether a sciatic nerve block is also used.

Femoral nerve block

The largest terminal nerve of the lumbar plexus, the femoral nerve, is formed from the posterior divisions of the ventral rami of the L2–4 nerve roots. The femoral nerve block provides excellent anesthesia in the femoral nerve distribution. Increasing LA injectant volume and application of pressure distal to the needle insertion are used in attempt to attain a "3-in-1" block, which includes coverage of the lateral femoral cutaneous nerve and the anterior portion of the obturator nerve. Numerous studies, however, have documented inconsistent results with the 3-in-1 block [83,84]. Nevertheless, it is a simple technique and offers excellent analgesia after knee surgery.

When used for knee arthroscopy, the femoral nerve block has high patient acceptance, a reduced incidence of pain requiring treatment in the PACU from 36% to 1.7%, and decreased length of hospital stay compared with GA [85]. Two studies comparing femoral nerve block with intra-articular LA injection have found that both methods provide good analgesia and similar pain VAS scores for up to 24 hours [86,87]. A combined femoral-sciatic nerve block using mepivacaine has been compared with propofol-remifentanil GA [88] and unilateral [89] and bilateral [90] SAB for knee arthroscopy. Reflecting the minimally painful nature of this procedure, patients in all groups reported low pain VAS scores at discharge, and fewer than 37% of patients required opioid analgesia in the first 24 hours after surgery. In these studies, the recovery advantages of the femoral-sciatic nerve block included earlier micturition by 95 minutes and sooner ambulation by 50 minutes.

A femoral nerve block with long-acting LA can provide up to 23 hours of analgesia after ACL repair and can assist with the comfortable and timely transition of ambulatory patients out of the hospital [91,92]. There is evidence that, when compared with placebo, femoral nerve block improves immediate postoperative analgesia [91,93], prolongs the time to first requested analgesic [93], and reduces 24-hour morphine consumption by 45% [93]. A continuous femoral nerve block provides the option to further prolong postoperative analgesia after ACL repair [94]. In a series comparing continuous femoral nerve versus fascia iliaca blocks, both techniques provided low postoperative pain VAS scores and opioid requirements [95].

Some studies, however, have failed to show significant postoperative analgesic benefit from a femoral nerve block after ACL reconstruction [96,97]. Investigators have hypothesized that this is the result of pain originating from the geniculate contributions of the sciatic nerve distribution [98,99]. Consequently, a combination femoral-sciatic nerve block is particularly useful for ACL repair using a hamstring graft, in which there is significant pain in the sciatic nerve distribution [100]. In a comparison of femoral-sciatic nerve block versus femoral nerve block alone for ACL repair, Williams et al [100] found that the combined femoral-sciatic nerve block was associated with reduced pain and analgesic requirements. More importantly, these benefits have facilitated ACL repair as an outpatient procedure [99,100] with a projected annual cost savings of $98,613 in an institution performing 250 procedures per year [101].

Investigators have reported the beneficial effects of femoral nerve block (without additional sciatic block) for patients undergoing TKA and other painful open knee procedures [102]. Because of the intensity and duration of pain that occur with these procedures, many reports involve the use of a continuous femoral nerve block. A number of studies have documented dense analgesia with up to 50% reduction in pain VAS scores for 48 hours [103,104], up to 64% lower postoperative opioid requirements [103,105–107], a reduced incidence of side effects [106], and a 20% shorter hospital stay [104] with femoral nerve catheters when compared with IVPCA. An additional benefit includes improved short-term postoperative rehabilitation and joint mobilization [104,106]. The continuous femoral nerve infusion of LA has been found to provide similar analgesia but fewer side effects than a single dose of intrathecal morphine [108], a single dose of epidural morphine [109], or a continuous infusion of epidural LA [104,106]. In an attempt to determine the best LA infusion regimen for continuous femoral nerve blocks used for TKA, Singelyn and Gouverneur [110] compared continuous infusion alone versus continuous infusion with intermittent boluses versus intermittent boluses alone. Reduced IVPCA opioid consumption was noted in the continuous infusion group that had a mean of 0 PCA attempts over 48 hours compared with 44 to 66 attempts in the other groups. The consumption of LA, however, was 32% to 58% lower with the intermittent bolus strategy. The continuous infusion with intermittent bolus modality provided intermediate LA consumption but was associated with the highest opioid consumption, contrasting with results from similar studies involving upper extremity infusions [22].

As discussed in relation to ACL repair, some authors have been unable to reproduce these beneficial results using femoral nerve block for TKA and have suggested that this may be because of the unblocked sciatic or obturator nerve contributions to the knee [111]. Cook et al [112] have documented improved postoperative analgesia as well as a 39% reduction in opioid consumption in the first 24 hours from a combined femoral-sciatic nerve block compared with femoral nerve block alone. When used with a continuous femoral nerve block, intermittent boluses or continuous infusion of LA through a sciatic nerve catheter can further extend postoperative analgesia in 67% [113] to 83% [114] of patients and reduce pain VAS scores by 67% [114]. Compared with SAB followed by postoperative parenteral opioids, femoral-sciatic nerve blocks are associated with a 2- to 8-hour prolongation in the time to first analgesic [115], decreased total opioid consumption of 53% to 63% in the first 24 hours [115,116], and reduced pain VAS scores of 42% to 54% [115,116]. Chelly et al [117] compared combined femoral-sciatic nerve block versus epidural analgesia and found a 20% reduction in the amount of opioid consumed, a 50% lower incidence of PONV, and an earlier discharge from the hospital in the femoral-sciatic nerve block group.

The safety and ease of performance of this technique make this one of the most commonly performed lower extremity PNBs. The femoral nerve block can provide excellent postoperative analgesia for major knee procedures, is a less invasive alternative to lumbar plexus block, and is a technique that preserves hip flexion. In the literature there is variability in the extent and duration of analgesia provided after major knee surgery. This variability likely reflects the different techniques used (single injection versus continuous infusion, with or without sciatic or obturator nerve block) and interpatient variability in the importance of the sciatic innervation of the knee.

Sciatic nerve block

Formed from the rami of L4–S3, the sciatic nerve is composed of three anatomically and functionally distinct components: the posterior femoral cutaneous, tibial, and common peroneal nerves. Numerous approaches have been described to achieve analgesia along the length of this nerve. These approaches can be divided into proximal (classic, Raj, anterior, lateral, and subgluteal) and distal (popliteal fossa) techniques.

The majority of publications on sciatic nerve block describe its use as an adjunct to femoral or lumbar plexus blocks for knee and hip procedures (see above). Other studies evaluate the use of a proximal sciatic nerve block as the primary technique for foot and ankle surgery, although the paucity of studies on this topic reflects the more common use of distal sciatic nerve block for these procedures. Long-acting LA can provide safe and effective pain relief for up to 16 hours after foot and ankle surgery [118]. Casati et al [119] documented a high success rate, low postoperative opioid requirements, and excellent patient satisfaction in a series of patients who underwent sciatic nerve block for foot and ankle procedures. Cooper et al [120] studied patients who had open cal-caneal fracture repair and compared postoperative analgesia from sciatic nerve block versus IVPCA. They documented reduced pain VAS scores for 24 hours in the block group and found equal analgesic efficacy in blocks administered pre- or postoperatively.

Continuous proximal sciatic nerve block can extend the duration of analgesia after painful orthopedic procedures on the distal lower extremity, although the number of studies investigating its use seems low given the excellent results it can provide. Significant analgesic benefit has been proven when continuous sciatic nerve block is provided pre- and postoperatively for patients undergoing below-knee amputation [121]. Both surgical and phantom limb pain can be reduced with this technique, with a resulting improvement in sleep. In a study examining continuous sciatic nerve block with 0.2% ropivacaine, di Benedetto et al [122] compared a continuous infusion regimen versus a strategy involving a continuous infusion with patient-controlled boluses. Both regimens provided similarly effective analgesia, with pain VAS scores lower than 30 mm for 24 hours; however, there was 42% less LA consumed in the continuous infu-sion with patient-controlled boluses group.

Overall, the lower number of studies on the use of proximal sciatic nerve blocks for distal lower extremity surgery is surprising given its efficacy. This block has the potential to provide potent postoperative analgesia after major foot and ankle procedures and continuous catheter techniques can safely prolong the duration of pain relief.

Popliteal fossa sciatic nerve block

In the popliteal fossa, the sciatic nerve divides into the tibial and common peroneal nerves. Popliteal fossa sciatic nerve block is accomplished 7 to 10 cm superior to the popliteal skin crease, before the divergence of these nerves. This distal sciatic nerve block is advantageous because it preserves hamstring muscle function, allowing easier ambulation; however, sensation to the posterior thigh remains because the posterior cutaneous nerve is spared.

Popliteal fossa sciatic nerve block with long-acting LA can provide analgesia of 20 hours after foot or ankle procedures [123]. In a series of 652 popliteal blocks performed by trainees and staff anesthesiologists for foot and ankle procedures, Singelyn et al [124] documented a superior success rate, with only 3% of patients requiring conversion to GA, and excellent patient tolerance of the initial block. High patient satisfaction was illustrated when 95% of patients described being completely satisfied with their anesthesia and analgesia, 4% conveyed satisfaction with moderate reservations, and 1% expressed major reservations with the technique. The safety of this block was highlighted in another large series by Provenzano et al [125]. This descriptive study involved 439 popliteal blocks performed primarily on outpatients, and the investigators found no postoperative neurologic sequelae. In a report by Hansen et al [126], a number of patients who had experience with GA for previous foot or ankle surgery volunteered that the popliteal block provided superior postoperative analgesia. None of the patients in this study required opioids in the PACU, and comfortable ambulatory discharge was facilitated. Further evidence of the analgesia provided by this block is found in two studies by McLeod et al [127,128]. In outpatients undergoing foot and ankle procedures, they compared the popliteal fossa sciatic nerve block versus ankle block [127] and versus sub-cutaneous LA infiltration [128]. The popliteal fossa sciatic nerve block provided 1080 to 1082 minutes of postoperative analgesia, significantly longer than either the ankle block (690 minutes) or subcutaneous infiltration (373 minutes). Four times as many patients experienced severe pain at home in the subset that received subcutaneous LA infiltration, and patient satisfaction was correspondingly lower in this group. In a study of outpatients, Vloka et al [129] described a novel use of popliteal block for patients undergoing short saphenous vein stripping. They compared a popliteal block with chloroprocaine versus SAB and found that the popliteal block facilitated more comfortable and prompt same-day discharge. This occurred because patients experienced less pain immediately postoperatively, spent half as long in PACU as SAB patients, and were discharged from the hospital more than 1 hour earlier than SAB patients. However, the use of a short-acting LA for the popliteal block failed to confer analgesic benefit after discharge.

Extending these analgesic advantages, continuous popliteal sciatic nerve block has been used for hospitalized and ambulatory patients. A continuous block with dilute bupivacaine [130,131] and ropivacaine [132,133] provides better analgesia [130–133] and 70% to 100% lower opioid requirements than placebo [130,131,133,134]. This technique provides such high-quality analgesia that 40% to 80% of patients do not require opioid analgesia for the duration of the LA infusion [130,133]. Fewer opioid-related side effects result [130,131,133,134], which was highlighted by a 90% reduction in the incidence of nausea and vomiting when continuous popliteal sciatic nerve block was compared with parenteral analgesics [131]. Additional benefits include a reduced number of sleep disturbances by 60% to 94% [132,133], a 50% shorter hospital length of stay [130], and a 40% lower incidence of hospital admissions among outpatients [130]. Consequently, this type of block resulted in reduced perioperative costs [130] and high patient satisfaction [130,133]. Challenges related to continuous popliteal sciatic nerve block include catheter kinking, breakage or dislodgement [130–133], and leakage of infusate from the catheter insertion site [132,133].

Despite its slow onset, the popliteal block provides effective analgesia for foot and ankle procedures. Although more proximal sciatic nerve block results in weakened hamstrings, the popliteal block preserves hamstring function and facilitates ambulation.

Paravertebral block

The paravertebral block is accomplished by an injection of LA as the spinal nerve roots exit the central neuraxis. The block is unique in that a single injection can block the ventral and dorsal rami as well as the gray and white rami communicans, thereby providing a dense sensory and sympathetic block. As a result, unilateral segmental analgesia can be provided for a variety of thoracic and abdominal surgical procedures.

The continuous paravertebral block has been extensively compared with the thoracic epidural for post-thoracotomy analgesia [135–137]. In a number of studies involving patients who underwent lung resection, paravertebral block provided analgesia of similar or better quality than the thoracic epidural. Paravertebral block was associated with fewer side effects, including a reduction in the incidence of hypotension (up to 67% with epidurals to zero with the paravertebral block), a decrease in the incidence of PONV by 80% [137], and an 85% lower rate of urinary retention [135]. Impressively, measures of pulmonary function were equal to or better than those seen in patients with thoracic epidurals [136,137]. Catala et al [138] investigated continuous thoracic paravertebral block infusion regimens and found that patients who received a continuous infusion of LA experienced 33% to 42% lower pain VAS scores from 4 to 48 hours postoperatively than patients who had intermittent boluses of 0.375% bupivacaine. Additional reports exist on the safe and effective use of single-injection and continuous paravertebral blocks for conventional [139] and minimally invasive [140,141] cardiac surgery as well as major vascular surgery [142].

Additionally, many investigators have documented the safe and effective use of paravertebral blocks for major and minor breast cancer procedures as well as cosmetic and reconstructive breast augmentation [143–149]. Long-acting LA can provide up to 23 hours of analgesia [143]. When compared with GA, paravertebral block results in 50% to 80% lower pain VAS scores [146,149], 48% to 95% reduced opioid consumption [145,146,149], and less painful restricted movement [146]. Further benefits include a 48% to 97% decreased incidence of PONV [145,146,149], a shorter hospital stay [145,149], and the enhanced ability to perform breast procedures on an outpatient basis [143,145]. The potential for cost savings are evident [143]. There are case reports describing the use of continuous paravertebral catheters for analgesia after breast cancer surgery [150], however, pain after resolution of single-injection paravertebral block is usually readily managed with oral analgesics.

Similar positive results have been obtained when paravertebral blocks are used for inguinal [151,152] and ventral [153] hernia repair as well as loop ileostomy closure [154]. When used for inguinal hernia repair, this technique provides up to 14 hours of postoperative analgesia and delays the time to the first dose of opioid by up to 22 hours [151]. A study by Naja et al [155] documents no need for opioid analgesia in the first 24 hours and no PONV among patients who had a paravertebral block for inguinal hernia repair. In this study, the length of hospital stay after paravertebral block was one half that after GA or SAB. This group also compared paravertebral block versus GA for ventral hernia repair [153]. They found that the paravertebral block resulted in lower pain VAS scores, diminished the number of patients requiring post-operative opioids from 90% to 0% in the first 24 hours, decreased incidence of PONV by 88%, and reduced length of hospital stay from 4.1 days to 2.3 days. However, the postoperative benefits of this technique over extended ilioinguinal-iliohypogastric block have not been as compelling [156].

Segmental analgesia achieved with paravertebral block has broad value, ranging from thoracic and breast surgery to inguinal and abdominal procedures. It has been extensively studied and has many advantages compared with thoracic epidural anesthesia and requires less to place. Given its multiple uses and excellent results, it may be one of the most underused PNBs.

Summary

This article reviews the extensive literature base on the use of PNBs for postoperative pain management. The discussion focuses on the advantages of individual blocks used for common surgical procedures. The technical aspects or side effects of each approach are found in standard reference texts.

Intense, site-specific analgesia results from PNBs. These blocks provide superior postoperative analgesia with fewer side effects than most other analgesic techniques, including parenteral opioids. As a result PONV, sedation, concentration difficulties, pruritus, and urinary retention are minimized. In addition, the return to important preoperative functions such as eating, drinking, ambulation, and sleeping is enhanced. These advantages facilitate a prompt recovery and discharge, achieve cost savings, and result in high patient satisfaction.

Nevertheless some benefits achieved from single-injection techniques are limited by the finite duration of the LA. Prolongation of these attributes can be achieved with a continuous catheter. The use of these modalities has also been supported by a number of studies illustrating that continuous lower extremity blocks provide analgesia of equal quality but with fewer side effects than continuous epidural infusions. Further advantages of continuous PNBs include the potential to enhance rehabilitation after major total joint arthroplasty and the potential to improve results of reimplantation procedures. Preliminary work on the use of continuous PNBs in outpatients has been promising and has the potential for significant cost savings and outcome improvement.

Despite these advantages, PNB techniques continue to be underused. This may be because of the limited number of regional anesthesia instructors available in teaching institutions in addition to a focus on GA by United States residency programs. A nationwide survey of third-year anesthesiology residents illustrated this problem [157] when the majority of sampled trainees expressed low confidence in their ability to perform most PNBs. To foster the continued use of these techniques for postoperative analgesia, it is essential to develop improved teaching modalities. Finally, although the beneficial analgesic effects of PNBs are well-demonstrated, additional research showing improved patient outcome may provide further impetus for their expanded use.

References

[1] Lanz E, Theiss D, Jankovic D. The extent of blockade following various techniques of brachial plexus block. Anesth Analg 1983;62(1):55–8.

[2] Hadzic A, Vloka JD, Kuroda MM, et al. The practice of peripheral nerve blocks in the United States: a national survey. Reg Anesth Pain Med 1998;23(3):241–6.

[3] Klein SM, Pietrobon R, Nielsen KC, et al. Peripheral nerve blockade with long-acting local anesthetics: a survey of the Society for Ambulatory Anesthesia. Anesth Analg 2002;94(1):71–6.

[4] Brown AR, Weiss R, Greenberg C, et al. Interscalene block for shoulder arthroscopy: comparison with general anesthesia. Arthroscopy 1993;9(3):295–300.

[5] Al-Kaisy A, McGuire G, Chan VW, et al. Analgesic effect of interscalene block using low-dose bupivacaine for outpatient arthroscopic shoulder surgery. Reg Anesth Pain Med 1998;23(5): 469–73.

[6] Kinnard P, Truchon R, St-Pierre A, et al. Interscalene block for pain relief after shoulder surgery: a prospective randomized study. Clin Orthop 1994;304:22–4.

[7] Arciero RA, Taylor DC, Harrison SA, et al. Interscalene anesthesia for shoulder arthroscopy in a community-sized military hospital. Arthroscopy 1996;12(6):715–9.

[8] Laurila PA, Lopponen A, Kanga-Saarela T, et al. Interscalene brachial plexus block is superior to subacromial bursa block after arthroscopic shoulder surgery. Acta Anaesthesiol Scand 2002;46(8):1031–6.

[9] Singelyn FJ, Lhotel L, Fabre B. Pain relief after arthroscopic shoulder surgery: a comparison of intraarticular analgesia, suprascapular nerve block, and interscalene brachial plexus block. Anesth Analg 2004;99(2):589–92.

[10] D'Alessio JG, Rosenblum M, Shea KP, et al. A retrospective comparison of interscalene block and general anesthesia for ambulatory surgery shoulder arthroscopy. Reg Anesth 1995;20(1): 62–8.

[11] Chelly JE, Greger J, Al Samsam T, et al. Reduction of operating and recovery room times and overnight hospital stays with interscalene blocks as sole anesthetic technique for rotator cuff surgery. Minerva Anestesiol 2001;67(9):613–9.

[12] Esteves S, Sa P, Figueiredo D, et al. Duration and quality of postoperative analgesia after brachial plexus block for shoulder surgery: ropivacaine 0.5% versus ropivacaine 0.5% plus clonidine. Rev Esp Anestesiol 2002;49(6):302–5.

[13] Iskandar H, Benard A, Ruel-Raymond J, et al. The analgesic effect of interscalene block using clonidine as an analgesic for shoulder arthroscopy. Anesth Analg 2003;96(1):260–2.

[14] Culebras X, Van Gessel E, Hoffmeyer P, et al. Clonidine combined with a long acting local anesthetic does not prolong postoperative analgesia after brachial plexus block but does induce hemodynamic changes. Anesth Analg 2001;92(1):199–204.

[15] Lee IO, Kim WK, Kong MH, et al. No enhancement of sensory and motor blockade by ketamine added to ropivacaine interscalene brachial plexus blockade. Acta Anaesthesiol Scand 2002;46(7):821–6.

[16] Flory N, Van-Gessel E, Donald F, et al. Does the addition of morphine to brachial plexus block improve analgesia after shoulder surgery? Br J Anaesth 1995;75(1):23–6.

[17] Tuominen M, Haasio J, Hekali R, et al. Continuous interscalene brachial plexus block: clinical efficacy, technical problems and bupivacaine plasma concentrations. Acta Anaesthesiol Scand 1989;33(1):84–8.

[18] Boezaart AP, de Beer JF, du Toit C, et al. A new technique of continuous interscalene nerve block. Can J Anaesth 1999;46(3):275–81.

[19] Klein SM, Grant SA, Greengrass RA, et al. Interscalene brachial plexus block with a continuous catheter insertion system and a disposable infusion pump. Anesth Analg 2000;91(6):1473–8.

[20] Ekatodramis G, Borgeat A, Huledal G, et al. Continuous interscalene analgesia with ropivacaine 2 mg/ml after major shoulder surgery. Anesthesiology 2003;98(1):143–50.

[21] Tuominen M, Pitkanen M, Rosenberg PH. Postoperative pain relief and bupivacaine plasma levels during continuous interscalene brachial plexus block. Acta Anaesthesiol Scand 1987; 31(4):276–8.

[22] Singelyn FJ, Seguy S, Gouverneur JM. Interscalene brachial plexus analgesia after open shoulder surgery: continuous versus patient-controlled infusion. Anesth Analg 1999;89(5): 1216–20.

[23] Borgeat A, Schappi B, Biasca N, et al. Patient-controlled analgesia after major shoulder surgery: patient-controlled interscalene analgesia versus patient-controlled analgesia. Anesthesiology 1997;87(6):1343–7.

[24] Denny NM, Barber N, Sildown DJ. Evaluation of an insulated Tuohy needle system for the placement of interscalene brachial plexus catheters. Anaesthesia 2003;58(6):554–7.

[25] Borgeat A, Kalberer F, Jacob H, et al. Patient-controlled interscalene analgesia with ropivacaine 0.2% versus bupivacaine 0.15% after major open shoulder surgery: the effects on hand motor function. Anesth Analg 2001;92(1):218–23.

[26] Borgeat A, Tewes E, Biasca N, et al. Patient-controlled interscalene analgesia with ropivacaine after major shoulder surgery: PCIA vs PCA. Br J Anaesth 1998;81(4):603–5.

[27] Casati A, Borghi B, Fanelli G, et al. Interscalene brachial plexus anesthesia and analgesia for open shoulder surgery: a randomized, double-blinded comparison between levobupivacaine and ropivacaine. Anesth Analg 2003;96(1):253–9.

[28] Klein SM, Steele SM, Nielsen KC, et al. The difficulties of ambulatory interscalene and intra-articular infusions for rotator cuff surgery: a preliminary report. Can J Anaesth 2003;50(3): 265–9.

[29] Ilfeld BM, Enneking FK. A portable mechanical pump providing over four days of patient-controlled analgesia by perineural infusion at home. Reg Anesth Pain Med 2002;27(1):100–4.

[30] Ilfeld BM, Morey TE, Wright TW, et al. Continuous interscalene brachial plexus block for postoperative pain control at home: a randomized, double-blinded, placebo-controlled study. Anesth Anal 2003;96(4):1089–95.

[31] Nielsen KC, Greengrass RA, Pietrobon R, et al. Continuous interscalene brachial plexus blockade provides good analgesia at home after major shoulder surgery-report of four cases. Can J Anaesth 2003;50(1):57–61.

[32] Wilson AT, Nicholson E, Burton L, et al. Analgesia for day-case shoulder surgery. Br J Anaesth 2004;92(3):414–5.

[33] Winnie AP, Collins VJ. The subclavian perivascular technique of brachial plexus anesthesia. Anesthesiology 1964;25(3):353–63.

[34] Bedder MD, Kozody R, Craig DB. Comparison of bupivacaine and alkalinized bupivacaine in brachial plexus anesthesia. Anesth Analg 1988;67(1):48–52.

[35] Vaghadia H, Chan V, Ganapathy S, et al. A multicentre trial of ropivacaine 7.5 mg x ml(-1) vs bupivacaine 5 mg x ml(-1) for supra clavicular brachial plexus anesthesia. Can J Anaesth 1999; 46(10):946–51.

[36] Cox CR, Checketts MR, Mackenzie N, et al. Comparison of S(-)-bupivacaine with racemic (RS)-bupivacaine in supraclavicular brachial plexus block. Br J Anaesth 1998;80(5):594–8.

[37] Eledjam JJ, Deschodt J, Viel EJ, et al. Brachial plexus block with bupivacaine: effects of added alpha-adrenergic agonists: comparison between clonidine and epinephrine. Can J Anaesth 1991;38(7):870–5.

[38] Candido KD, Franco CD, Khan MA, et al. Buprenorphine added to the local anesthetic for brachial plexus block to provide postoperative analgesia in outpatients. Reg Anesth Pain Med 2001;26(4):352–6.

[39] Viel EJ, Eledjam JJ, De La Coussaye JE, et al. Brachial plexus block with opioids for postoperative pain relief: comparison between buprenorphine and morphine. Reg Anesth 1989; 14(6):274–8.

[40] Franco CD, Vieira ZE. 1,001 subclavian perivascular brachial plexus blocks: success with a nerve stimulator. Reg Anesth Pain Med 2000;25(1):41–6.

[41] Desroches J. The infraclavicular brachial plexus block by the coracoid approach is clinically effective: an observational study of 150 patients. Can J Anaesth 2003;50(3):253–7.

[42] Salazar CH, Espinosa W. Infraclavicular brachial plexus block: variation in approach and results in 360 cases. Reg Anesth Pain Med 1999;24(5):411–6.

[43] Hadzic A, Arliss J, Kerimoglu B, et al. A comparison of infraclavicular nerve block versus general anesthesia for hand and wrist day-case surgeries. Anesthesiology 2004;101(1):127–32.

[44] Ilfeld BM, Morey TE, Enneking FK. Continuous infraclavicular brachial plexus block for postoperative pain control at home: a randomized, double-blinded, placebo-controlled study. Anesthesiology 2002;96(6):1297–304.

[45] Ilfeld BM, Morey TE, Enneking FK. Continuous infraclavicular perineural infusion with clonidine and ropivacaine compared with ropivacaine alone: a randomized, double-blinded, controlled study. Anesth Analg 2003;97(3):706–12.

[46] Ilfeld BM, Morey TE, Enneking FK. Infraclavicular perineural local anesthetic infusion: a comparison of three dosing regimens for postoperative analgesia. Anesthesiology 2004; 100(2):395–402.

[47] Stan TC, Krantz MA, Solomon DL, et al. The incidence of neurovascular complications following axillary brachial plexus block using a transarterial approach: prospective study of 1,000 consecutive patients. Reg Anesth 1995;20(6):486–92.

[48] Koscielniak-Nielsen ZJ, Rotboll-Nielsen P, Rassmussen H. Patients' experiences with multiple stimulation axillary block for fast-track ambulatory hand surgery. Acta Anaesthesiol Scand 2002;46(7):789–93.

[49] Thompson GE, Rorie DK. Functional anatomy of the brachial plexus sheaths. Anesthesiology 1983;59(2):117–22.

[50] Partridge BL, Katz J, Benirschke K. Functional anatomy of the brachial plexus sheath: implications for anesthesia. Anesthesiology 1987;66(6):743–7.

[51] Urban MK, Urquhart B. Evaluation of brachial plexus anesthesia for upper extremity surgery. Reg Anesth 1994;19(3):175–82.

[52] Davis WJ, Lennon RL, Wedel DJ. Brachial plexus anesthesia for outpatient surgical procedures on an upper extremity. Mayo Clin Proc 1991;66(5):470–3.

[53] Pearce H, Lindsay D, Leslie K. Axillary brachial plexus block in two hundred consecutive patients. Anaesth Intensive Care 1996;24(4):453–8.

[54] Koscielniak-Nielsen ZJ, Stens-Pedersen HL, Lippert FK. Readiness for surgery after axillary block: single or multiple injection techniques. Eur J Anaesthesiol 1997;14(2):164–71.

[55] Coventry DM, Barker KF, Thomson M. Comparison of two neurostimulation techniques for axillary brachial plexus blockade. Br J Anaesth 2001;86(1):80–3.

[56] Bouaziz H, Narchi P, Mercier FJ, et al. The use of a selective axillary nerve block for outpatient hand surgery. Anesth Analg 1998;86(4):746–8.

[57] Singelyn FJ, Dangoisse M, Bartholomee S, et al. Adding clonidine to mepivacaine prolongs the duration of anesthesia and analgesia after axillary brachial plexus block. Reg Anesth 1992;17(3):148–50.

[58] Singelyn FJ, Gouverneur JM, Robert A. A minimum dose of clonidine added to mepivacaine prolongs the duration of anesthesia and analgesia after axillary brachial plexus block. Anesth Analg 1996;83(5):1046–50.

[59] Kapral S, Gollmann G, Waltl B, et al. Tramadol added to mepivacaine prolongs the duration of an axillary brachial plexus blockade. Anesth Analg 1999;88(4):853–6.

[60] Robaux S, Blunt C, Viel E, et al. Tramadol added to 1.5% mepivacaine for axillary brachial plexus block improves postoperative analgesia dose-dependently. Anesth Analg 2004;98(4): 1172–7.

[61] Candido KD, Winnie AP, Ghaleb AH, et al. Buprenorphine added to the local anesthetic for axillary brachial plexus block prolongs postoperative analgesia. Reg Anesth Pain Med 2002; 27(2):162–7.

[62] Karakaya D, Buyukgoz F, Baris S, et al. Addition of fentanyl to bupivacaine prolongs anesthesia and analgesia in axillary brachial plexus block. Reg Anesth Pain Med 2001;26(5):434–8.

[63] Nishikawa K, Kanaya N, Nakayama M, et al. Fentanyl improves analgesia but prolongs the onset of axillary brachial plexus block by peripheral mechanism. Anesth Analg 2000;91(2): 384–7.

[64] Bourke DL, Furman WR. Improved postoperative analgesia with morphine added to axillary block solution. J Clin Anesth 1993;5(2):114–7.

[65] Chan VW, Peng PW, Kaszas Z, et al. A comparative study of general anesthesia, intravenous regional anesthesia, and axillary block for outpatient hand surgery: clinical outcome and cost analysis. Anesth Analg 2001;93(5):1181–4.

[66] McCartney CJ, Brull R, Chan VW, et al. Early but no long-term benefit of regional compared with general anesthesia for ambulatory hand surgery. Anesthesiology 2004;101(2):461–7.

[67] Ebert B, Braunschweig R, Reill P. Quantification of variations in arm perfusion after plexus anesthesia with color doppler sonography. Anaesthesist 1995;44(12):859–62.

[68] Bergman BD, Hebl JR, Kent J, et al. Neurologic complications of 405 consecutive continuous axillary catheters. Anesth Analg 2003;96(1):247–52.

[69] Mezzatesta JP, Scott DA, Schweitzer SA, et al. Continuous axillary brachial plexus block for postoperative pain relief: intermittent bolus versus continuous infusion. Reg Anesth 1997;22(4): 357–62.

[70] Rawal N, Allvin R, Axelsson K, et al. Patient-controlled regional analgesia (PCRA) at home: controlled comparison between bupivacaine and ropivacaine brachial plexus analgesia. Anesthesiology 2002;96(6):1290–6.

[71] Parkinson SK, Mueller JB, Little WL, et al. Extent of blockade with various approaches to the lumbar plexus. Anesth Analg 1989;68(3):243–8.

[72] Jankowski CJ, Hebl JR, Stuart MJ, et al. A comparison of psoas compartment block and spinal and general anesthesia for outpatient knee arthroscopy. Anesth Analg 2003;97(4): 1003–9.

[73] Matheny JM, Hanks GA, Rung GW, et al. A comparison of patient-controlled analgesia and continuous lumbar plexus block after anterior cruciate ligament reconstruction. Arthroscopy 1993;9(1):87–90.

[74] Luber MJ, Greengrass R, Vail TP. Patient satisfaction and effectiveness of lumbar plexus and sciatic nerve block for total knee arthroplasty. J Arthroplasty 2001;16(1):17–21.

[75] Kaloul I, Guay J, Cote C, et al. The posterior lumbar plexus (psoas compartment) block and the three-in-one femoral nerve block provide similar postoperative analgesia after total knee replacement. Can J Anaesth 2004;51(1):45–51.

[76] de Visme V, Picart F, Le Jouan R, et al. Combined lumbar and sacral plexus block compared with plain bupivacaine spinal anesthesia for hip fractures in the elderly. Reg Anesth Pain Med 2000;25(2):158–62.

[77] Biboulet P, Morau D, Aubas P, et al. Postoperative analgesia after total-hip arthroplasty: comparison of intravenous patient-controlled analgesia with morphine and single injection of femoral nerve or psoas compartment block; a prospective, randomized, double-blind study. Reg Anesth Pain Med 2004;29(2):102–9.

[78] Hevia-Sanchez V, Bermejo-Alvarez MA, Hevia-Mendez A, et al. Posterior block of lumbar plexus for postoperative analgesia after hip arthroplasty. Rev Esp Anestesiol 2002;49(10): 507–11.

[79] Stevens RD, Van Gessel E, Flory N, et al. Lumbar plexus block reduces pain and blood loss associated with total hip arthroplasty. Anesthesiology 2000;93(1):115–21.

[80] Buckenmaier III CC, Xenos JS, Nilsen SM. Lumbar plexus block with perineural catheter and sciatic nerve block for total hip arthroplasty. J Arthroplasty 2002;17(4):499–502.

[81] Capdevila X, Macaire P, Dadure C, et al. Continuous psoas compartment block for post-operative analgesia after total hip arthroplasty: new landmarks, technical guidelines, and clinical evaluation. Anesth Analg 2002;94(6):1606–13.

[82] Turker G, Uckunkaya N, Yavascaoglu B, et al. Comparison of the catheter-technique psoas compartment block and the epidural block for analgesia in partial hip replacement surgery. Acta Anaesthesiol Scand 2003;47(1):30–6.

[83] Lang SA, Yip RW, Chang PC, et al. The femoral 3-in-1 block revisited. J Clin Anesth 1993; 5(4):292–6.

[84] Marhofer P, Nasel C, Sitzwohl C, et al. Magnetic resonance imaging of the distribution of local anesthetic during the three-in-one block. Anesth Analg 2000;90(1):119–24.

[85] Patel NJ, Flashburg MH, Paskin S, et al. A regional anesthetic technique compared to general anesthesia for outpatient knee arthroscopy. Anesth Analg 1986;65(2):185–7.

[86] Goranson BD, Lang S, Cassidy JD, et al. A comparison of three regional anaesthesia techniques for outpatient knee arthroscopy. Can J Anaesth 1997;44(4):371–6.

[87] De Andres J, Bellver J, Barrera L, et al. A comparative study of analgesia after knee surgery with intraarticular bupivacaine, intraarticular morphine, and lumbar plexus block. Anesth Analg 1993;77(4):727–30.

[88] Casati A, Cappelleri G, Berti M, et al. Randomized comparison of remifentanil-propofol with a sciatic-femoral nerve for out-patient knee arthroscopy. Eur J Anaesthesiol 2002;19(2): 109–14.

[89] Cappelleri G, Casati A, Fanelli G, et al. Unilateral spinal anesthesia or combined sciatic-femoral nerve block for day-case knee arthroscopy: prospective, randomized comparison. Minerva Anestesiol 2000;66(3):131–6.

[90] Casati A, Cappelleri G, Fanelli G, et al. Regional anaesthesia for outpatient knee arthroscopy: a randomized clinical comparison of two different anaesthetic techniques. Acta Anaesthesiol Scand 2000;44(5):543–7.

[91] Mulroy MF, Larkin KL, Batra MS, et al. Femoral nerve block with 0.25% or 0.5% bupivacaine improves postoperative analgesia following outpatient arthroscopic anterior cruciate ligament repair. Reg Anesth Pain Med 2001;26(1):24–9.

[92] Edkin BS, McCarty EC, Spindler KP, et al. Analgesia with femoral nerve block for anterior cruciate ligament reconstruction. Clin Orthop 1999;369:289–95.

[93] Peng P, Claxton A, Chung F, et al. Femoral nerve block and ketorolac in patients undergoing anterior cruciate ligament reconstruction. Can J Anaesth 1999;46(10):919–24.

[94] Lynch J, Trojan S, Arhelger S, et al. Intermittent femoral nerve blockade for anterior cruciate ligament repair: use of a catheter technique in 208 patients. Acta Anaesthesiol Belg 1991; 42(4):207–12.

[95] Morau D, Lopez S, Biboulet P, et al. Comparison of continuous 3-in-1 and fascia Iliaca compartment blocks for postoperative analgesia: feasibility, catheter migration, distribution of sensory block, and analgesic efficacy. Reg Anesth Pain Med 2003;28(4):309–14.

[96] Schwarz SK, Franciosi LG, Ries CR, et al. Addition of femoral 3-in-1 blockade to intra-articular ropivacaine 0.2% does not reduce analgesic requirements following arthroscopic knee surgery. Can J Anaesth 1999;46(8):741–7.

[97] Frost S, Grossfeld S, Kirkley A, et al. The efficacy of femoral nerve block in pain reduction for outpatient hamstring anterior cruciate ligament reconstruction: a double-blind, prospective, randomized trial. Arthroscopy 2000;16(3):243–8.

[98] Mansour NY, Bennetts FE. An observational study of combined continuous lumbar plexus and single-shot sciatic nerve blocks for post-knee surgery analgesia. Reg Anesth 1996;21(4): 287–91.

[99] Nakamura SJ, Conte-Hernandez A, Galloway MT. The efficacy of regional anesthesia for outpatient anterior cruciate ligament reconstruction. Arthroscopy 1997;13(6):699–703.

[100] Williams BA, Kentor ML, Vogt MT, et al. Femoral-sciatic nerve blocks for complex out-

patient knee surgery are associated with less postoperative pain before same-day discharge: a review of 1,200 consecutive cases from the period 1996–1999. Anesthesiology 2003;98(5): 1206–13.

[101] Williams BA, Kentor ML, Vogt MT, et al. Economics of nerve block pain management after anterior cruciate ligament reconstruction: potential hospital cost savings via associated postanesthesia care unit bypass and same-day discharge. Anesthesiology 2004;100(3):697–706.

[102] Ng HP, Cheong KF, Lim A, et al. Intraoperative single-shot "3-in-1" femoral nerve block with ropivacaine 0.25%, ropivacaine 0.5% or bupivacaine 0.25% provides comparable 48-hr analgesia after unilateral total knee replacement. Can J Anaesth 2001;48(11):1102–8.

[103] Edwards ND, Wright EM. Continuous low-dose 3-in-1 nerve blockade for postoperative pain relief after total knee replacement. Anesth Analg 1992;75(2):265–7.

[104] Singelyn FJ, Deyaert M, Joris D, et al. Effects of intravenous patient-controlled analgesia with morphine, continuous epidural analgesia, and continuous three-in-one block on post-operative pain and knee rehabilitation after unilateral total knee arthroplasty. Anesth Analg 1998;87(1):88–92.

[105] Dahl JB, Christiansen CL, Daugaard JJ, et al. Continuous blockade of the lumbar plexus after knee surgery–postoperative analgesia and bupivacaine plasma concentrations: a controlled clinical trial. Anaesthesia 1988;43(12):1015–8.

[106] Capdevila X, Barthelet Y, Biboulet P, et al. Effects of perioperative analgesic technique on the surgical outcome and duration of rehabilitation after major knee surgery. Anesthesiology 1999;91(1):8–15.

[107] Serpell MG, Millar FA, Thomson MF. Comparison of lumbar plexus block versus conventional opioid analgesia after total knee replacement. Anaesthesia 1991;46(4):275–7.

[108] Tarkkila P, Tuominen M, Huhtala J, et al. Comparison of intrathecal morphine and continuous femoral 3-in-1 block for pain after major knee surgery under spinal anaesthesia. Eur J Anaesthesiol 1998;15(1):6–9.

[109] Schultz P, Anker-Moller E, Dahl JB, et al. Postoperative pain treatment after open knee surgery: continuous lumbar plexus block with bupivacaine versus epidural morphine. Reg Anesth 1991;16(1):34–7.

[110] Singelyn FJ, Gouverneur JM. Extended "three-in-one" block after total knee arthroplasty: continuous versus patient-controlled techniques. Anesth Analg 2000;91(1):176–80.

[111] Hirst GC, Lang SA, Dust WN, et al. Femoral nerve block: single injection versus continuous infusion for total knee arthroplasty. Reg Anesth 1996;21(4):292–7.

[112] Cook P, Stevens J, Gaudron C. Comparing the effects of femoral nerve block versus femoral and sciatic nerve block on pain and opiate consumption after total knee arthroplasty. J Arthroplasty 2003;18(5):583–6.

[113] Weber A, Fournier R, Van Gessel E, et al. Sciatic nerve block and the improvement of femoral nerve block analgesia after total knee replacement. Eur J Anaesthesiol 2002;19(11): 834–6.

[114] Ben-David B, Schmalenberger K, Chelly JE. Analgesia after total knee arthroplasty: is continuous sciatic blockade needed in addition to continuous femoral blockade? Anesth Analg 2004;98(3):747–9.

[115] McNamee DA, Convery PN, Milligan KR. Total knee replacement: a comparison of ropivacaine and bupivacaine in combined femoral and sciatic block. Acta Anaesthesiol Scand 2001;45(4):477–81.

[116] Allen JG, Denny NM, Oakman N. Postoperative analgesia following total knee arthroplasty: a study comparing spinal anesthesia and combined sciatic femoral 3-in-1 block. Reg Anesth Pain Med 1998;23(2):142–6.

[117] Chelly JE, Greger J, Gebhard R, et al. Continuous femoral blocks improve recovery and outcome of patients undergoing total knee arthroplasty. J Arthroplasty 2001;16(4):436–45.

[118] Taboada M, Alvarez J, Cortes J. The effects of three different approaches on the onset time of sciatic nerve blocks with 0.75% ropivacaine. Anesth Analg 2004;98(1):242–7.

[119] Casati A, Fanelli G, Borghi B, et al. Ropivacaine or 2% mepivacaine for lower limb peripheral

nerve blocks. Study Group on Orthopedic Anesthesia of the Italian Society of Anesthesia, Analgesia, and Intensive Care. Anesthesiology 1999;90(4):1047–52.

[120] Cooper J, Benirschke S, Sangeorzan B, et al. Sciatic nerve blockade improves early postoperative analgesia after open repair of calcaneus fractures. J Orthop Trauma 2004;18(4): 197–201.

[121] Smith BE, Fischer HB, Scott PV. Continuous sciatic nerve block. Anaesthesia 1984;39(2): 155–7.

[122] di Benedetto P, Casati A, Bertini L. Continuous subgluteus sciatic nerve block after orthopedic foot and ankle surgery: comparison of two infusion techniques. Reg Anesth Pain Med 2002; 27(2):168–72.

[123] Rongstad K, Mann RA, Prieskorn D, et al. Popliteal sciatic nerve block for postoperative analgesia. Foot Ankle Int 1996;17(7):378–82.

[124] Singelyn FJ, Gouverneur JM, Gribomont BF. Popliteal sciatic nerve block aided by a nerve stimulator: a reliable technique for foot and ankle surgery. Reg Anesth 1991;16(5):278–81.

[125] Provenzano DA, Viscusi ER, Adams Jr SB, et al. Safety and efficacy of the popliteal fossa nerve block when utilized for foot and ankle surgery. Foot Ankle Int 2002;23(5):394–9.

[126] Hansen E, Eshelman MR, Cracchiolo III A. Popliteal fossa neural blockade as the sole anesthetic technique for outpatient foot and ankle surgery. Foot Ankle Int 2000;21(1):38–44.

[127] McLeod DH, Wong DH, Vaghadia H, et al. Lateral popliteal sciatic nerve block compared with ankle block for analgesia following foot surgery. Can J Anaesth 1995;42(9):765–9.

[128] McLeod DH, Wong DH, Claridge RJ, et al. Lateral popliteal sciatic nerve block compared with subcutaneous infiltration for analgesia following foot surgery. Can J Anaesth 1994;41(8): 673–6.

[129] Vloka JD, Hadzic A, Mulcare R, et al. Combined popliteal and posterior cutaneous nerve of the thigh blocks for short saphenous vein stripping in outpatients: an alternative to spinal anesthesia. J Clin Anesth 1997;9(8):618–22.

[130] White PF, Issioui T, Skrivanek GD, et al. The use of a continuous popliteal sciatic nerve block after surgery involving the foot and ankle: does it improve the quality of recovery? Anesth Analg 2003;97(5):1303–9.

[131] Singelyn FJ, Aye F, Gouverneur JM. Continuous popliteal sciatic nerve block: an original technique to provide postoperative analgesia after foot surgery. Anesth Analg 1997;84(2): 383–6.

[132] Zaric D, Boysen K, Christiansen J, et al. Continuous popliteal sciatic nerve block for outpatient foot surgery–a randomized, controlled trial. Acta Anaesthesiol Scand 2004;48(3):337–41.

[133] Ilfeld BM, Morey TE, Wang RD, et al. Continuous popliteal sciatic nerve block for postoperative pain control at home: a randomized, double-blinded, placebo-controlled study. Anesthesiology 2002;97(4):959–65.

[134] Chelly JE, Greger J, Casati A, et al. Continuous lateral sciatic blocks for acute postoperative pain management after major ankle and foot surgery. Foot Ankle Int 2002;23(8):749–52.

[135] Matthews PJ, Govenden V. Comparison of continuous paravertebral and extradural infusions of bupivacaine for pain relief after thoracotomy. Br J Anaesth 1989;62(2):204–5.

[136] Perttunen K, Nilsson E, Heinonen J, et al. Extradural, paravertebral and intercostal nerve blocks for post-thoracotomy pain. Br J Anaesth 1995;75(5):541–7.

[137] Richardson J, Sabanathan S, Jones J, et al. A prospective, randomized comparison of preoperative and continuous balanced epidural or paravertebral bupivacaine on post-thoracotomy pain, pulmonary function and stress responses. Br J Anaesth 1999;83(3):387–92.

[138] Catala E, Casas JI, Unzueta MC, et al. Continuous infusion is superior to bolus doses with thoracic paravertebral blocks after thoracotomies. J Cardiothorac Vasc Anesth 1996;10(5): 586–8.

[139] Canto M, Sanchez MJ, Casas MA, et al. Bilateral paravertebral blockade for conventional cardiac surgery. Anaesthesia 2003;58(4):365–70.

[140] Ganapathy S, Murkin JM, Boyd DW, et al. Continuous percutaneous paravertebral block for minimally invasive cardiac surgery. J Cardiothorac Vasc Anesth 1999;13(5):594–6.

[141] Dhole S, Mehta Y, Saxena H, et al. Comparison of continuous thoracic epidural and para-vertebral blocks for postoperative analgesia after minimally invasive direct coronary artery bypass surgery. J Cardiothorac Vasc Anesth 2001;15(3):288–92.

[142] Richardson J, Vowden P, Sabanathan S. Bilateral paravertebral analgesia for major abdominal vascular surgery: a preliminary report. Anaesthesia 1995;50(11):995–8.

[143] Weltz CR, Greengrass RA, Lyerly HK. Ambulatory surgical management of breast carcinoma using paravertebral block. Ann Surg 1995;222(1):19–26.

[144] Greengrass R, O'Brien F, Lyerly K, et al. Paravertebral block for breast cancer surgery. Can J Anaesth 1996;43(8):858–61.

[145] Coveney E, Weltz CR, Greengrass R, et al. Use of paravertebral block anesthesia in the surgical management of breast cancer: experience in 156 cases. Ann Surg 1998;227(4):496–501.

[146] Pusch F, Freitag H, Weinstabl C, et al. Single-injection paravertebral block compared to general anaesthesia in breast surgery. Acta Anaesthesiol Scand 1999;43(7):770–4.

[147] Klein SM, Bergh A, Steele SM, et al. Thoracic paravertebral block for breast surgery. Anesth Analg 2000;90(6):1402–5.

[148] Terheggen MA, Wille F, Borel Rinkes IH, et al. Paravertebral blockade for minor breast surgery. Anesth Analg 2002;94(2):355–9.

[149] Naja MZ, Ziade MF, Lonnqvist PA. Nerve-stimulator guided paravertebral blockade vs. general anaesthesia for breast surgery: a prospective randomized trial. Eur J Anaesthesiol 2003; 20(11):897–903.

[150] Buckenmaier III CC, Klein SM, Nielsen KC, et al. Continuous paravertebral catheter and outpatient infusion for breast surgery. Anesth Analg 2003;97(3):715–7.

[151] Klein SM, Greengrass RA, Weltz C, et al. Paravertebral somatic nerve block for outpatient inguinal herniorrhaphy: an expanded case report of 22 patients. Reg Anesth Pain Med 1998; 23(3):306–10.

[152] Weltz CR, Klein SM, Arbo JE, et al. Paravertebral block anesthesia for inguinal hernia repair. World J Surg 2003;27(4):425–9.

[153] Naja Z, Ziade MF, Lonnqvist PA. Bilateral paravertebral somatic nerve block for ventral hernia repair. Eur J Anaesthesiol 2002;19(3):197–202.

[154] Kalady MF, Fields RC, Klein S, et al. Loop ileostomy closure at an ambulatory surgery facility: a safe and cost-effective alternative to routine hospitalization. Dis Colon Rectum 2003;46(4): 486–90.

[155] Naja MZ, el Hassan MJ, Oweidat M, et al. Paravertebral blockade vs general anesthesia or spinal anesthesia for inguinal hernia repair. Middle East J Anesthesiol 2001;16(2):201–10.

[156] Klein SM, Pietrobon R, Nielsen KC, et al. Paravertebral somatic nerve block compared with peripheral nerve blocks for outpatient inguinal herniorrhaphy. Reg Anesth Pain Med 2002; 27(5):476–80.

[157] Smith MP, Sprung J, Zura A, et al. A survey of exposure to regional anesthesia techniques in American anesthesia residency training programs. Reg Anesth Pain Med 1999;24(1):11–6.

ELSEVIER
SAUNDERS

Anesthesiology Clin N Am
23 (2005) 163–184

ANESTHESIOLOGY
CLINICS OF
NORTH AMERICA

Postoperative Pain Management in Children

Susan T. Verghese, MD[a,b], Raafat S. Hannallah, MD[a,b,*]

[a]*The George Washington University Medical Center, Washington, DC, USA*
[b]*Division of Anesthesiology, Children's National Medical Center, 111 Michigan Avenue, Northwest,
Washington, DC 20010, USA*

Awareness and treatment of postoperative pain in children has improved over the past few years. Numerous clinical practice guidelines and policy statements have been published on the subject of pediatric pain [1]. Children suffer postoperative pain in the same way as adults. Frequently, factors such as fear, anxiety, coping style, and lack of social support can exaggerate the physical pain in children further. The need for analgesics following surgery depends upon the nature of the procedure and the pain threshold of the patient. It does not depend on the age, or on whether the child is an inpatient or an outpatient.

Pain assessment is a critical component of pain management. Assessing pain in young children, however, can be challenging. Self-reporting is only possible in older children or those with considerable cognitive and communicative abilities. Therefore, several tools and pain assessment scales should be available to provide qualitative and quantitative information and documentation of pain (Figs. 1, 2). The measurement of pain in infants, young children, and children with developmental disabilities who are unable to self-report is particularly challenging and merits increased attention [1].

The increased awareness of the need to provide better postoperative analgesia in children has stimulated the introduction of several treatment modalities into pediatric anesthesia practice. The current trend is to use regional blocks or local infiltration whenever possible to supplement general anesthesia during

* Corresponding author. Children's National Medical Center, Washington, DC 20010.
E-mail address: rhannall@cnmc.org (R.S. Hannallah).

0889-8537/05/$ – see front matter © 2005 Elsevier Inc. All rights reserved.
doi:10.1016/j.atc.2004.11.008   *anesthesiology.theclinics.com*

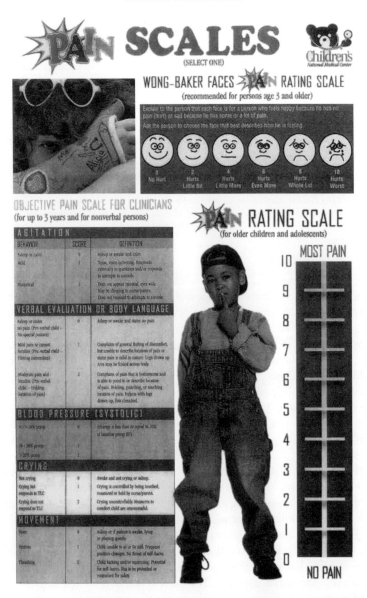

Fig. 1. Pain scales. At Children's National Medical Center (CNMC), staff has a choice among three different scales to assess a child's pain. The Objective Pain Scale (OPS) is used for children up to 3 years of age or nonverbal children. The Wong-Baker Faces Rating Scale is used for patients age 3 and over, and the Lineal Analogue Pain Scale is used for older children and adolescents.

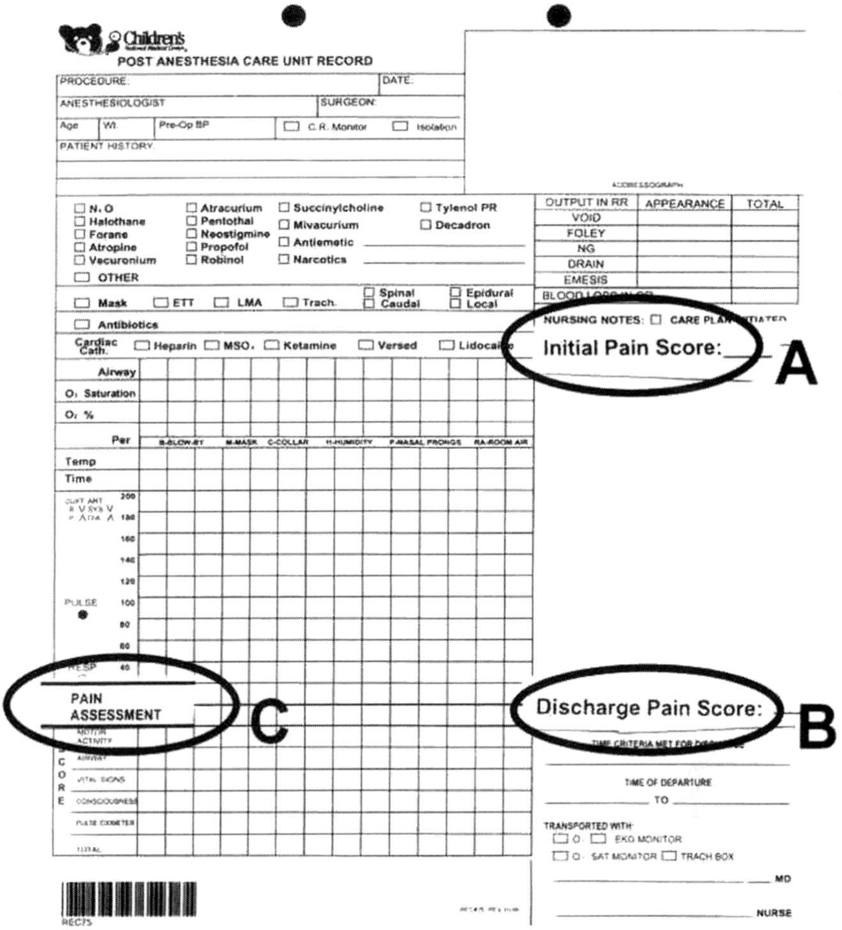

Fig. 2. PACU record at CNMC. Pain is assessed and a pain score documented when the child arrives in PACU (*A*), upon discharge (*B*), and every time vital signs are recorded (*C*). Similar assessments and documentation are made on the Pediatric Flow Sheet for in-patients at minimum every 8 hours.

surgery, and to use a multi-modal approach to systemic analgesia to limit the need for opioids during recovery.

Nonopioid analgesics

Acetaminophen

Acetaminophen is the most commonly used mild analgesic for pediatric outpatients. Recent 24-hour pharmacokinetics studies have changed the traditional dosing guidelines for acetaminophen in children [2]. For young children, the initial dose often is administered rectally (up to 45 mg/kg) before awakening from anesthesia [3]. Supplemental doses can be given orally (10 to 15 mg/kg) or rectally (20 mg/kg) every 4 to 6 hours (not on an as needed basis) to maintain adequate blood level (10 to 20 μg/mL) and therefore effective analgesia [4].

Recent studies have examined the serum concentrations of acetaminophen that are associated with analgesia. Anderson et al [4] demonstrated good analgesia and opioid-sparing effects in children with serum concentrations over 10.5 μg/mL. Other studies, however, failed to prove the analgesic value of the recommended doses of acetaminophen in children following tonsillectomy or cleft palate repair [5,6]. Acetaminophen may be combined with codeine for more effective control of moderately severe pain or discomfort. Acetaminophen with codeine elixir contains 120 mg acetaminophen and 12 mg codeine per 5 mL. The usual dose is 5 mL for children between the ages of 3 and 6 years, and 10 mL for the 7- to 12-year-old age group [7].

Nonsteroidal Anti-inflammatory drugs

Nonselective nonsteroidal anti-inflammatory drugs (NSAIDs) (eg, ketorolac) have proved effective in relieving postoperative pain following a range of operations in children. Ketorolac is the only intravenous (IV) form of NSAID available in the United States. Early administration immediately following induction seems to provide optimal postoperative analgesia. Several studies have demonstrated the analgesic and opioid-sparing effects of ketorolac, which may reduce the incidence of opioid-related adverse effects such as respiratory depression, nausea, and vomiting in children [14]. IV ketorolac (0.5 mg/kg) also has been shown to reduce the frequency and severity of postoperative bladder spasms after ureteral reimplant procedures in children [15]. These spasms can be extremely uncomfortable, can occur in spite of regional analgesic blockade, and are treated poorly with most opioid analgesics. Ketorolac appears to suppress bladder contractions and increase bladder capacity by lowering bladder prostaglandins level, thereby reducing the C fiber-mediated bladder pain and hyperactivity.

Like many other NSAIDs, however, ketorolac has some troubling adverse effects, with reported instances of decreased bone repair after osteotomy, bronchospasm, acute renal failure, and possibly increased surgical bleeding secondary to altered platelet function [16]. Several recent articles reported an increased incidence of postoperative hemorrhage in patients who received ketorolac following tonsillectomy [17,18]. A recent quantitative systemic review of 25 studies with data from 970 patients examined the risk of bleeding after tonsillectomy when NSAIDs were used. Of four bleeding endpoints (intraoperative blood loss, postoperative bleeding, hospital admission, and reoperating because of bleeding), only reoperation happened significantly more frequently with NSAIDs. Compared with opioids, NSAIDs were equianalgesic, with less risk of postoperative nausea and vomiting (PONV) [18]. More studies are needed to determine the optimal dose and route of administration of ketorolac, and its efficacy as an analgesic following more painful surgical procedures in children.

Cyclo-oxygenase (COX-2)-specific inhibitors

The development of selective COX-2 inhibitors that can alleviate pain and inflammation without inhibiting the platelet function that is mediated by the COX-1-derived prostanoids promises to be valuable in pediatric patients. Only oral preparations are available in the United States (celecoxib and valdecoxib). (Please see article elsewhere in this issue.) The IV preparation (parecoxib, a prodrug of valdecoxib) is available in other countries. Pediatric studies with COX-2-specific inhibitors are limited. Pickering et al [19] compared the analgesic effectiveness of acetaminophen alone with acetaminophen combined with ibuprofen or rofecoxib. The addition of ibuprofen, but not rofecoxib, to acetaminophen reduced the need for early analgesia following tonsillectomy by 50% compared with acetaminophen alone. Joshi et al [20], on the other hand, studied 66 patients, aged 3 to 11 years, scheduled to undergo tonsillectomy. They found that a single preoperative dose of rofecoxib (1 mg/kg) resulted in less vomiting and lower 24-hour pain scores in pediatric patients undergoing an elective tonsillectomy. More pediatric trials are going to be forthcoming to establish the place of this class of drugs in postoperative pain management in children.

Dextromethorphan

Dextromethorphan, a popular antitussive ingredient, is an isomer of codeine analog levorphanol. Its analgesic effect is through noncompetitive N-methyl-D-aspartate (NMDA) receptor antagonism. Several authors reported on the preoperative use of dextromethorphan for control of postadenotonsillectomy pain with mixed results. Dawson et al [12] reported a 34% reduction in the need for IV morphine during the first 6 hours after surgery in children who received a single 1 mg/kg dose of dextromethorphan preoperatively. There was no difference, however, in oral analgesic consumption or type of diet tolerated from controls beyond 6 hours. Conversely, Rose et al [13] questioned the efficacy of dextromethorphan in reducing postadenotonsillectomy pain in patients who received preoperative morphine and acetaminophen analgesia. The attraction of dextromethorphan lies in the lack of activity at the mu receptors, and therefore lack of undesirable opioid adverse effects such as respiratory depression, and PONV. More work, however, is needed to confirm its efficacy in this patient population.

Tramadol

Tramadol, a synthetic analog of codeine, is an analgesic agent with a dual mechanism of action, including a weak activity at the mu–opioid receptors and inhibition of the reuptake of the neurotransmitters norepinephrine and serotonin.

Tramadol's lack of sedation and minimal effects on respiration may offer a distinct advantage over the typical opioid analgesics for relief of postoperative pain in children [8]. Of note, tramadol is not a controlled drug. An IV dose of tramadol 1 to 2 mg/kg has been shown to be a suitable alternative to IV morphine in post-tonsillectomy patients [9]. Oral tramadol has been shown to have the same analgesic efficacy as oral diclofenac for post-tonsillectomy pain in patients 11 years and older, without the adverse effects of NSAIDs [10]. Another study with oral tramadol demonstrated a dose-ranging effect, with patients receiving a 2 mg/kg dose requiring 42% fewer rescue analgesics than those who received a 1 mg/kg dose [8]. The most troubling adverse effect of tramadol is increased incidence of PONV. This is more likely with postoperative oral administration than with intraoperative IV use [9]. Unfortunately, the use of ondansetron to treat PONV results in inhibition of tramadol analgesia, probably because of reduction of binding of the 5-HT$_3$ receptors at the spinal level [11].

Potent opioid analgesics

When opioids are indicated in the immediate recovery period, a short-acting drug usually is chosen. IV use allows more accurate titration of the dose and avoids the use of standard dosages based on weight, which may lead to under-medication or relative overdose. Fentanyl, up to a dose of 2 μg/kg, is the authors' drug of choice for IV use. Meperidine (0.5 mg/kg) and codeine (1.0 to 1.5 mg/kg) can be used intramuscularly if an IV route is not established. Intramuscular codeine tends to result in less vomiting than other opioids, especially morphine [21]. Children, however, are so fearful of intramuscular injections that they often will deny pain to avoid the therapeutic, but equally painful, injection. Nasal administration of fentanyl has been shown to result in an analgesic blood level comparable to that following IV use [22], which makes it useful for children who do not have, or have lost, their IV access [23].

Other modalities of opioid administration (eg, transdermal or oral trans-mucosal) have been developed. These, however, often are used in children with chronic pain and not usually indicated for postoperative analgesia.

Intravenous patient/parent/nurse-controlled analgesia in children

Intravenous patient-controlled analgesia (IV-PCA) is considered one of the most effective techniques for postoperative analgesia in adults. IV-PCA provides effective pain treatment, adjusts the dose according to individual needs, and allows the patients to be in control of their pain management decisions. The use of this technique recently has expanded to most adolescents, and even young children. Not only does IV-PCA provide consistent opioid blood levels, but it also pares children the pain of IM injections that used to be used for postoperative opioid administration routinely.

An IV-PCA-based analgesic regimen requires an appropriate IV opioid loading dose to initiate adequate analgesia. Morphine is the most commonly used opioid for pediatric IV-PCA. The dose is based on the child's body weight. The optimum bolus dose (usually 0.02 mg/kg) is the minimum dose required to produce satisfactory analgesia without causing significant adverse effects. Lockout periods should provide sufficient time for the improved analgesia to be noted. Although there is no correct or optimal lockout period, a range of 5 to 10 minutes usually is prescribed.

Protocols with and without background infusion have been used successfully in children. The addition of background infusion to on-demand IV-PCA may improve the overall quality of analgesia and allow better sleep quality with less bolus requirements at night. Some authors, however, have suggested that the use of background infusion may increase the total dose of opioid used, and therefore increase the incidence of opioid-related adverse effects such as excessive sedation, nausea, and respiratory depression, without apparent improved pain scores [24]. More recently, Yildiz et al [25] reported that by decreasing the bolus dose by 50%, the total opioid (meperidine) consumption was actually lower when a background infusion was added as compared with bolus dosing alone, with no statistical differences in pain, sedation, and nausea scores between the two regimens.

Initially, pediatric IV-PCA was reserved for adolescents and older children. More recently, however, these restrictions have been relaxed. Many young children today are familiar with electronic game operations at a very young age, and can grasp the concept of pushing a button to take away the pain. Rather than have rigid age-limit criteria on prescribing IV-PCA, the technique should be available to any child who understands the concept. Most 6- or 7-year-old children of average intelligence should be able to operate the IV-PCA devices effectively. Some children as young as 5 years of age have been able to successfully use IV-PCA. The maturity of the child, the familiarity with the equipment and hospital environment, and the support of the parents are factors that can encourage early use. There are even reports of children as young as 3 years of age, who met all these criteria, and were able to use the IV-PCA device on their own [26].

Morphine is the most commonly used opioid for PCA in children. It has a reasonably long duration of actin and mild sedative effect. Like all opioids, however, morphine can cause nausea, vomiting, pruritus, and can decrease gastrointestinal function, and possibly urinary retention. When morphine is contraindicated, or if dose-limiting adverse effects are encountered, fentanyl or hydromorphone can be used. Fentanyl has faster onset and shorter duration than morphine. When children are expected to have constant pain, a background infusion usually is required. In situations of intermittent severe pain of short duration, fentanyl boluses are particularly effective, owing to the rapid onset and short duration of action.

Hydromorphone, which is a hydrogenated ketone of morphine, has greater potency (7 to 10 times that of morphine), and frequently is used as an alternative to morphine. Although hydromorphone has not been demonstrated to be superior to morphine in terms of analgesic efficacy or adverse effect profile, it frequently is tolerated well by some children who have difficulty tolerating morphine [27]. The addition of NSAID drugs such as ketorolac to the morphine IV-PCA regimen has been shown to decrease the morphine requirements and the opioid-related adverse effects [28].

A variation on the use of PCA technology in children is that of nurse- or parent-assisted PCA [29]. The technique is controversial because of concerns regarding the risk of overdose and the potential for respiratory depression if someone other than the patient is allowed to initiate bolus doses. Advocates of this approach maintain that it allows young children, and those who are physically or cognitively impaired to receive the same PCA benefits as older children [29]. Children are started on small-dose continuous opioid infusion. The protocol allows the bolus doses of opioid to be administered by a nurse or parent to treat acute exacerbations of pain. In a series of 240 treatments in 212 patients, there was a 1.7% incidence of apnea and episodes of desaturation requiring treatment with naloxone [29]. These findings reinforce the need for treatment paradigms and close patient monitoring to minimize the risk and allow for effective intervention when someone other than the patient activates IV-PCA devices.

It is the authors' view that nurse-assisted PCA is a misnomer. Nurse-controlled analgesia is simply an alternative delivery system of controlled drugs by nursing staff that allows them to work around the rigid policies regarding handling of these drugs that can cause delay in pain relief [30]. Using the PCA pump, the nurse can administer a pre-calculated and programmed analgesic dose immediately once the assessment of pain is made without leaving the patient's bedside. The alternative is having to go to a medicine cabinet, obtain the drug, calculate the dose, get a witness, and then administer it (frequently intramuscularly) long after the child's need is established. When properly employed, the use of IV-PCA devices to allow timely administration of opioids by the nurse is an excellent patient care convenience and safety initiative. Parent-controlled analgesia, on the other hand, needs further evaluation before it can be recommended on a wider scale.

Weaning children from IV-PCA is similar to the approach in adults. It usually is based on documented decreasing bolus demands and ability to tolerate oral fluids. If a background infusion is used, it usually is ceased first. The total daily opioid doses before weaning can be used to calculate the appropriate equivalent of oral analgesics.

Epidural/caudal blocks

Single-shot caudal analgesia is the most useful and popular pediatric regional block used today [31]. Extensive clinical experience attests to the ease of performance, reliability, and safety, especially in patients weighing over 10 kg

[32]. This block is deceptively simple to perform, however, and one must have respect for the rare but potentially serious complications that can occur with any regional technique. Single-shot caudal blocks are ideally suited for surgical procedures below the level of the umbilicus [33]. Analgesia for higher dermatomes can be achieved at the expense of a larger dose of local anesthetic. The addition of a caudal catheter can allow for continuous infusion or repeated administration of medications, prolonging the analgesia for as long as necessary.

Single-shot caudal analgesia

Three variables determine the quality, duration, and extent of a caudal block: volume, total dose, and concentration of the local anesthetic. There is no general agreement, however, on whether age or weight is the best criterion for selecting a dose to achieve the desired level of caudal analgesia in children. Busoni and Andreuccetti evaluated the correlation of spread of the local anesthetic to age and weight [34]. They noted that age and weight were predictors of the desired level of analgesia, but weight was a better predictor in newborns and infants, whereas age was a better guide in older children.

Clinically, the most workable formula is that suggested by Armitage [35]. It correlated the level of block with the volume of local anesthetic injected. For sacral or a T-10 level, the volume is 0.5 mL/kg is used, while for a lower or midthoracic levels, the volume is 1 and 1.25 mL/kg respectively. Because there is no opportunity to repeat a single-shot block, the initial dose must be large enough to produce the required level of analgesia. Armitage noted that children may be very distressed if they cannot move or feel their legs and that it is important to avoid using concentrations of local anesthetic agents strong enough to cause motor blockade.

It is difficult to assess the effectiveness of the caudal block by testing for sensory levels in an anesthetized child. The ability to decrease the concentration of inhaled anesthetic without using opioids during surgery often is considered to indicate a successful block. In addition, laxity of the patient's anal sphincter as evidenced during placement of an acetaminophen suppository after the block has set in can be used as a test to confirm the effectiveness of the caudal block in children [36]. The presence of a lax anal sphincter at the end of surgery correlates significantly with the reduced administration of opioids intraoperatively and in the PACU. A tight sphincter at the end of surgery may suggest the need to repeat the block before the child awakens, or consider alternate methods of postoperative analgesia.

Mazoit et al [37] studied the pharmacokinetics of bupivacaine after caudal anesthesia in infants receiving 2.5 mg/kg of bupivacaine and found that serum levels were in the range of 0.5 to 1.9 μg/mL, with peak plasma levels occurring 10 to 60 minutes after administration. Eyres et al [38] measured plasma bupivacaine concentrations after caudal injection of 3 mg/kg of 0.25% bupivacaine in 45 children whose ages ranged from 4 months to 12 years and found mean blood levels ranging from 1.2 to 1.4 μg/mL, which are well below the limits projected to be toxic in adults. In all studies, the peak plasma levels of bupivacaine were less than those considered toxic in adults.

Bromage [39] attempted to quantitate the duration of caudal analgesia in children by recording the time that elapsed before the block level had receded by at least two spinal segments. When bupivacaine alone was used, that time was 2 hours; the time was slightly longer if an epinephrine-containing local anesthetic solution was used. Bromage also noted that the total duration of action in the lower sacral segments was considerably longer than the time that elapsed before recession began. This observation correlates well with clinical experience, where bupivacaine caudal analgesia, as judged by the time elapsing before the child requires supplemental analgesia, may persist for 4 or 5 hours.

The main disadvantage of a single-shot caudal block is the limited duration of action (90 to 120 minutes with bupivacaine) [39]. Many investigators have attempted to prolong the analgesic effects of a single-shot caudal block by combining local anesthetic drug with other additives. Addition of preservative-free morphine to local anesthetics has been noted to prolong the duration of analgesia after major surgical procedures [40]. Jamali et al [41] reported on the use of clonidine as an adjunct for pediatric caudal analgesia. They compared bupivacaine alone (0.25%, 1 mL/kg); with bupivacaine and epinephrine (1:200,000); and with bupivacaine and clonidine (1 μg/kg) for postoperative analgesia. Adding clonidine to the caudal analgesic mixture more than doubled the analgesic time. There were no differences in respiratory rate, oxygen saturation values, or hemodynamic parameters among the three groups. There was also no difference in sedation or sleep time among the three groups. In children undergoing longer surgical procedures below the umbilicus, a repeat caudal block can be done at the end of surgery. If prolonged operative or postoperative analgesia is required, a caudal catheter can be inserted for the administration of repeated bolus doses or a continuous infusion in pediatric patients undergoing perineal or lower abdominal or lower extremity surgery.

High caudal blocks

A higher level of blockade (up to T4) may be necessary to block the peritoneal stimulation arising from spermatic cord traction in children undergoing orchidopexy or during umbilical hernia repair. A high volume aids the spread of the local anesthetic in the epidural space and increases the duration of postoperative analgesia. Increasing the volume of 0.25% bupivacaine to more than 1 mL/kg blocks the signs of the peritoneal stimulation but can result in motor weakness of lower extremities. This is especially marked when epinephrine is added to the bupivacaine solution. Wolf et al [42] demonstrated that children who received caudal blocks performed with 0.125% bupivacaine at the completion of surgery had postoperative analgesia that was just as effective as that produced by 0.25% bupivacaine but with less evidence of motor weakness. The advantage of using 0.125% bupivacaine was that these patients were able to ambulate better than the children whose caudal blocks were performed with the more concentrated solution. It is important to note that the local anesthetic must be diluted with preservative-free normal saline solution. The total mg/kg dosage always should be checked to ensure that it is within the acceptable safe dose of the drug. In a recent study of healthy children undergoing orchidopexy, a caudal block performed with a higher volume of dilute (0.2%) bupivacaine was more effective in blocking the peritoneal stimulation during spermatic cord traction than the lower volume of the more concentrated (0.25%) solution [43]. A significant point in this study was that the same total dose of local anesthetic was used in all children, and there was no change in the quality of postoperative analgesia [43].

Continuous epidural anesthesia

The most common sites of epidural catheter insertion are caudal (by means of sacrococcygeal ligament), lumbar (L3-4 vertebrae), and thoracic (T 7-11 vertebrae). Epidural catheter placement allows repeated injections or the use of continuous infusions to provide prolonged blockade. Placement of the epidural catheter in congruence with the surgical incision allows the local anesthetics to be placed close to the site of action and to obtain the desired effect with minimal doses.

Caudal
The caudal space can be entered by the same technique as in the single-shot caudal technique by inserting either a Tuohy or a Crawford epidural needle or an 18-G IV catheter through the sacrococcygeal membrane. After confirming that there is no blood or cerebrospinal fluid on aspiration, the measured length of caudal catheter is threaded into the desired location. The bevel of the needle should be pointed posteriorly to advance the catheter easily. The advantage of using continuous caudal block with general anesthesia is that it reduces the requirements of intraoperative inhaled anesthetics and opioids, lessening the need for postoperative mechanical ventilation, especially in neonates and formerly premature infants with pulmonary problems. Caudal epidural anesthesia by means of a catheter has been used as the sole mode of anesthesia in formerly premature infants having inguinal hernia repair without any postoperative problems [44]. In another study of 20 premature, high-risk infants for abdominal or thoracic surgery under combined caudal epidural and general anesthesia, epidurography confirmed 17 of the catheters to be in the desired location. In two patients, however, the catheters were misplaced within the dura, epidural vessel lumen, and one was coiled within the epidural space [45].

It is possible to advance the caudal catheter cephalad to a thoracic or high lumbar position in infants and children. The catheter should not be forced but smoothly and gently threaded into the desired position, and the position of the catheter tip should be confirmed radiologically.

The caudal approach to thoracic epidural anesthesia in children was reported to show the catheter tip to be within two vertebrae of the target position by radiologic confirmation in 17 out of 20 children [46]. Thoracic epidural catheters have been placed by means of the caudal canal using electrical nerve stimulation guidance and electrocardiographic guidance in 20 infants [47,48]. Despite the lack of reports of infection with caudal catheters in children, daily inspection and strict asepsis with tape and clean bio-occlusive barrier dressing of the catheter site are essential. The incidence of epidural catheter tip colonization was increased with the caudal route of insertion, and the bacteria differed from those cultured from the lumbar insertion site in a study of 91 children. A higher incidence of gram-negative bacteria was cultured from the caudal catheter tips than from the lumbar epidural catheter tips [49]. In some patients, tunneling the catheter under the skin to a higher position has been used to minimize contamination [50]. Difficulty in keeping the catheter insertion site free of fecal contamination has led many pediatric anesthesiologists to place lumbar and thoracic epidural catheters instead.

Lumbar

Epidural blockade to T10 (thoracic dermatome corresponding to the umbilicus) provides analgesia for surgery in the lower limb, perineal, urologic, and inguinal areas. A higher level up to T4–T6 (thoracic dermatome corresponding to the nipple line) is necessary for abdominal and lower thoracic surgery. Continuous lumbar epidurals can be performed successfully in small children. In 20 neonates undergoing major thoracoabdominal surgeries, lumbar epidural anesthesia was used intraoperatively and continued for 72 hours postoperative analgesia. There were no complications, and all but one were extubated awake at the end of the surgery in the operating room [51]. Radiological imaging is useful with this type of anesthesia in very small infants to confirm the position of the catheter [52]. A review of epidural anesthesia in 240 neonates showed an incidence of one intravascular migration of catheter, one dural puncture, and one convulsion. Intraoperative analgesia was effective in all, and most patients had intermittent top-up instead of continuous infusion [53].

Thoracic

In older children and adults it is appropriate for an experienced anesthesiologist to place thoracic epidural catheters for pain control during and after extensive thoracoabdominal surgeries. The spinous processes in the thoracic area are longer and slant downward at a sharper angle; additionally, the interspaces are narrower. The introducer needle therefore needs to be angled more cephalad to approach the interspace. Continuous thoracic epidural infusions placed preoperatively (T3–T8 level) have been used in children undergoing pectus repair for intra- and postoperative analgesia with excellent results [54]. A thoracic epidural blockade is essential for pain control in the perioperative period after the newer minimally invasive repair of the pectus deformity (the Nuss procedure), where a retrosternal metal bar is placed in the chest thoracoscopically. In this procedure, although there is no cartilage resection or osteotomy, the pain from the bar placement is sufficient to warrant a well-established thoracic epidural blockade before surgery and has been used successfully in children as young as

7 years of age [55]. In a retrospective review of 220 children undergoing pediatric cardiac surgery under general anesthesia supplemented with regional anesthesia techniques, Peterson et al [56] showed that thoracic epidural catheter use was associated with the lowest incidence of adverse effects. The safety of insertion and maintenance of thoracic epidural anesthesia in 63 infants and children was reported to be very high with no incidence of dural puncture [57]. Lumbar and low thoracic catheters can be threaded up to block higher thoracic levels if the site of the operation is higher. A very high block (T1–T4), however, also can result in bradycardia, hypotension, and reduced cardiac output by blocking the cardiac sympathetic outflow from the vasomotor center. Placement of thoracic epidural catheters in children should be done only by anesthesiologists who are thoroughly experienced in placing lumbar epidural catheters in children and clearly not by beginners. Unlike adults, epidural catheters are placed in children when they are asleep or deeply sedated and therefore, eliciting paresthesia is not possible [58]. The risk of spinal cord injury is real, and extreme care should be taken to avoid it during a thoracic epidural placement [59].

Patient-controlled epidural anesthesia

Epidural analgesia can be administered as continuous infusion or as patient-controlled epidural anesthesia (PCEA) in older children and teenagers who can understand how to use the PCA devices. In addition to self-administered boluses, which allow patients a certain amount of autonomy over their pain control, a continuous background infusion always is used in PCEA. PCEA usually is used after extensive abdominal, thoracic surgeries (eg, pectus repair) or extensive lower limb and spine surgeries [60]. Orders for PCEA should have, in addition to the drug concentration (local anesthetic and opioid- usually fentanyl), volume and basal infusion rate, bolus dose, lockout period, and the number of hourly boluses. Because the time needed for a bolus dose to produce a change is longer with epidural compared with IV drug administration, the lockout interval is longer, usually 15 minutes compared with 5 to 8 minutes.

The efficacy of this modality of pain treatment was evaluated in a recent study of 128 children, and satisfactory analgesia without serious toxicity or adverse effects was reported in children as young as 5 years of age [61]. In another study of 48 children, both continuous epidural anesthesia (CEA) and PCEA with 0.2% ropivacaine provided adequate pain relief in the first 48 hours after orthopedic surgery. Adequate analgesia, however, was obtained with 50% less volume infused with PCEA compared with CEA [62]. This is a potential advantage if the technique is going to be used in a younger patient for a longer period of time.

The use of percutaneously inserted subcutaneously tunneled epidural catheters for prolonged analgesia in pediatric patients has been found to be a safe and effective method of providing analgesia in children suffering pain from end-stage malignancies [63].

Bupivacaine toxicity and convulsions have occurred in children receiving large doses of bupivacaine by means of continuous caudal or epidural infusions. Berde [64] suggests that for epidural bupivacaine infusions, after a loading dose of 2 to 2.5 mg/kg, not to exceed infusion rates of 0.4 to 0.5 mg/kg per hour for older infants, toddlers, and children, or 0.2 to 0.25 mg/kg per hour for neonates.

A combination of a dilute bupivacaine solution (0.1%) and fentanyl 2 μg/mL has been found effective. The dosing schedule depends on the proximity of the catheter tip to the dermatomal level of the incision. If catheter tips can be placed close to the dermatomes involved in surgery, Berde recommends an infusion rate of 0.2 to 0.3 mL/kg per hour [64]. If the catheter tip is positioned at lumbar or caudal levels for upper abdominal surgery, hydrophilic opioids (eg, morphine or hydromorphone) should be used. Appropriate postoperative monitoring of these patients is essential.

Local anesthetics/adjuncts

Although local anesthetics are used extensively in infants and children, most have not been studied systematically, or even approved (by the Food and Drug Administration) for use in patients younger than 12 years of age. Generally, the same drugs that are used in adults also are used in children. Because of several anatomic and developmental differences, infants and children can be at increased risk for toxicity. Relatively larger volumes of local anesthetics are used for caudal and epidural blockade. Elimination can be delayed in neonates because of decreased protein binding. Because most blocks are performed with the children anesthetized or heavily sedated, test dosing is not usually practical or sensitive. Detection of accidental intravascular (or intraosseous) injection is extremely difficult. In experienced hands, however, local anesthetic toxicity is extremely rare in infants and children. Still, seizures, dysrhythmias, and cardiovascular collapse have been reported.

Bupivacaine

Bupivacaine is the most commonly used drug for regional anesthesia in infants and children. The drug, however, has a toxicity profile among the worst of the amide local anesthetics; in particular, the ratio of the cardiotoxic to the convulsant dose for bupivacaine is lower than for most other local anesthetics. Cardiac toxicity from bupivacaine, including myocardial depression and dysrhythmias, can be refractory to treatment. The toxic plasma concentration of bupivacaine is 4 μg/mL. The maximum recommended single bolus dose of bupivacaine is 2.5 to 3.0 mg/kg. The maximum recommended infusion rate for bupivacaine is 0.4 to 0.5 mg/kg per hour (10 to 12 mg/kg per day) in older infants and children, and 0.2 to 0.25 mg/kg per hour (5 to 6 mg/kg per day) in neonates [64]. Most of the reports of frank convulsions associated with bupivacaine infusions occurred during infusions in excess of recommended limits.

The presence of free versus bound bupivacaine in the plasma is of critical importance in examining the risk of bupivacaine toxicity, especially in infants. The principal binding protein for bupivacaine is α_1-acid glycoprotein. In adults, bupivacaine is approximately 95% bound to plasma proteins, and only 5% of the measured bupivacaine concentration is available to produce toxic reactions in the myocardium and central nervous system.

Levels of α_1-acid glycoprotein, and thus bupivacaine free fractions, in older infants and children are comparable to the values seen in adults. On the other hand, α_1-acid glycoprotein levels in neonates and infants younger than 6 months can be less than 50% of those seen in children and adults, and free bupivacaine concentrations can exceed 20%. Levels of α_1-acid glycoprotein can be particularly low in premature infants, but levels increase during early infancy and approach adult values by 6 months of age [65].

Are the new local anesthetics better?

Two new local anesthetics, ropivacaine and levobupivacaine, have become available recently. Both drugs are enantiomerically pure compounds rather than racemic mixtures of two stereoisomers. Both are purported to have anesthetic potency equivalent to bupivacaine while having lower toxicity and less unwanted motor blockade [66].

Ropivacaine has an anesthetic potency equivalent to bupivacaine and a toxic threshold higher than that of bupivacaine. Ropivacaine is reported to produce less motor block than equivalent concentrations of bupivacaine. Ropivacaine undergoes slower absorption from the caudal epidural space in children compared with bupivacaine, possibly because of its intrinsic vasoconstrictor properties. Ropivacaine has been shown in several animal models to have a higher threshold for toxicity than bupivacaine. The fatal dose of ropivacaine in sheep has been shown to be almost twice that of bupivacaine (7.3 versus 3.7 mg/kg). In human volunteers, larger doses of ropivacaine are tolerated compared with bupivacaine before the development of symptoms of toxicity [67].

In studies comparing ropivacaine with bupivacaine in adults, controversies remain about the supposed lower potency of ropivacaine. To obtain an equianalgesic effect, a higher concentration seems to be required, thus partially reducing the advantage of lower toxicity and leading to a similar therapeutic ratio. These data are different from the pediatric experience, where 0.2% ropivacaine has an equianalgesic effect with 0.25% bupivacaine, and the safe therapeutic window is wider [68].

Although specific dosage recommendations for ropivacaine use in children have not been published, given potency comparable to bupivacaine, it seems reasonable to follow the dosage guidelines for bupivacaine when administering ropivacaine to infants and children. Ropivacaine concentrations used for caudal and epidural anesthesia in children typically range from 0.2 to 0.25% in a volume of 1 mL/kg. Loading doses of 0.2% ropivacaine for epidural anesthesia in infants and children range from 0.5 to 0.85 mL/kg. Caudal or epidural anesthesia with comparable concentrations and volumes of ropivacaine or bupivacaine produces equivalent analgesia [69].

Levobupivacaine is the levorotatory enantiomer of racemic bupivacaine. Numerous studies in animals have confirmed the lower toxic potential of levobupivacaine compared with dexbupivacaine. The toxicity of levobupivacaine may be intermediate to those of racemic bupivacaine and ropivacaine. Studies of the effects of IV infusion of levobupivacaine and racemic bupivacaine in sheep found that convulsions occurred sooner, lasted longer, and required a lower dose after infusion of bupivacaine racemate compared with levobupivacaine [70].

As is the case for ropivacaine, no specific dosage limits have been published for levobupivacaine in infants and children; however, given potency comparable to that of racemic bupivacaine, it seems sensible to follow the dosage limits for bupivacaine when administering levobupivacaine to infants and children. In adults, the peak plasma concentration of levobupivacaine is approximately 20% to 25% greater than that of bupivacaine racemate after epidural or IV administration of identical doses. The degree of protein binding of levobupivacaine in infants and children is not known. Despite higher plasma concentrations of levobupivacaine, the plasma concentration of free (unbound) levobupivacaine is lower than that of bupivacaine racemate because of greater protein binding of the levorotatory enantiomer.

Use of adjunctive agents

One of the major challenges in pediatric regional anesthesia is to balance the efficacy of the block with the safety of the patient. Single-injection blocks have limited duration. Using concentrated local anesthetic solutions, which may be necessary to achieve adequate analgesia, can result in unwanted motor blockade. Using more dilute solutions may result in partially effective blocks. To circumvent these problems, various additives have been used to improve the quality of blocks without increasing the total dose of the local anesthetic drugs [71]. Although it is clear that the extended duration of analgesia that can be achieved is significant, it is not clear that this results in improved patient outcome, or outweighs persistent concerns about the potential for neurotoxicity of some of the additives [71,72].

Epinephrine

Epinephrine reduces the systemic uptake of the local anesthetic drugs, and through its alpha-2 adrenergic stimulating properties, enhances the duration and quality of peripheral and neuro-axial blocks. The effect is less pronounced with bupivacaine than it is with more hydrophilic drugs such as lidocaine. Unfortunately, most commercially premixed epinephrine-containing local anesthetic solutions have a lower pH than plain solutions. This may delay the uptake of the drug across neural membranes [73].

Sodium bicarbonate

Addition of 0.1 mL of a standard 8.4% solution of sodium bicarbonate to 20 mL solution of 0.25% bupivacaine will raise the pH of the local anesthetic from 5.49 to 7.04. Several studies have shown that the elevation of the pH of local anesthetics results in more rapid onset of action and enhanced quality and duration of block [74]. This approach is particularly useful when commercial epinephrine-containing bupivacaine is used, or to enhance the effect of a very dilute solution of bupivacaine.

Neuraxial opioids

Neuraxial administration of opioids results in excellent and long-lasting analgesia. Most opioids have been administered in the epidural space of children with the same lipophilic/hydrophilic considerations as in adults [75]. Delayed respiratory depression is always possible, whether the opioid is administered by means of the caudal, epidural, or spinal routes, especially in young infants. This is particularly true with concomitant administration of systemic opioids. Thus neuraxial administration of opioids requires specific routines and protocols for their safe use in children. Other adverse effects include vomiting, urinary retention, postoperative ileus, and pruritus.

Alpha-2-agonists

The addition of the alpha-2-agonist clonidine to local anesthetic solutions has been shown to enhance the duration and quality of central and peripheral nerve blocks [76]. The exact mechanism responsible for this analgesic action is not known. Possible explanations include the possibility that the entire effect of clonidine could be caused by systemic uptake. Alternatively, a spinal or peripheral mechanism of action has been proposed. Support for the spinal effect lies in the fact that alpha-2-adrenoreceptors that are believed to be associated with spinal modulation or inhibition of pain transmission have been identified in the dorsal horn of the spinal cord. Support for a peripheral effect of clonidine is in the observations that peripheral alph-2 receptors of subtype-C have been implicated in producing analgesia, and that administration of clonidine together with local anesthetics has been found to improve the quality of peripheral nerve blocks.

Clinically, the addition of clonidine (1 to 2 µg/kg) to a single-injection bolus of a local anesthetic consistently has been shown to substantially prolong the duration of caudal blockade. The addition of clonidine in doses of approximately 0.1 µg/kg per hour significantly enhances the analgesic quality of continuous epidural infusions. The main advantage of clonidine (versus opioids) is the negligible risk of respiratory depression. There is a higher incidence of mild-to-moderate sedation with clonidine. Although this may be undesirable in ambulatory patients, it may be advantageous following major surgery in hospitalized children.

S-ketamine

The analgesic effect of caudal ketamine is believed to result from the interaction with NMDA or opioid receptors at the spinal level. Studies have shown that low-dose epidural ketamine combined with morphine produces superior analgesia when compared with epidural ketamine administered alone [77]. As with clonidine, the main advantage of using epidural ketamine is the lack of respiratory depression. Using a bolus dose of up to 1 mg/kg of caudal or epidural preservative-free ketamine, the risk of psychological adverse effects appears to be low. There are insufficient data to recommend the use of continuous epidural infusions of S-ketamine in children. This is probably the result of the difficulties in obtaining preservative-free ketamine, and by ongoing concerns about potential neurotoxicity [71].

Neostigmine

Caudal neostigmine, 20 to 50 μg/kg, provides dose-dependent analgesia. Doses exceeding 30 μg/kg, however, are associated with a higher incidence of nausea and vomiting [78]. A single caudal injection of neostigmine 2 μg/kg combined with 0.2% ropivacaine offers an advantage over ropivacaine alone for postoperative pain relief in preschool children undergoing genitourinary surgery [79].

Tramadol

Tramadol is a unique analgesic with mu-1 agonist activity. Its analgesic effect is assumed to lack respiratory depression while providing prolonged analgesia after epidural administration in adults and children. A comparative study evaluated the effect of administering 1.5 mg/kg of tramadol alone, 0.25% bupivacaine alone, or a combination of the two drugs by means of the caudal route in a volume of 1 mL/kg in children undergoing hernia operation. The combination of tramadol 1.5 mg/kg with 0.25% bupivacaine provided the maximum duration of postoperative analgesia compared with children who received either the bupivacaine or the tramadol alone [80].

Summary

There is increased awareness of the need for effective postoperative analgesia in infants and young children. Pain assessment is a critical component of pain management. A multi-modal approach to preventing and treating pain usually is used to minimize adverse effects of individual drugs or techniques [81]. Mild nonopioid analgesics are safe and effective for minor surgery. Opioids should be added when indicated. Proper dosing and monitoring are essential to ensure safety. Regional analgesia must be considered unless contraindicated. Bupivacaine, a long-acting well-studied local anesthetic, is used most commonly in children. The extreme rarity of major toxicity from local anesthetics suggests that widespread replacement of bupivacaine with the newer drugs ropivacaine or levobupivacaine is probably not necessary for routine practice. These newer drugs, however, may be specifically indicated in situations where prolonged infusions are planned, in neonates, in patients with impaired hepatic function, and for anesthetic techniques requiring a large mass of a local anesthetic drug.

References

[1] O'Rouke D. The measurement of pain in infants, children, and adolescents: from policy to practice. Phys Ther 2004;84:560–70.

[2] Birmingham PK, Tobin MJ, Fisher DM, et al. Initial and subsequent dosing of rectal acetaminophen in children—a 24-hour pharmacokinetic study of new dose recommendations. Anesthesiology 2001;94:385–9.

[3] Montgomery CJ, McCormack JP, Reichert CC, et al. Plasma concentrations after high-dose (45 mg.kg-1) rectal acetaminophen in children. Can J Anaesth 1995;42:982–6.

[4] Anderson BJ, Holford NH, Woollard GA, et al. Perioperative pharmacodynamics of acetaminophen analgesia in children. Anesthesiology 1999;90:411–21.

[5] Romsing J, Hertel S, Harder A, et al. Examination of acetaminophen for outpatient management of postoperative pain in children. Paediatr Anaesth 1998;8:235–9.

[6] Bremerich DH, Neidhart G, Heimann K, et al. Prophylactically-administered rectal acetaminophen does not reduce postoperative opioid requirements in infants and small children undergoing elective cleft palate repair. Anesth Analg 2001;92:907–12.

[7] Hannallah RS. Outpatient anesthesia. In: Coté C, Todres D, editors. A practice of anesthesia for infants and children. 3rd edition. Philadelphia: WB Saunders Company; 2001. p. 55–67.

[8] Finkel JC, Rose JB, Schmitz ML, et al. An evaluation of the efficacy and tolerability of oral tramadol hydrochloride tablets for the treatment of postsurgical pain in children. Anesth Analg 2002;94:469–73.

[9] Engelhardt T, Steel E, Johnston G, et al. Tramadol for pain relief in children undergoing tonsillectomy: a comparison with morphine. Paediatr Anaesth 2003;13:249–52.

[10] Courtney MJ, Cabraal D. Tramadol vs diclofenac for post-tonsillectomy analgesia. Arch Otolaryngol Head Neck Surg 2001;127:385–8.

[11] Arcioni R, Rocca MD, Romano S, et al. Ondansetron inhibits the analgesic effects of tramadol: a possible 5-HT$_3$ spinal receptor involvement in acute pain in humans. Anesth Analg 2002; 94:1553–7.

[12] Dawson GS, Seidman P, Ramadan HH. Improved postoperative pain control in pediatric adenotonsillectomy with dextromethorphan. Laryngoscope 2001;111:1223–6.

[13] Rose JB, Guy R, Cohen DE, et al. Preoperative oral dextromethorphan does not reduce pain or analgesic consumption in children after adenotonsillectomy. Anesth Analg 1999;88:749–53.

[14] Hall SC. Tonsillectomies, ketorolac, and the march of progress. Can J Anaesth 1996;43:544–8.

[15] Park JM, Houck CS, Sethna NF, et al. Ketorolac suppresses postoperative bladder spasms after pediatric ureteral reimplantation. Anesth Analg 2000;91:11–5.

[16] Splinter WM, Rhine EJ, Roberts DW, et al. Ketorolac tromethamine increases bleeding after tonsillectomy in children. Can J Anaesth 1996;43:560–3.

[17] Marret E, Flahault A, Samama CM, et al. Effects of postoperative, nonsteroidal, anti-inflammatory drugs on bleeding risk after tonsillectomy. Anesthesiology 2003;98:1497–502.

[18] Moiniche S, Romsing J, Dahl JB, et al. Nonsteroidal anti-inflammatory drugs and the risk of operative site bleeding after tonsillectomy: a quantitative systemic review. Anesth Analg 2003;96:68–77.

[19] Pickering AE, Bridge HS, Nolan J, et al. Double-blind, placebo-controlled analgesic study of ibuprofen or rofecoxib in combination with paracetamol for tonsillectomy in children. Br J Anaesth 2002;88:72–7.

[20] Joshi W, Connelly NR, Reuben SS, et al. An evaluation of the safety and efficacy of administering rofecoxib for postoperative pain management. Anesth Analg 2003;97:35–8.

[21] Semple D, Russell S, Doyle E, et al. Comparison of morphine sulphate and codeine phosphate in children undergoing adenotonsillectomy. Paediatr Anaesth 1999;9:135–8.

[22] Galinkin JL, Fazi LM, Cuy RM, et al. Use of intranasal fentanyl in children undergoing myringotomy and tube placement during halothane and sevoflurane anesthesia. Anesthesiology 2000;93:1378–83.

[23] Finkel JF, Cohen IT, Hannallah RS, et al. The effect of intranasal fentanyl on the emergence characteristics after sevoflurane anesthesia in children undergoing surgery for bilateral myringotomy tube placement. Anesth Analg 2001;92:1164–8.

[24] Peters JWB, Hoekstra BIENG, Abu-Saad HH, et al. Patient-controlled analgesia in children and adolescents: a randomized controlled trial. Paediatr Anaesth 1999;9:235–41.

[25] Yildiz K, Tercan E, Dogru K, et al. Comparison of patient-controlled analgesia with and without a background infusion after appendectomy in children. Paediatr Anaesth 2003;13:427–31.

[26] Rusy LM, Olsen DJ, Farber NE. Successful use of patient-controlled analgesia in pediatric patients 2 and 3 years old: two case reports. Am J Anesthesiol 1997;24:212–4.

[27] McDonald AJ, Cooper MG. Patient-controlled analgesia —an appropriate method for pain control in children. Paediatr Drugs 2001;3:273–84.

[28] Sutter KA, Shaw BA, Gerardi JA, et al. Comparison of morphine patient-controlled analgesia with and without ketorolac for postoperative analgesia in pediatric orthopedic surgery. Am J Orthop 1999;28:351–8.

[29] Monitto CL, Greenberg RS, Kost-Byerly S, et al. The safety and efficacy of parent-/nurse-controlled analgesia in patients less than six years of age. Anesth Analg 2000;91:573–9.

[30] Kanagasundaram SA, Cooper MG, Lane LJ. Nurse-controlled analgesia using a patient-controlled analgesia device: an alternative strategy in the management of severe cancer pain in children. J Paediatr Child Health 1997;33:352–5.

[31] Rice LJ, Hannallah RS. Pediatric regional anesthesia. In: Motoyama EK, editor. Smith's anesthesia for infants and children. 5th edition. St. Louis (MO): Mosby; 1990. p. 393–425.

[32] Dalens B, Hasnouai A. Caudal anesthesia in pediatric surgery—success rate and adverse effects in 750 consecutive patients. Anesth Analg 1989;68:83–6.

[33] Hannallah RS, Broadman LM, Belman AB, et al. Comparison of caudal and ilioinguinal/iliohypogastric nerve blocks for control of post-orchiopexy pain in pediatric ambulatory surgery. Anesthesiology 1987;66:832–4.

[34] Busoni P, Andreuccetti T. The spread of caudal analgesia in children—a mathematical model. Anaesth Intensive Care 1986;14:140–4.

[35] Armitage EN. Local anaesthetic techniques for prevention of postoperative pain. Br J Anaesth 1986;58:790–800.

[36] Verghese S, Mostello L, Patel RI, et al. Testing the anal sphincter tone predicts the effectiveness of caudal analgesia in children. Anesth Analg 2002;94:1161–4.

[37] Mazoit JX, Denson DD, Samii K. Pharmacokinetics of bupivacaine following caudal anesthesia in infants. Anesthesiology 1988;68:387–91.

[38] Eyres RL, Hastings C, Brown TCK. Plasma bupivacaine concentrations in children during caudal epidural analgesia. Anaesth Intensive Care 1983;11:20–2.

[39] Bromage PR. Aging and epidural dose requirements. Br J Anaesth 1969;41:1016–22.

[40] Krane EJ, Jacobson LE, Lynn AM, et al. Caudal morphine for postoperative analgesia in children: a comparison with caudal bupivacaine and intravenous morphine. Anesth Analg 1987;66:647–53.

[41] Jamali S, Monin S, Begon C, et al. Clonidine in pediatric caudal anesthesia. Anesth Analg 1994;78:663–6.

[42] Wolf AR, Valley RD, Fear DW, et al. Bupivacaine for caudal analgesia in infants and children: the optimal effective concentration. Anesthesiology 1988;69:102–6.

[43] Verghese S, Hannallah R, Rice L, et al. Caudal anesthesia in children: effect of volume vs. concentration of bupivacaine in blocking spermatic cord traction response during orchidopexy. Anesth Analg 2002;95:1219–24.

[44] Tobias JD, Rasmussen GE, Holcomb III GW, et al. Continuous caudal anesthesia with chloroprocaine as an adjunct to general anaesthesia in neonates. Can J Anaesth 1996;43:69–72.

[45] Van Nierck J, Bax-Vermeire BM, Geurts JW, et al. Epidurography in premature infants. Anaesthesia 1990;45:722–5.

[46] Gunter GB, Eng C. Thoracic epidural anesthesia via the caudal approach in children. Anesthesiology 1992;76:935–8.

[47] Tsui BC, Tarkkila P, Gupta S, et al. Confirmation of caudal needle placement using nerve stimulation. Anesthesiology 1999;91:374–8.

[48] Tsui BCH, Seal R, Koller J. Thoracic epidural catheter placement via the caudal approach in infants by using electrocardiographic guidance. Anesth Analg 2002;95:326–30.

[49] Mc Neely JK, Trentadue NC, Rusy LM, et al. Culture of bacteria for lumbar and caudal epidural catheters used for postoperative analgesia in children. Reg Anesth 1997;22:428–31.

[50] Bubeck J, Boos K, Krause H, et al. Subcutaneous tunneling of caudal catheters reduces the rate of bacterial colonization to that of lumbar epidural catheters. Anesth Analg 2004; 99:689–93.

[51] Vas L, Naregal P, Sanzgiri S, et al. Some vagaries of neonatal lumbar epidural anaesthesia. Paediatr Anaesth 2000;10:114–5.

[52] Valairucha S, Seefelder C, Houck CS, et al. Thoracic epidural catheters placed by the caudal route in infants: the importance of radiographic confirmation. Paediatr Anaesth 2002;12:424–8.

[53] Bosenberg AT. Epidural analgesia for major neonatal surgery. Paediatr Anaesth 1998;8:114–5.

[54] McBride WJ, Dicker R, Abajian JC, et al. Continuous thoracic epidural infusions for postoperative analgesia after pectus deformity repair. J Pediatr Surg 1996;31(11):105–7.

[55] Fukunaga T, Kitamura S, Kinouchi K, et al. Anesthetic management for the correction of pectus excavatum using pectus bar under video assistance. Masui 2001;50:171–4.

[56] Peterson KL, De Campil WM, Pike NA, et al. A report of 220 cases of regional anesthesia in pediatric cardiac surgery. Anesth Analg 2000;90:1014–9.

[57] Tobias JD, Lowe S, O' Dell N, et al. Thoracic epidural anaesthesia in infants and children. Can J Anaesth 1993;40:810–2.

[58] Krane EJ, Dalens BJ, Murat I, et al. The safety of epidurals placed during general anesthesia. Reg Anesth Pain Med 1998;23:433–8.

[59] Kasai T, Yaegashi K, Hirose M, et al. Spinal cord injury in a child caused by an accidental dural puncture with a single-shot thoracic epidural needle. Anesth Analg 2003;96:65–7.

[60] Arms DM, Smith JT, Osteyee J, et al. Postoperative analgesia for pediatric spine surgery. Orthopedics 1998;21:539–44.

[61] Birmingham PK, Wheeler M, Suresh S, et al. Patient-controlled epidural analgesia in children: can they do it? Anesth Analg 2003;96:686–91.

[62] Antok E, Bordet F, Duflo F, et al. Patient-controlled epidural analgesia versus continuous epidural infusion with ropivacaine for postoperative analgesia in children. Anesth Analg 2003; 97:1608–11.

[63] Aram L, Krane EJ, Kozloski LJ, et al. Tunneled epidural catheters for prolonged analgesia in pediatric patients. Anesth Analg 2001;92:1432–8.

[64] Berde CB. Convulsions associated with pediatric regional anesthesia. Anesth Analg 1992; 75:164–6.

[65] Lerman J, Strong HA, Le Dez KM, et al. Effects of age on the serum concentration of alpha-1 acid glycoprotein and the binding of lidocaine in pediatric patients. Clin Pharmacol Ther 1989;46:219–25.

[66] De Negri P, Ivani G, Tirri T, et al. A comparison of epidural bupivacaine, levobupivacaine, and ropivacaine on postoperative analgesia and motor blockade. Anesth Analg 2004;99:45–8.

[67] Nancarro C, Rutten AJ, Runciman WB, et al. Myocardial and cerebral drug concentrations and the mechanisms of death after fatal intravenous doses of lidocaine, bupivacaine, and ropivacaine in the sheep. Anesth Analg 1989;69:276–83.

[68] Ivani G. Ropivacaine: is it time for children? Paediatr Anaesth 2002;12:383–7.

[69] Gunter JB. Benefits and risks of local anesthetics in infants and children. Paediatr Drugs 2002; 4:649–72.

[70] Huang YF, Pryor ME, Mather LE, et al. Cardiovascular and central nervous system effects of intravenous levobupivacaine and bupivacaine in sheep. Anesth Analg 1998;86:797–804.

[71] Ansermino MK, Basu R, Vandebeek C, et al. Nonopioid additives to local anaesthetics for caudal blockade in children: a systematic review. Paediatr Anaesth 2003;13:561–73.

[72] de Beer DAH, Thomas ML. Caudal additives in children—solutions or problems? Br J Anaesth 2003;90:487–98.

[73] Robinson J, Fernando R, Sun Wai WY, et al. Chemical stability of bupivacaine, lidocaine and epinephrine in pH-adjusted solutions. Anaesthesia 2000;55:853–8.

[74] Capogna G, Celleno D, Laudano D, et al. Alkalinization of local anesthetics. Which block which local anesthetic? Reg Anesth 1995;20:369–77.

[75] Rosen KR, Rosen DA. Caudal epidural morphine for control of pain following open-heart surgery in children. Anesthesiology 1989;70:418–21.

[76] Eisenach JJC, De Kock MM, Klimscha WM. Alpha sub 2-adrenergic agonists for regional anesthesia: a clinical review of clonidine (1964–1995). Anesthesiology 1996;85:655–74.

[77] Marhofer P, Krenn CG, Plochl W, et al. S(+) ketamine for caudal block in paediatric anaesthesia. Br J Anaesth 2000;84:341–5.

[78] Batra YK, Arya VK, Mahajan R, et al. Dose response study of caudal neostigmine for postoperative analgesia in paediatric patients undergoing genitourinary surgery. Paediatr Anaesth 2003;13:515–21.

[79] Turan A, Memis D, Basaran UN, et al. Caudal ropivacaine and neostigmine in pediatric surgery. Anesthesiology 2003;98:719–22.

[80] Senel AC, Akyol A, Dohman D, et al. Caudal bupivacaine–tramadol combination for post-operative analgesia in pediatric herniorrhaphy. Acta Anaesthesiol Scand 2001;45:786–9.

[81] Verghese ST. Caudal/epidural anesthesia in children. Parts 1 and 2. In: Eisenkraft JB, editor. Progress in anesthesiology. San Antonio (TX): Dannemiller Memorial Educational Foundation; 2004. p. 99–108, 1127–36.

ELSEVIER
SAUNDERS

Anesthesiology Clin N Am
23 (2005) 185–202

ANESTHESIOLOGY
CLINICS OF
NORTH AMERICA

Multimodal Analgesia Techniques and Postoperative Rehabilitation

Girish P. Joshi, MB, BS, MD, FFARCSI

Perioperative Medicine and Ambulatory Anesthesia, University of Texas,
Southwestern Medical Center, 5323 Harry Hines Blvd, Dallas, TX 75390-9068, USA

Advances in our understanding of the pathophysiology of postoperative pain have led to the development of effective perioperative analgesic regimens [1]. It is now well recognized that pain is a complex and multifactorial phenomenon and therefore requires a multimodal therapy [1]. The concept of multimodal or "balanced" analgesia suggests that combinations of several analgesics of different classes and different sites of analgesic administration rather than single analgesic or single technique provide superior pain relief with reduced analgesic-related side effects [1–3].

It has been assumed that multimodal analgesia regimens will improve pain relief, reduce opioid requirements, and opioid-related side effects and thus will improve surgical outcome. However, although numerous studies [3–8] have shown opioid sparing effects of multimodal analgesia techniques, this method has not resulted in reduced opioid-side effects. Furthermore, the improved pain relief from multimodal analgesia techniques has not translated into improved postoperative outcome [4–8]. The reasons for the lack of improved postoperative outcome are not yet clear. Reasons may in part be inappropriate combinations of analgesics or techniques. The combinations used may not be rational, because they may not block the different types of pain responses resulting from surgical insult (ie, inability to block nociceptive as well as inflammatory pain responses). Another reason may be the use of analgesic techniques that may improve pain relief at rest but may not control movement-evoked pain (dynamic pain relief). Most importantly, even though dynamic pain relief is achieved, it is not always integrated with a multimodal postoperative rehabilitation program [5–8].

E-mail address: girish.joshi@utsouthwestern.edu

This article reviews the analgesic options for postoperative pain management and their benefits and limitations, but it is not intended to provide detailed discussion on individual analgesic techniques because they are covered elsewhere in this issue. In addition, the optimal analgesic combinations are suggested, and the role of multimodal rehabilitation techniques in improving surgical outcome is discussed.

Analgesia options for multimodal techniques

In addition to opioids, the analgesic modalities available for postoperative pain management include regional or local analgesia techniques such as epidural analgesia and peripheral nerve blocks as well as wound infiltration and intra-articular or intracavity administration of local anesthetics. In addition, cyclo-oxygenase (COX) enzyme blockers such as acetaminophen, nonsteroidal anti-inflammatory drugs (NSAIDs) or COX-2– specific inhibitors are becoming popular. Recently, there has been an increased interest in using analgesic adjuncts such as N-methyl-D-aspartate (NMDA) receptor antagonists (eg, ketamine and dextromethorphan), α_2 agonists (eg, clonidine and dexmedetomidine), anti-convulsants (eg, gabapentin and pregabalin), and corticosteroids.

Opioids

Opioids are efficacious analgesics that are particularly suited for moderate to severe postoperative pain. However, they are limited by their significant side effects. Opioid use has been associated with dose-related adverse effects including nausea, vomiting, sedation, dizziness, drowsiness, bladder dysfunction, and constipation, all of which may contribute to a delayed recovery [9]. Opioids also reduce gastrointestinal motility and contribute to postoperative ileus. In addition, opioids affect sleep patterns, which may increase postoperative fatigue [10]. Furthermore, recent data [11,12] suggest that clinically relevant tolerance to opioids can occur within hours of their use, which may reduce their analgesic efficacy.

Although opioids, particularly when administered through an intravenous patient-controlled analgesia (IV-PCA) system, improve patient satisfaction, they do not improve postoperative morbidity or reduce hospital stay [13,14]. The lack of improved outcome with opioids, irrespective of the route of administration, may be related to their inability to reduce surgical stress responses. Furthermore, although opioids reduce spontaneous pain (rest pain), their ability to control dynamic pain is limited [14]. Recent evidence suggests that dynamic pain may contribute to postoperative physiologic impairment, and dynamic pain has also been identified as a major risk factor in the development of chronic persistent postoperative pain.

Therefore, it is now well recognized that opioids should be used sparingly. The concept of opioid-free or opioid-reduced analgesia is receiving increasing attention [15]. Thus, it is recommended that nonopioid analgesics and techniques be used as the first line of therapy and that opioids should be reserved for more severe pain that is not adequately controlled with nonopioids.

Epidural analgesia

Epidural analgesia provides superior dynamic pain relief and reduces the endocrine-metabolic stress response to surgery, which may prevent postoperative organ dysfunction and reduce morbidity. As a consequence, epidural analgesia may reduce postoperative complications and enhance rehabilitation [16–20]. However, numerous meta-analyses and systematic reviews [21] have reported conflicting results. These controversial findings may be the result of an inadequate number of appropriately designed randomized, controlled trials and the inclusion of studies with numerous variables that influence the efficacy of epidural analgesia (eg, the choice of analgesic, catheter surgical incision congruence, and duration of analgesia) in the same analysis. Importantly, the value of epidural analgesia in improving postoperative outcome and reducing hospital stay remains controversial [5–8].

The lack of consistently improved outcome with epidural analgesia may in part be caused by incongruence between the epidural catheter site and surgical injury and the use of a predominantly opioid-based rather than local anesthetic-based epidural solution. An optimum epidural analgesia technique includes catheter placement in a location congruent to the surgical incision dermatome (eg, thoracic epidural for thoracic and upper abdominal surgery or lumbar epidural for lower limb surgery) and an infusion consisting of a local anesthetic with or without low-dose opioid that is administered for at least 24 to 48 hours. The use of adjuncts (eg, epinephrine, clonidine, and ketamine) along with the local anesthetic solution remains controversial, and its routine use is not recommended at this time.

It is now recognized that the inflammatory responses to injury (eg, increase in cytokines) are not modified by neural blockade. Current evidence [22] suggests that the combination of COX-2 inhibitors (ie, NSAIDs and COX-2– specific inhibitors) with epidural analgesia (both initiated preoperatively and continued during the postoperative and rehabilitative phase) reduces postoperative pain and opioid consumption and reduces the recovery time.

Continuous peripheral nerve blocks and paravertebral blocks

Peripheral nerve blocks provide superior dynamic pain relief and should also reduce surgical stress and enhance rehabilitation. Because these techniques provide site-specific analgesia, they are associated with fewer side effects compared with other analgesic techniques [23]. However, the duration of analgesia after a single-shot technique is limited. In fact, the abrupt termination of the analgesic effect may lead to an increased perception of pain after the recovery from the neural blockade [24]. In addition, single-shot techniques may not have any long-term benefits compared with general anesthesia [25]. Continuous peripheral nerve blocks should prolong the benefits of single-shot peripheral nerve blocks and thus should form the basis of postoperative pain management whenever possible. Similarly, continuous paravertebral blocks provide segmental analgesia, which may be similar to thoracic epidural analgesia but with lower incidence of side effects such as hypotension and urinary retention. Continuous peripheral nerve blocks and paravertebral blocks have a major role in pain management because they enhance ambulation, reduce opioid-related side effects, facilitate early hospital discharge, and expedite the return to daily living. However, these techniques have been underused. The use of continuous peripheral nerve blocks and paravertebral blocks is reviewed elsewhere in this issue.

Concerns regarding continuous peripheral nerve blockade include patient injury related to the insensate extremity, particularly after discharge. Catheter migration, potential local anesthetic toxicity, masking of surgical-related nerve injury, and compartment syndrome are other concerns. There is clearly a need for a refinement of peripheral nerve block techniques and the development of more effective methods for continuous administration. The availability of longer-acting, slow-release preparations that incorporate local anesthetics into liposomes (or microspheres), which extend the duration of action, should enhance the efficacy of local anesthetic techniques. However, these agents are not yet available for clinical use. Most importantly, there is a need for larger, well-designed studies showing improved postoperative outcomes with continuous peripheral nerve blocks and continuous paravertebral blocks.

Acetaminophen

Acetaminophen is a widely used over-the-counter analgesic and antipyretic drug; however, it is underused in the perioperative period. Although the mechanism of action of acetaminophen is poorly understood, it is believed to act by the inhibition of the COX-3 isoenzyme and subsequent reduced prostanoid release in the central nervous system [26–28]. In addition, there is some suggestion that it acts on the opioidergic system and NMDA receptors.

Acetaminophen is devoid of some of the side effects of nonselective NSAIDs, such as impaired platelet aggregation, gastrointestinal ulceration and hemorrhage, and cardiorenal adverse effects [29,30]. Furthermore, unlike nonselective NSAIDs and COX-2–specific inhibitors, acetaminophen does not have clinically significant effects on bone and ligament healing [29,30]. Although it is generally considered safe, acetaminophen is associated with liver and gastrointestinal toxicity at high doses [31–33]. It is a weak analgesic, and therefore it is only suitable for the treatment of mild pain [29,30]. Furthermore, it has a weak anti-inflammatory activity and may not be suitable for blocking inflammatory pain response [26].

The availability of injectable forms of acetaminophen (prodrug, propacetamol, and paracetamol) has expanded our knowledge of the pharmacodynamics of acetaminophen, such as the relationship between peak concentrations and clinical efficacy [34]. Recently, a ready-to-use intravenous formulation of paracetamol has been made available in Europe. Intravenous paracetamol, 1 g, has similar analgesic efficacy as propacetamol, 2 g, the prodrug of acetaminophen. The initial dose of injectable acetaminophen may be administered intraoperatively and may be followed by an oral administration after the patient is discharged. Compared with oral formulations, parenteral acetaminophen has a predictable onset and duration of action [34]. In addition, oral acetaminophen may be less efficacious because intraoperative opioids as well as inhaled anesthetics delay gastric emptying and reduce gastrointestinal absorption of orally administered drugs [35,36].

Acetaminophen has a favorable efficacy-side effect profile and is therefore recommended as the first-line analgesic. Although acetaminophen is a weak analgesic and may not be adequate as the sole analgesic, it may be combined with other analgesics to provide superior analgesia and reduce opioid requirements [37,38]. However, acetaminophen displays an analgesic ceiling effect similar to NSAIDs and COX-2–specific inhibitors [39]. Importantly, patients should be warned that commonly used opioid combinations consist of acetaminophen.

Nonsteroidal anti-inflammatory drugs and cyclooxygenase-2–specific inhibitors

The nonselective (traditional) NSAIDs are one of the most widely used analgesics [40,41]. With the introduction of parenteral preparations of NSAIDs (eg, ketorolac, diclofenac, and ketoprofen), these drugs have become more popular in the management of postoperative pain. The mechanism of the NSAID analgesic effect is the inhibition of the COX-2 enzyme. It has been increasingly apparent that, in an inflammatory model, the COX-2 enzyme plays an important role in peripheral and central sensitization [1]. Emerging evidence [1] from animal studies indicates that the early and sustained inhibition of the COX-2 enzyme may prevent the damaging modifications to neuronal function that would otherwise result in postoperative morbidity.

Therefore, the nonspecific NSAIDs should reduce sensitization of nociceptors, attenuate inflammatory pain response, prevent central sensitization, and thus improve postoperative pain relief. The other potential advantages of NSAIDs include reduced opioid requirements and possibly opioid-related side effects. Macario and Lipman [42] compiled randomized, controlled trials of ketorolac versus placebo with opioids given for breakthrough pain that were published in English-language journals from 1986 to 2001. They found that 70% of patients in control groups experienced moderate-to-severe pain at 1 hour postoperatively, whereas 36% of the control patients had moderate-to-severe pain 24 hours postoperatively. Although ketorolac was efficacious, analgesia was improved in patients receiving a combination of ketorolac and opioids. Depending on the type of surgery, ketorolac reduced opioid dose requirements by a mean of 36%

(range 0%–73%), but this did not result in a concomitant reduction in opioid side effects (eg, nausea and vomiting). This may have resulted from the studies having sample sizes that were inadequate for detecting differences in the incidence of opioid-related side effects. The risk for adverse events increased with high doses, with prolonged therapy (>5 days), and in the elderly. The authors concluded that although ketorolac appears to be safe, it should be used at the lowest dose necessary.

Despite numerous benefits [40–42], nonselective NSAIDs are not routinely used because of concerns regarding their potential side effects such as impaired coagulation (and increased perioperative bleeding), gastric irritation (particularly when these drugs are administered in fasting patients), and renal dysfunction [43]. NSAIDs should not be used in patients with pre-existing coagulation defects or those undergoing certain surgical procedures (eg, tonsillectomy and plastic surgery). Similarly, this group of drugs should be avoided in patients with pre-existing renal dysfunction, hypovolemia, cardiac failure, sepsis, or end-stage liver disease [44]. Finally, NSAIDs should be used with caution in the elderly and in clinical situations in which prostaglandins have proven therapeutic benefits, such as circulatory insufficiency, myocardial ischemia, and coronary vasospasm [45].

A large prospective, randomized multicenter European trial [46] evaluated the risks of death, increased surgical site bleeding, gastrointestinal bleeding, acute renal failure, and allergic reactions with the short-term use (≤5 days) of appropriate doses of ketorolac compared with diclofenac or ketoprofen. Of the 11,245 patients included in the study, 5634 patients received ketorolac, and 5611 patients received one of the comparators. In the 30-day postoperative follow-up, 155 (1.38%) patients experienced a serious adverse outcome, with 19 (0.17%) deaths, 117 (1.04%) with surgical site bleeding, 12 (0.12%) with allergic reactions, 10 (0.09%) with acute renal failure, and four (0.04%) patients with gastrointestinal bleeding [46]. There were no differences between ketorolac and ketoprofen or diclofenac. Postoperative anticoagulants increased equally the risk of surgical site bleeding with both ketorolac and the comparators. Other risk factors for serious adverse outcomes were age, American Society of Anesthesiologists physical status, and the type of surgical procedure (eg, plastic, ear, nose and throat, gynecological, and urological surgery). The authors concluded that the side effect profile of ketorolac is similar to other injectable nonselective NSAIDs, provided the contraindications to its use are observed [46].

Thus, although the overall adverse events with nonselective NSAIDs are not increased in the perioperative period, the contraindications to their use are numerous [43–47]. Therefore, the limitations of nonselective NSAIDs prevent their use even when they would otherwise be desirable. The development of COX-2–specific inhibitors, a new group of anti-inflammatory and analgesic drugs, which selectively target COX-2 while sparing COX-1, were developed to obtain the therapeutic benefits of NSAIDs while overcoming their limitations (see elsewhere in this issue). Although COX-2–specific inhibitors seem to have analgesic efficacy that is similar to nonselective NSAIDs, they may have an advantage over nonselective NSAIDs because they do not affect platelet function and reduce the risk of gastrointestinal ulceration [48–51]. Because of the lack of antiplatelet effects and improved gastrointestinal tolerability, COX-2–specific inhibitors may be safely administered preoperatively.

Until recently, three COX-2–specific inhibitors, celecoxib, rofecoxib, and valdecoxib, were available in the United States. However, rofecoxib was recently removed from the market because of concerns over its association with an increased risk of cardiovascular events. Parecoxib is the first injectable COX-2–specific inhibitor approved in Europe for the short-term treatment of moderate to severe postoperative pain. It is currently undergoing Phase III clinical trials for approval by the US Food and Drug Administration [52,53]. The perioperative dosage of celecoxib is initially 400 mg, followed by 200 mg twice per day, whereas the dosage for valdecoxib is initially 40 mg, followed by 20 mg twice per day. Of note, the COX-2–specific inhibitors also exhibit a "ceiling effect" with respect to their maximum analgesic effect, similar to nonspecific NSAIDs. Furthermore, the currently available COX-2–specific inhibitors (ie, celecoxib and valdecoxib) are contraindicated in patients with a history of sulphonamide allergy, and the cardiorenal precautions with these drugs are similar to those of nonselective NSAIDs.

Nitric oxide-releasing derivatives of acetaminophen and nonsteroidal anti-inflammatory drugs

The nitric oxide (NO) moiety significantly improves the analgesic effects of acetaminophen and NSAIDs, possibly because of the involvement of NO in the nociceptive process [54,55]. NO modulates spinal and sensory neuron excitability through multiple mechanisms. In particular, the moiety stimulates the formation of cGMP by guanylyl cyclase in neurons and, depending on the expression of cGMP-gated ion channels, may result in an increased or reduced neuronal excitability [54,55]. Moreover, NO is involved in inflammatory processes associated with neuropathic pain subsequent to peripheral nerve injury. In addition, animal studies [56–58] indicate that the gastrointestinal mucosal damage, prostaglandin release, and changes in mucosal blood flow associated with some analgesics are significantly reduced because of NO-dependent mechanisms. This has lead to the development of combinations of a nitrate with a conventional analgesic, the NO-releasing analgesics [56–58]. The NO-donating analgesics should have enhanced efficacy and an improved side effect profile compared with their parent drug. There is increasing evidence suggesting that NO-donating NSAIDs (eg, NO-aspirin, NO-naproxen, NO-flurbiprofen, NO-diclofenac, NO-ibuprofen, and NO-acetaminophen) have anti-inflammatory and antinociceptive effects similar to that of their parent compound but without the adverse effects such as gastrointestinal toxicity and hepato-tocixity, because of the protective effects of NO on the gastric mucosa and hepatocytes. For example, NCX-701 is an NO-releasing derivative of acetamino-phen, synthesized for the potential treatment of inflammation and pain [59].

N-methyl-D-aspartate receptor antagonists

Recently, excitatory neurotransmitters acting through NMDA receptors have been incriminated in the development and maintenance of hyperalgesia and allodynia and persistent postoperative pain. [1]. Although the analgesic properties of ketamine have been well known for a long time, the precise mechanisms are still unclear. In addition to its effects on the NMDA receptor [60], ketamine may also act on several receptor systems such as opioidergic and cholinergic as well as monoaminergic systems and may have local anesthetic effects through the sodium channel blockade. Therefore, ketamine may play a role in perioperative pain management [61–63]. However, the optimal dose and route of administration of ketamine remain controversial.

Low-dose ketamine (0.25–0.5 mg/kg, IV, or 25–50 μg/kg/min infusion) reduces opioid consumption, prolongs analgesia, and improves pain relief prevents tolerance to opioids. De Kock et al [64] found that intravenous but not epidurally administered ketamine reduced mechanical hyperalgesia surrounding the surgical wound, reduced early morphine consumption, and diminished the incidence of residual pain as expressed by analgesic requirements until the sixth postoperative month. These findings correlate with those of Zahn and Brennan [65] who reported the lack of neuraxial effects of ketamine in a rat postoperative model. Similarly, the administration of ketamine with IV-PCA morphine does not appear to provide any benefit over IV-PCA morphine alone. However, because of the lack of consistent benefits and possibility of side effects (eg, hemodynamic and psychotomimetic effects), ketamine may be reserved for situations in which routine analgesics are ineffective or limited by their side effects.

α₂ Receptor agonists

$α_2$ Receptor agonists (eg, clonidine and dexmedetomidine) provide sedative and analgesia sparing effects through central actions in the locus ceruleus and in the dorsal horn of the spinal cord, respectively [66]. When administered orally, intravenously, or transdermally, clonidine may reduce opioid requirements and improve analgesia. Similarly, the addition of clonidine to the local anesthetic solution for neuraxial or peripheral nerve blocks may enhance and prolong analgesia. However, the analgesic benefits of clonidine remain controversial. In addition, clonidine is limited by its side effects, including bradycardia, hypotension, and excessive sedation.

Compared with clonidine, dexmedetomidine is more selective and has a shorter duration of action. When used in the perioperative period, it has anesthetic and opioid sparing effects. Dexmedetomidine does not cause respiratory depression, despite its potent sedative effects. Because of its opioid sparing effects [67], it is increasingly used in patients at high risk of airway obstruction and respiratory depression associated with opioids (eg, patients with sleep apnea and morbid obesity). Initial studies recommended a loading dose of dexmedetomidine, 1 μg/kg, followed by an infusion of 0.4 μg/kg/h. However, this regimen may increase cardiovascular side effects (bradycardia and hypotension). Therefore, the avoidance of a loading dose may be preferred. Of note, most studies have evaluated the use of dexmedetomidine in the intraoperative or immediate postoperative period, therefore its long-term benefits are not yet clear.

Gabapentin and pregabalin

Gabapentin and pregabalin are structural analogs of γ-aminobutyric acid and can be used for the treatment of persistent neuropathic pain [68]. Although the mechanisms of action of gabapentin and pregabalin are not clear, it is believed they act through the modulation of the $\alpha_2\delta$-1 subunit of the voltage-dependent calcium channels in the dorsal horn of the spinal cord [69]. Recent studies have evaluated the efficacy of gabapentin in the management of postoperative pain. Fassoulaki et al [70] compared the analgesic effects of gabapentin, 1200 mg, and mexiletine, 600 mg, after breast surgery for cancer. They found that both gabapentin and mexiletine equally reduced analgesic requirements at rest; however, gabapentin was more effective in reducing pain after movement. Similarly, Dirks et al [71] reported that gabapentin, 1200 mg, before surgery reduced postoperative morphine requirements and movement-related pain after radical mastectomy. Pregabalin, 300 mg orally, has been shown to reduce pain after third molar extraction [72]. However, gabapentin and pregabalin cause dizziness and somnolence. Studies with larger sample sizes and optimal dosing regimens are required before gabapentin or pregabalin can be recommended in the perioperative period.

Glucocorticoids

Glucocorticoids have anti-inflammatory properties, block the COX and lipooxygenase enzymes, and have the potential to reduce pain and to improve postoperative outcome by reducing the inflammatory response to surgical stress. Recently, preoperative dexamethasone (4–8 mg, IV) has been shown to have analgesic effects and to reduce postoperative nausea and vomiting. Although no side effects have been observed with a single dose of dexamethasone in large studies [73], there is a potential for increased gastrointestinal side effects as well as delayed wound healing.

Optimal multimodal analgesia techniques

An ideal analgesic combination would reduce the intensity of movement-evoked pain and the surgical stress response, improve postoperative outcome, and reduce the need for hospitalization. Another potential benefit of multimodal analgesia techniques is the reduction of analgesic-related adverse effects. It is crucial to reduce not only major adverse effects (eg, respiratory depression with opioids) but also minor, so-called annoying, side effects because patients usually choose pain relief for less upsetting or less severe side effects [74]. Most importantly, an optimal analgesic technique would be individualized to each patient's needs and specific to a surgical procedure.

Kehlet and Dahl [2] reported improvement in postoperative analgesia using multimodal analgesia techniques. Almost a decade after their initial report, Kehlet et al [3] reassessed the benefits of multimodal analgesia and found that combining different analgesics improved postoperative analgesia. However, they did not find any reduction in analgesic adverse effects. Jin and Chung [4] analyzed randomized, controlled trials published up until 2000, evaluating the effects of multimodal analgesia on postoperative pain relief and recovery profile after outpatient and inpatient surgery. They too found that multimodal analgesia techniques improved postoperative pain relief in both outpatients and inpatients. However, an improvement in recovery profile (eg, reduced discharge time, early mobilization, and early convalescence) was not consistently observed. They noted that, unfortunately, not all studies evaluated postoperative recovery profile.

Although initially it was assumed that multimodal analgesia would reduce the incidence of adverse effects, most studies have not been able to validate these assumptions [2–4]. For example, the use of NSAIDs has been shown to reduce opioid requirements by 20% to 40%. However, these studies have not shown a consistent reduction in opioid-related side effects [2–4]. Similarly, commonly used combinations of acetaminophen and NSAIDs have not been shown to reduce opioid side effects [38]. Unfortunately, most studies evaluating multimodal analgesia techniques are inadequately powered to detect a reduction in side effects, or they have not adequately evaluated analgesic side effects. For example, most commonly, only the incidence of side effects is evaluated but not their severity or resultant patient distress (ie, bothersomeness). However, more recent studies have used a symptom distress scale, which examines opioid side effects in much greater detail and provides information on clinically meaningful events [52,53]. It appears that an optimal analgesic technique should be potent enough to reduce opioid requirements by at least 30% to reduce opioid side effects [75].

How does one determine optimal analgesic combinations? With numerous analgesic options, it can be difficult for clinicians to decide on the optimal number and type of analgesic combination for a specific surgical procedure. The choice of analgesic combination is generally based on the type, efficacy, and side effect profile of the analgesic modality for a specific surgical procedure.

Neural blockade should be used whenever possible. The choice of the local anesthetic technique would depend on the type of surgical procedure. For example, for minor outpatient surgical procedures, local anesthetic infiltration of the surgical wound, intracavity, or field blocks may be adequate. For more extensive ambulatory surgical procedures, peripheral nerve block or paravertebral blocks may be preferred. Continuous peripheral nerve or paravertebral blocks provide prolonged analgesia after discharge and may be used, particularly after extensive painful outpatient surgical procedures requiring rigorous rehabilitation.

For major surgical procedures in hospitalized patients (eg, thoracic surgery, upper abdominal surgery, major vascular surgery, and hip and knee surgery), continuous epidural analgesia with local anesthetic-opioid combinations may be beneficial. Continuous peripheral nerve or paravertebral blocks provide site-specific analgesia and may be excellent alternatives to central neuraxial techniques. In fact, these techniques may be superior to central neuraxial techniques because of their superior adverse effect profile.

In addition to regional analgesic techniques, all patients may receive oral or parenteral NSAIDs or COX-2–specific inhibitors, with or without acetaminophen if there are no contraindications. Furthermore, there may be a benefit in combining epidural or peripheral analgesia with COX-2–specific inhibitors in improving analgesia and reducing local anesthetic requirements and associated side effects (eg, reduced sympathetic blockade and motor blockade). For inpatients in whom neuraxial or peripheral analgesia cannot be performed, IV-PCA with opioid combined with NSAIDs or COX-2–specific inhibitors should be considered. For outpatient surgical procedures, nonopioid analgesics may be supplemented with oral opioids (eg, hydrocodone, oxycodone, and tramadol).

Furthermore, the number and type of analgesic combinations could also be determined based on the possibility of the patient in developing significant or persistent postoperative pain [76–79]. For example, patients at high risk of development of persistent postoperative pain may benefit from administration of corticosteroids, ketamine, α_2 agonists, and gabapentin along with the regional analgesia, NSAIDs, and opioids. This hypothesis needs to be confirmed in well-designed studies in patients undergoing surgical procedures that pose a high risk of persistent postoperative pain (eg, mastectomy and thoracotomy). Because of significant variations in the degree of postoperative pain among patients undergoing similar surgical procedures, it would be helpful to identify the patients who are most likely to have severe postoperative pain. This should allow for more aggressive analgesic therapy in this high-risk patient population.

Multimodal analgesia as a part of preemptive analgesia techniques

The concept of preemptive analgesia (ie, analgesic intervention made before noxious stimuli) to prevent the establishment of peripheral and central sensitization and thus amplification and prolongation of pain has been overwhelmingly demonstrated in animal studies using inflammatory models [1,80]. Thus, an optimal preemptive analgesic technique would start before the surgical injury and continue until the response to pain is resolved. However, clinical studies evaluating preemptive (or preventative) analgesia provide conflicting results [81–84]. Recently published articles [82,84] that have critically reviewed clinical studies related to the preemptive effect of analgesic therapies report modest or equivocal benefits from preemptive analgesia. One of the reasons for the failure of clinical studies to show benefits may be because of an inappropriate definition of this concept [81,84]. Furthermore, most clinical trials were of short duration and evaluated unimodal analgesia techniques (eg, local anesthesia alone or NSAIDs alone) rather than multimodal analgesia techniques. Also, preemptive analgesic techniques have not targeted the different analgesic pathways simultaneously. Interestingly, animal studies using the incisional model have not been able to show a benefit of preemptive analgesia. Nevertheless, the timing of analgesic administration is crucial and should depend on the pharmacokinetics of the analgesic. Therefore, it would be beneficial to administer analgesics preoperatively or intraoperatively so that their peak analgesic effect occurs just before emergence from anesthesia.

Multimodal approach to shorten convalescence

In addition to providing dynamic pain relief and reduced surgical stress responses, a prerequisite to improve surgical outcome and shorten postoperative convalescence and debility is the implementation of a multimodal and multi-disciplinary rehabilitation therapy [5–8]. This involves changes in current anesthesia practice emphasizing preoperative optimization, patient selection and education, improved perioperative monitoring, early resuscitation, more responsive fluid therapy (ie, avoidance of hypovolemia and hypervolemia), maintenance of normothermia, and prevention of postoperative nausea and vomiting [8]. In addition, the surgical stress response (and associated organ dysfunction) may be reduced by modern surgical techniques such as microscopic and minimally invasive surgery, which reduce tissue handling, trauma, and blood loss [8]. Furthermore, modifications of traditional postoperative care regimens (ie, avoidance of tubes, catheters, drains, and restrictions), prevention of postoperative hypoxemia, improved sleep, early oral feeding (avoidance of semi-starvation and fatigue), and early mobilization are necessary parts of a fast-track rehabilitation program [8].

Available data indicate that patients who are a part of a clinical pathway using multimodal rehabilitation therapy may have a reduced length of stay, a lower incidence of complications, and improved pain control [85–89]. Kehlet and Wilmore [6] reviewed the effects of modifying perioperative care in noncardiac surgical patients on morbidity and mortality. They found that the introduction of these newer approaches to perioperative care (ie, fast-track surgery or accelerated care programs) reduced postoperative morbidity and mortality and concluded that the application of this new concept should reduce the need for postoperative hospitalization and allow more surgical procedures to be performed on an outpatient basis. Thus, the success of a fast-track surgery program requires a multidisciplinary approach involving anesthesiologists, surgeons, nurses, and physical therapists.

Future considerations

Although the concept of multimodal analgesia has been well accepted and included in our current pain management plan, it has not resulted in improved postoperative outcome (eg, improved function and return to daily living and reduced incidence of persistent postoperative pain). Many studies have insufficient study design because of an inappropriate combination of analgesic techniques or inadequate duration of analgesia. Therefore, more studies are necessary to identify optimal analgesic combinations and optimal administration techniques with greater efficacy, improved safety, and the ability to improve postoperative outcome.

Future therapies may be directed more specifically to the pathophysiologic pain process [1]. In addition to currently used analgesics, future multimodal analgesic techniques may also include the use of α_2-adrenergic agonists, NMDA receptor antagonists, anticonvulsants, and glucocorticoids. Furthermore, bradykinin, substance P antagonists, and leukotriene synthesis blockers may also be used as part of a balanced analgesia regimen. The role of these analgesic techniques needs to be clarified by further investigation and clinical experience, which also focuses on patient outcome.

Future outcome studies are required to evaluate whether the introduction of multimodal analgesia techniques, which optimize dynamic pain relief, integrated with an accelerated multimodal rehabilitation (recovery) program would improve postoperative outcome, reduce hospital stay, and shorten convalescence [8]. Future postoperative multimodal strategies will need to be patient-specific and procedure-specific [89–91], both of which are integrated with clinical pathways and acute pain services [92,93]. Such individualized analgesic regimens should reduce postoperative pain intensity, morbidity, and the need for hospitalization as well as allow an early return to daily living.

Summary

Although the management of postoperative pain poses some unique challenges for the practitioner, an important reason for suboptimal pain management is the inadequate or improper application of available information and analgesic therapies. Multimodal analgesia techniques, including regional analgesic techniques, acetaminophen, nonspecific NSAIDs or COX-2–specific inhibitors, and opioids, have become standard practice. The choice of analgesic combinations should depend not only on their analgesic efficacy but also on the side effect profile of these combinations. Thus, even if a certain analgesic regimen provides superior pain relief, it may not be clinically beneficial if it is also associated with more adverse events.

Although it is clear that multimodal analgesia techniques improve postoperative pain relief, there are insufficient data on the optimal multimodal regimen for a particular patient undergoing a particular surgical procedure.

Nevertheless, regional analgesia techniques have evolved as a critical component of a multimodal approach to achieving the goal of dynamic pain relief with improved outcomes. Other nonopioid analgesics (eg, acetaminophen and non-specific NSAIDs or COX-2–specific inhibitors) should be used, assuming there are no contraindications, at their ceiling doses, administered on a round-the-clock schedule of dosing. Opioids should be used as "rescue" analgesics on an as-needed basis because opioid-related side effects can retard patients' postoperative recovery. In addition, nonpharmacologic interventions should become a standard component of multimodal analgesia techniques. However, there is a need for the development of an evidence-based approach to reliable, comprehensive, individualized analgesic plans for specific surgical procedures.

Finally, because surgical morbidity is multifactorial, a multimodal approach to perioperative care is required to achieve a significant improvement in post-operative outcome and reduce convalescence. Therefore, it is important that a multidisciplinary approach be used to manage postoperative care as a con-tinuum from the preoperative period through the convalescence period.

References

[1] Woolf CJ. Pain: moving from symptom control towards mechanism-specific pharmacologic management. Ann Intern Med 2004;140:441–51.

[2] Kehlet H, Dahl JB. The value of "multimodal" or "balanced analgesia" in postoperative pain treatment. Anesth Analg 1993;77:1048–56.

[3] Kehlet H, Werner M, Perkins F. Balanced analgesia: what is it and what are its advantages in postoperative period? Drugs 1999;58:793–7.

[4] Jin F, Chung F. Multimodal analgesia for postoperative pain control. J Clin Anesth 2001; 13:524–39.

[5] Kehlet H, Holte K. Effect of postoperative analgesia on surgical outcome. Br J Anaesth 2001;87:62–72.

[6] Kehlet H, Wilmore DW. Multimodal strategies to improve surgical outcome. Am J Surg 2002;183:630–41.

[7] Kehlet H, Dahl JB. Anaesthesia, surgery, and challenges for postoperative recovery. Lancet 2003;362:1921–8.

[8] Kehlet H. Effect of postoperative pain treatment on outcome–current status and future strategies. Langenbecks Arch Surg 2004;389:244–9.

[9] Wheeler M, Oderda GM, Ashburn MA, et al. Adverse events associated with postoperative opioid analgesia: a systemic review. J Pain 2002;3:159–80.

[10] Kay DC, Eisenstein RB, Jansinki DR. Morphine effects on human REM state, waking state and NREM sleep. Psychopharmacologia 1969;14:404–16.

[11] Chia YY, Liu K, Wang JJ, et al. Intraoperative high dose fentanyl induces postoperative fentanyl tolerance. Can J Anaesth 1999;46:872–7.

[12] Guignard B, Bossard AE, Coste C, et al. Acute opioid tolerance: intraoperative remifentanil increases postoperative pain and morphine requirement. Anesthesiology 2000;93:409–17.

[13] Ballantyne JC, Carr DB, Chalmers TC, et al. Postoperative patient-controlled analgesia: meta-analysis of initial randomized control trials. J Clin Anesth 1993;5:182–93.

[14] Walder B, Schafer M, Henzi I, et al. Efficacy and safety of patient-controlled opioid analgesia for acute postoperative pain: a quantitative systematic review. Acta Anaesthesiol Scand 2001; 45:795–804.

[15] Kehlet H, Rung GW, Callesen T. Postoperative opioid analgesia: time for reconsideration? J Clin Anesth 1996;8:441–5.

[16] Balantyne JC, Carr DB, deFerranti S, et al. The comparative effects of postoperative analgesic therapies on pulmonary outcome: cumulative meta-analyses of randomized, controlled trials. Anesth Analg 1998;86:598–612.

[17] Rodgers A, Walker N, Schug S, et al. Reduction of postoperative mortality and morbidity with epidural or spinal anaesthesia: results from an overview of randomised trials. BMJ 2000; 321:1493–504.

[18] Rigg JR, Jamrozik K, Myles PS, et al. Epidural anaesthesia and analgesia and outcome of major surgery: a randomised trial. Lancet 2002;359:1276–82.

[19] Carli F, Mayo N, Klubien K, et al. Epidural analgesia enhances functional exercise capacity and health-related quality of life after colonic surgery: results of a randomized trial. Anesthesiology 2002;97:540–9.

[20] Block BM, Liu SS, Rowlingon AJ, et al. Efficacy of postoperative epidural analgesia: a meta-analysis. JAMA 2003;290:2455–63.

[21] De Leon-Casasola OA. When it comes to outcome, we need to define what a perioperative epidural technique is. Anesth Analg 2003;96:315–8.

[22] Buvanendran A, Kroin JS, Tuman KJ, et al. Effects of perioperative administration of a selective cyclooxygenase 2 inhibitor on pain management and recovery of function after knee replacement: a randomized controlled trial. JAMA 2003;290:2411–8.

[23] Capdevila X, Barthelet Y, Biboulet P, et al. Effects of perioperative analgesia technique on the surgical outcome and duration of rehabilitation. Anesthesiology 1999;91:8–15.

[24] Wilson AT, Nicholson E, Burton L, et al. Analgesia for day-case shoulder surgery. Br J Anaesth 2004;92:414–5.

[25] McCartney CJL, Brull R, Chan VWS, et al. Early but no long-term benefit of regional compared general anesthesia for ambulatory hand surgery. Anesthesiology 2004;101:461–7.

[26] Botting RM. Mechanism of action of acetaminophen: is there a cyclooxygenase 3? Clin Infect Dis 2000;5(Suppl 31):S202–10.

[27] Chandrasekharan NV, Dai H, Roos KLT, et al. COX-3, a cyclooxygenase-1 variant inhibited by acetaminophen and other analgesic/antipyretic drugs: cloning, structure, and expression. Proc Natl Acad Sci U S A 2002;15:13926–31.

[28] Schwab JM, Beiter T, Linder JU, et al. COX-3-a virtual pain target in humans? FASEB J 2003;17:2174–5.

[29] Kehlet H, Werner MU. Role of paracetamol in the acute pain management. Drugs 2003;63: 15–22.

[30] Graham GG, Graham RI, Day RO. Comparative analgesia, cardiovascular and renal effects of celecoxib, rofecoxib and acetaminophen (paracetamol). Curr Pharm Des 2002;8:1063–75.

[31] Ostapowicz G, Fontana RJ, Schiodt FV, et al. Results of a prospective study of acute liver failure at 17 tertiary care centers in the United States. Ann Intern Med 2002;137:947–54.

[32] Garcia Rodriguez LA, Hernandez-Diaz S. Relative risk of upper gastrointestinal complications among users of acetaminophen and nonsteroidal anti-inflammatory drugs. Epidemiology 2001; 12:570–6.

[33] Rahme E, Pettitt D, LeLorier J. Determinants and sequelae associated with utilization of acetaminophen versus traditional nonsteroidal antiinflammatory drugs in an elderly population. Arthritis Rheum 2002;46:3046–54.

[34] Holmer Pettersson P, Owall A, Jakobsson J. Early bioavailability of paracetamol after oral or intravenous administration. Acta Anaesthesiol Scand 2004;48:867–70.

[35] Mushambi MC, Rowbotham DJ, Bailey SM. Gastric emptying after minor gynaecological surgery: the effect of anaesthetic technique. Anaesthesia 1992;47:287–9.

[36] Yuan CS, Foss JF, O'Connor M, et al. Effects of low-dose morphine on gastric emptying in healthy volunteers. J Clin Pharmacol 1998;38:1017–20.

[37] Romsing M, Moiniche S, Dahl JB. Rectal and parenteral paracetamol, and paracetamol in combination with NSAIDs for postoperative analgesia. Br J Anaesth 2002;88:215–26.

[38] Hyllested M, Jones S, Pedersen JL, et al. Comparative effects of paracetamol, NSAIDs or their combination in postoperative pain management: a quantitative review. Br J Anaesth 2002; 88:199–214.

[39] Hahn TW, Mogensen T, Lund LS, et al. Analgesic effect of i.v. paracetamol: possible ceiling effect of paracetamol in postoperative pain. Acta Anaesthesiol Scand 2003;47:138–45.

[40] Dahl JB, Kehlet H. Non-steroidal anti-inflammatory drugs: rationale use in severe post-operative pain. Br J Anaesth 1991;66:703–12.

[41] McCrory CR, Lindahl SG. Cyclooxygenase inhibition for postoperative analgesia. Anesth Analg 2002;95:169–76.

[42] Macario A, Lipman A. Ketorolac in the era of cyclo-oxygenase-2 selective nonsteroidal anti-inflammatory drugs: a systematic review of efficacy, side effects, and regulatory issues. Pain Med 2001;2:336–51.

[43] Kehlet H, Dahl JB. Are perioperative nonsteroidal anti-inflammatory drugs ulcerogenic in the short term? Drugs 1992;44(Suppl 5):S38–41.

[44] Kenny GNC. Potential renal, haematological and allergic adverse effects associated with non-steroidal anti-inflammatory drugs. Drugs 1992;44(Suppl 5):S31–7.

[45] Camu F, Van Lersberghe C, Lauwers MH. Cardiovascular risks and benefits of perioperative nonsteroidal anti-inflammatory drug treatment. Drugs 1992;44(Suppl 5):S42–51.

[46] Forrest JB, Camu F, Greer IA, et al. Ketorolac, diclofenac, and ketoprofen are equally safe for pain relief after major surgery. Br J Anesth 2002;88:227–33.

[47] Moiniche S, Romsing J, Dahl JB, et al. Non-steroidal anti-inflammatory drugs and the risk of operative bleeding after tonsillectomy-a quantitative systematic review. Anesth Analg 2003; 96:68–71.

[48] Gilron I, Milne B, Hong M. Cyclooxygenase-2 inhibitors in postoperative pain management. Anesthesiology 2003;99:1198–208.

[49] Gajraj NR. Cycloxygenase-2 inhibitors in postoperative pain management. Anesth Analg 2003;96:1720–38.

[50] Romsing J, Moiniche S. A systemic review of COX-2 inhibitors compared with traditional NSAIDs, or different COX-2 inhibitors for post-operative pain. Acta Anaesthesiol Scand 2004;48:525–46.

[51] Joshi GP. Valdecoxib for the management of chronic and acute pain. Expert Rev Neuro-therapeutics 2005;5:11–24.

[52] Joshi GP, Viscus E, Gan TJ, et al. Effective treatment of laparoscopic cholecystectomy pain with intravenous followed by oral COX-2 specific inhibitor. Anesth Analg 2004;98:336–42.

[53] Gan TJ, Joshi GP, Viscus E, et al. Presurgical parenteral and oral COX-2 specific inhibitors improve quality of recovery following laparoscopic cholecystectomy. Anesth Analg 2004;98: 1665–73.

[54] Luo ZD, Cizkova D. The role of nitric oxide in nociception. Curr Rev Pain 2000;4:459–66.

[55] Riedel W, Neeck G. Nociception, pain, and antinociception: current concepts. Z Rheumatol 2001;60:404–15.

[56] Fiorucci S, Antonelli E, Burgaud JL, et al. Nitric oxide-releasing NSAIDs: a review of their current status. Drug Saf 2001;24:801–11.

[57] Kulkarni SK, Jain NK, Singh A. Nitric oxide-releasing NSAIDs: a new dimension in nonsteroidal antiinflammatory drugs. Drugs Future 2001;26:485–9.

[58] Keeble JE, Moore PK. Pharmacology and potential therapeutic applications of nitric oxide-releasing non-steroidal anti-inflammatory and related nitric oxide-donating drugs. Br J Pharmacol 2002;137:295–310.

[59] Joshi GP. Update NCX-701 (nitro-acetaminophen). Curr Opin Investig Drugs 2004;5:755–9.

[60] Stubhaug A, Breivik H, Eide PK, et al. Mapping of punctuate hyperalgesia surrounding a surgical a surgical incision demonstrates that ketamine is a powerful suppressor of central sensitization to pain following surgery. Acta Anaesthesiol Scand 1997;41:1124–32.

[61] Schmid RL, Sandler AN, Katz J. Use and efficacy of low-dose ketamine in the manage-ment of acute postoperative pain: a review of current techniques and outcomes. Pain 1999;82: 111–25.

[62] McCartney CJ, Sinha A, Katz J. A qualitative systematic review of the role of N-methyl-D-aspartate receptor antagonists in preventative analgesia. Anesth Analg 2004;98:1385–400.

[63] Subramaniam K, Subramaniam B, Steinbrook RA. Ketamine as adjuvant analgesic to opioids: a qualitative and quantitative systematic review. Anesth Analg 2004;99:482–95.

[64] De Kock M, Lavand'homme P, Waterloos H. 'Balanced analgesia' in the perioperative period: is there a place for ketamine? Pain 2001;92:373–80.

[65] Zahn PK, Brennan TJ. lack of effect of intrathecally administered N-methyl-D-aspartate receptor antagonists in a rat model for postoperative pain. Anesthesiology 1998;88:143–56.

[66] Maze M, Tranquilli W. Alpha-2 adrenoceptor agonists: defining he role in clinical anesthesia. Anesthesiology 1991;74:581–605.

[67] Arain SR, Ruehlow RM, Uhrich TD, et al. The efficacy of dexmedetomidine versus morphine for postoperative analgesia after major surgery. Anesth Analg 2004;98:153–8.

[68] Gilron I. Is gabapentin a broad-spectrum analgesic? Anesthesiology 2002;97:537–9.

[69] Gee NS, Brown JP, Dissanayake VU, et al. The novel anticonvulsant drug, gabapentin (Neurontin), binds to the alpha2delta subunit of a calcium channel. J Biol Chem 1996;271:5768–76.

[70] Fassoulaki A, Patris K, Sarantopoulos C, et al. The analgesic effect of gabapentin and mexiletine after breast surgery for cancer. Anesth Analg 2002;95:985–91.

[71] Dirks J, Fredensborg BB, Christensen D, et al. A randomized study of the effects of single dose of gapapentin versus placebo on postoperative pain and morphine consumption after mastectomy. Anesthesiology 2002;97:560–4.

[72] Hill CM, Balkenohl M, Thomas DW, et al. Pregabalin in patients with postoperative dental pain. Eur J Pain 2001;5:119–24.

[73] Holte K, Kehlet H. Perioperative single-dose glucocorticoid administration-pathophysiological effects in clinical implications. J Am Coll Surg 2002;195:694–711.

[74] Gan TJ, Lubarsky DA, Flood EM, et al. Patient preferences for acute pain treatment. Br J Anaesth 2004;92:681–8.

[75] Gan TJ, Joshi GP, Zhao SZ, et al. Presurgical intravenous parecoxib sodium and follow-up oral valdecoxib for pain management after laparoscopic cholecystectomy surgery reduces opioid requirements and opioid-related adverse effects. Acta Anaesthesiol Scand 2004;48:1194–207.

[76] Perkins FM, Kehlet H. Chronic pain as an outcome of surgery: a review of predictive factors. Anesthesiology 2000;93:1123–33.

[77] Macrae WA. Chronic pain after surgery. Br J Anaesth 2001;87:88–98.

[78] Reuben SS. Preventing the development of complex regional pain syndrome after surgery. Anesthesiology 2004;101:1215–24.

[79] Gottschalk A, Raja SN. Severing the link between acute and chronic pain: the anesthesiologist's role in preventative medicine. Anesthesiology 2004;101:1063–5.

[80] Woolf CJ, Salter MW. Neuronal plasticity: increasing the pain in pain. Science 2000;288:1765–9.

[81] Kissin I. Preemptive analgesia. Anesthesiology 2000;93:1138–43.

[82] Moiniche S, Kehlet H, Dahl JB. A qualitative and quantitative systemic review of preemptive analgesia for postoperative pain relief. Anesthesiology 2002;96:725–41.

[83] Hogan QH. No preemptive analgesia: is that so bad? Anesthesiology 2002;96:526–7.

[84] Ochroch EA, Mardini IA, Gottschalk A. What is the role of NSAIDs in pre-emptive analgesia? Drug 2004;63:2709–23.

[85] Barratt SM, Smith RC, Kee AJ, et al. Multimodal analgesia and intravenous nutrition preserves total body protein following major upper gastrointestinal surgery. Reg Anesth Pain Med 2002;27:15–22.

[86] Cousins MJ. Postoperative multimodal analgesia and intravenous nutrition. Reg Anesth Pain Med 2002;27:536.

[87] Brodner G, Van Aken H, Hertle L, et al. Multimodal perioperative management-combining thoracic epidural analgesia, forced mobilization, and oral nutrition-reduces hormonal and metabolic stress and improves convalescence after major urologic surgery. Anesth Analg 2001;92:1594–600.

[88] Neal JM, Wilcox RT, Allen HW, et al. Near total esophagectomy: the influence of standard-ized multimodal management and intraoperative fluid restriction. Reg Anesth Pain Med 2003; 28:328–34.

[89] Ashburn MA, Caplan A, Carr DB, et al. Practice guidelines for acute pain management in the perioperative setting. Anesthesiology 2004;100:1573–81.

[90] Rosenquist RW, Rosenberg J. Postoperative pain guidelines. Reg Anesth Pain Med 2003;28: 279–88.

[91] Rowlingson JC, Rawal N. Postoperative pain guidelines–targeted to the site of surgery. Reg Anesth Pain Med 2003;28:265–7.

[92] Werner MU, Søholm L, Rotbøll-Nielsen P, et al. Does an acute pain service improve postoperative outcome? Anesth Analg 2002;95:1361–72.

[93] Rawal N. Acute pain services revisited-good from far, far from good? Reg Anesth Pain Med 2002;27:117–21.

ELSEVIER
SAUNDERS

Anesthesiology Clin N Am
23 (2005) 203–210

ANESTHESIOLOGY
CLINICS OF
NORTH AMERICA

Procedure-Specific Postoperative Pain Management

Henrik Kehlet, MD, PhD

*Section for Surgical Pathophysiology 4074, The Juliane Marie Centre Rigshospitalet,
2100 Copenhagen, Denmark*

Despite a significant improvement over the last decade in our understanding of acute (and chronic) pain mechanisms [1] and the establishment of acute pain services [2,3], recently updated studies continue to report that postoperative pain management is not satisfactory [4,5]. In addition, publications of guidelines for acute pain management [6], the introduction of "pain as the fifth vital sign," and the incorporation of the standards advocated by the Joint Commission for Accreditation of Health Care Organization apparently have not been effective and have not translated into improved postoperative analgesia. Furthermore, because the provision of sufficient dynamic pain relief is a prerequisite for successful postoperative recovery and reduced morbidity, which may have major economic implications, it is surprising and disappointing that pain management has not improved [7].

A recent approach to helping clinicians choose analgesics for postoperative analgesia has been the Oxford League Tables. The Oxford League tables express the number of patients who achieve analgesia sufficiently to observe a maximal pain response of at least 50% ($\geq$50% maximum total pain relief) compared with a placebo group (ie, the number needed to treat [NNT] values) [8]. The League tables, in a simplified manner, may provide considerable help to the clinician in choosing an analgesic agent; however, the tables are derived from a variety of surgical procedures (predominantly dental procedures).

Although, some investigators have claimed that there may be no systematic differences in the estimate of analgesic efficacy between dental and other post-surgical pain models [9], other investigators have emphasized that analgesic effects may vary substantially between pain models [10,11]. For example, the

E-mail address: henrik.kehlet@rh.dk

analgesic effects of aspirin may vary among postoperative, postpartum, and dental surgery settings [10,11]. Additionally, an analysis of existing data on the efficacy of acetaminophen in relation to the magnitude of surgery has demonstrated a significantly lower efficacy in orthopedic procedures compared with dental surgery, whereas its level of efficacy in minor gynecological procedures was judged to be between the two (Gray, Kehlet, Bonnet, and Rawal, unpublished data, 2005). Furthermore, a comparison among acetaminophen and nonsteroidal anti-inflammatory drugs (NSAIDs) or a combination of the two [12] suggests that the larger the surgical injury (and therefore pain) the smaller will be the difference in the analgesic efficacy between acetaminophen and NSAIDs. This contrasts with the findings in small-scale surgical injury in which it has been repeatedly demonstrated that NSAIDs have a better efficacy than acetaminophen [8,12]. Finally, the clinical relevance of a 50% decrease in pain may be different when decreasing from 80 to 40 than from 30 to 15 on a 100-point visual analog scale. Therefore, the recommendations based on the League tables may not necessarily be valid in all types of surgery.

Why do we need procedure-specific evidence?

As discussed above, the suboptimal provision of acute pain management may depend on many factors, and one may therefore question whether a new set of guidelines could be helpful in improving postoperative pain management or whether other organizational or economic factors need to be considered instead [2,3].

In this context, we propose that procedure-specific acute pain management guidelines may be helpful because the pain intensity and its consequences may be procedure-related [13–15]. Although the intensity of the acute pain state is expected to be related to the magnitude of the operation, this may not necessarily be so. When the size of the injury is considered, dental pain with a smaller injury may be relatively more painful compared with the pain observed in relation to the magnitude of tissue injury after hip replacement. However, the consequences of the injury and pain may be entirely different between these procedures because stress responses and organ dysfunctions resulting from the injury are different. Thus, pulmonary dysfunction may not present a problem associated with pain after dental or superficial operations compared with the significant reduction in pulmonary function in relation to pain after abdominal or hip replacement procedures. Therefore, an invasive analgesic technique that provides more efficient pain relief may be considered the treatment of choice for operations in which the stress-reducing effects and the improvement in organ functions may be important in addition to pain relief [16]; a good example is the use of continuous epidural analgesia for thoracic and major abdominal surgery. Thus, the choice of analgesic treatment should depend on the type of surgical procedure.

Another argument for procedure-specific pain guidelines is the fact that some analgesic modalities may only apply to certain surgical procedures. For example, intraperitoneal and intra-articular treatments only apply to abdominal and joint operations, respectively. On the other hand, analgesics such as acetaminophen, NSAIDs, and cyclooxygenase (COX)-2 inhibitors may be used in all types of surgery. Obviously, local anesthetic techniques must be related to the site of injury, but one needs to consider the side effects of nerve blockade with predominant motor function compared with their role in pain perception.

The risk-benefit ratio of different analgesics may also vary according to the surgical procedure. Thus, the clinical effects of opioid sparing (which are variable between analgesics) may also depend on the effects of the surgical injury. Opioid-related side effects such as nausea and vomiting occur more often in some operations than others (eg, head, neck, ear, gynecological, and abdominal surgical procedures are associated with a higher incidence of nausea and vomiting and opioid-related side effects than orthopedic and superficial procedures). Therefore, the recommendation of an analgesic based on its overall opioid-sparing effects may not necessarily translate to a similar reduction of opioid-related side effects in all types of surgery.

Similarly, the risk and clinical implications of postoperative bleeding associated with certain analgesics are also procedure-specific. For example, the inhibition of platelet aggregation and therefore the risk of bleeding associated with NSAIDs would be more relevant in operations that pose a risk of bleeding (eg, a tonsillectomy). Therefore, analgesics with no effects on platelet function (eg, acetaminophen and COX-2 specific inhibitors) may be preferable in these but not in other operations.

Postoperative pain may also depend on the choice of surgical technique (ie, the type of minimal invasive surgery or site and type of incision in open procedures). The technique of minimal invasive surgery can modify pain, as do horizontal and curved incisions, which may lower the intensity of postoperative pain compared with vertical incisions. Therefore, the choice of an adjuvant analgesic treatment should be made in relation to the surgical technique as well as surgical approach.

When these arguments are combined with the potential shortcomings of the League tables (ie, the use of NNT values) for choosing an analgesic for a given surgical procedure, it is possible that one of the reasons for continued suboptimal provision of postoperative pain management is the use of generalized guidelines. Clinicians need information in which the choice of analgesic technique includes the consideration of the operation and is based on the available evidence from that particular surgical procedure. Unfortunately, no such procedure-specific information on the choice of postoperative analgesic technique has been available in any major anesthesia, surgical, or pain textbooks.

Initiatives to provide procedure-specific pain management guidelines

To date, based on the above considerations and shortcomings of more generalized pain guidelines [6], two initiatives have been undertaken to provide procedure-specific guidelines [14,15]. Both of these guidelines are available on public Internet websites. One source is from the United States Veteran's Health Administration, in collaboration with the United States Department of Defense and the University of Iowa (www.oqp.med.va.gov/cpg/cpg.htm) [14], and the other is from a group of European anesthesiologists and surgeons, the Prospect Working Group (www.postoppain.org) [15].

The procedure-specific guidelines of the United States Veteran's Health Administration have been constructed based on a systematic review of the literature in a variety of procedures and has been interpreted by a consensus group to provide guidelines for the overall recommendations for specific analgesic interventions [14]. This group plans to update the guidelines every 3 years. The website, however, does not provide a complete list of appropriate references and

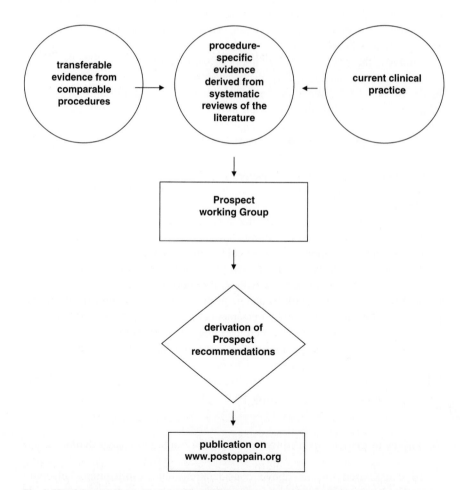

Fig. 1. Development of procedure-specific guidelines for postoperative pain management. (*From* the Prospect Working Group guidelines. Available at: www.postoppain.org; with permission.)

Box 1. An example of procedure-specific postoperative pain management guidelines (laparoscopic cholecystectomy)

Preoperative analgesia

Clonidine may be recommended based on its analgesia to side-effect ratio, depending on confirmation of benefits identified in preliminary trials (C).[a]
Dexamethasone (5–8 mg) is recommended as an antiemetic (A) and analgesic (B).

Intraoperative analgesia

Anesthetic techniques
Combined epidural and general anesthesia is not recommended for routine anesthetic management because the risks out-weigh the benefits; however, in certain high-risk pulmonary patients, it can be justified (A).

Operative techniques
Low pressure CO_2 pneumoperitoneum is recommended (A).
Warmed CO_2 pneumoperitoneum is not recommended (A).
Peritoneal lavage after CO_2 pneumoperitoneum is recommended (C).
Suction after CO_2 pneumoperitoneum is recommended (C).
Gasless techniques are not recommended (C).
Helium pneumoperitoneum is not recommended (C).
N_2O pneumoperitoneum is not recommended on safety grounds, despite potential analgesic effects (B).
Microlaparoscopic techniques cannot be currently recommended for analgesic benefits because of inconsistent findings (B).
Radially expanding or cutting trocars are not recommended for analgesic benefits because of inconsistent findings (B).

Analgesics
Clonidine may be recommended (C) based on its analgesia to side-effects ratio, depending on confirmation of benefits identified in preliminary trials.
Incisional local anesthetic infiltration is recommended at the end of surgery (A). Combined incisional and intraperitoneal local anesthetics are recommended (C) provided the dose is monitored to prevent toxicity.

Despite analgesic effects (C), interpleural local anesthetics are not recommended because of the invasive nature of the technique.

Intraperitoneal local anesthetics are recommended, although the effects are of limited duration (A). Combined incisional and intraperitoneal local anesthetics are recommended (C) provided the dose is monitored to prevent toxicity.

Long-acting potent opioids (morphine, meperidine) are not recommended for routine analgesia because of side effects during recovery (A). Short-acting potent opioids are recommended (A).

Weak opioids, including tramadol, are not recommended for intraoperative analgesia (A).

Postoperative analgesics

Postoperative epidural analgesia is recommended only in pulmonary high-risk patients and/or if laparoscopic cholecystectomy is converted to open surgery with a large incision (A), based on transferable evidence from other abdominal procedures.

Ketamine is not recommended as a single agent, based on transferable evidence (B).

Metamizole cannot be recommended because of limited efficacy data together with the risk of potential adverse events and interactions with NSAIDs (C).

NSAIDs are recommended (A). COX-2-specific inhibitors may be preferred in at-risk patients (eg, those with a history of gastroduodenal ulcer and risk of surgical bleeding) (C).

Potent opioids should be avoided where possible for first-line analgesia because of side effects, but short-acting potent opioids can be used in patients who experience severe pain in addition to the use of other agents (A).

Weak opioids, including tramadol, are recommended when NSAIDs or COX-2 inhibitors plus acetaminophen is not sufficient (A).

Acetaminophen is recommended for routine pain therapy as a component of multimodal analgesia based on transferable evidence (A).

Up to 6 hours postoperatively including the post anesthesia care unit (PACU)

Nonopioid analgesia with NSAIDs or COX-2-specific inhibitors combined with acetaminophen should be continued in the

PACU. Weak opioids are added for mild pain, and small doses of short-acting potent opioids are added for severe pain. In patients with severe pain, consider starting with a combination of NSAIDs/COX-2-specific inhibitors plus short-acting potent opioids.

Beyond 6 hours postoperatively

Nonopioid analgesic treatment with NSAIDs/COX-2-specific inhibitors and acetaminophen should be continued and supplemented with weak opioids if needed. The use of potent opioids is rarely necessary beyond 6 hours postoperatively. In patients with more severe pain, consider starting with a combination of NSAIDs/COX-2 inhibitors plus potent opioids.

[a] A–C, level of evidence (Cochrane).
Modified from Prospect Working Group guidelines. Available at: www.postoppain.org; with permission.

thereby does not allow individual choices or recommendations to be made based on local circumstances, regulatory issues, and economic considerations.

The Prospect Working Group guidelines have been constructed based on the available evidence from the type of surgery considered, and the specific data and publications from randomized clinical studies are provided on its website (Fig. 1) [15]. A systematic review of the literature for a particular procedure is performed using the Cochrane Collaboration, which includes randomized studies that assess the effects of analgesic, anesthetic, and operative techniques on postoperative pain. In addition, qualitative and quantitative (meta-analyses) outcomes are generated. The procedure-specific evidence together with transferable evidence from randomized studies in similar types of procedures (eg, knee arthroplasty data used as transferable evidence for hip arthroplasty) form the basis for the group's recommendations. Readers are presented with all the available evidence and are therefore able to make decisions based on their practice and do not necessarily need to follow the Prospect group's recommendations. This may be important because availability, costs, and organizational factors must be considered because all opportunities may not necessarily be available in all locations and countries. The choice of analgesic management may be further complicated because indications and contraindications are not uniform among countries. Therefore, the information based on the Prospect website may be more useful worldwide because the procedure-specific evidence is available with or without the recommendations from the expert group. An example of procedure-specific recommendations for analgesia after laparoscopic cholecystectomy is presented in Box 1 [15].

Summary

The existence of two procedure-specific guidelines may be helpful for clinicians. Presently, the guidelines provided by the group in the Unites States cover most types of procedures, whereas the European Prospect guidelines represent a more detailed information site but have so far covered only laparoscopic cholecystectomy and abdominal hysterectomy. However, toward the end of 2004, two additional procedures will be available on the website from the Prospect group (colonic resection and hip replacement), and guidelines for inguinal herniotomy and thoracotomy will follow in early 2005.

References

[1] Woolf CJ. Pain: moving from symptom control towards mechanism-specific pharmacologic management. Ann Intern Med 2004;140:441–51.

[2] Rawal N. Acute pain services revisited – good from far, far from good? Reg Anesth Pain Med 2002;27:117–21.

[3] Werner MU, Søholm L, Rotbøll-Nielsen P, et al. Does an acute pain service improve postoperative outcome? Anesth Analg 2002;95:1361–72.

[4] Apfelbaum JL, Chen C, Shilpa S, et al. Postoperative pain experience: results from a national survey suggest postoperative pain continues to be undermanaged. Anesth Analg 2003; 97:534–40.

[5] Dolin SJ, Cashman JN, Bland JM. Effectiveness of acute postoperative pain management: evidence from published data. Br J Anaesth 2002;89:409–23.

[6] Ashburn MA, Caplan A, Carr DB, et al. Practice guidelines for acute pain management in the perioperative setting. Anesthesiology 2004;100:1573–81.

[7] Kehlet H, Dahl JB. Anaesthesia, surgery and challenges in postoperative recovery. Lancet 2003;362:1921–8.

[8] Moore A, Edvards J, Barden J, et al. Bandolier's little book of pain. Oxford: Oxford University Press; 2003.

[9] Barden J, Edwards JE, McQuay HJ, et al. Pain and analgesic response after third molar extraction and other postsurgical pain. Pain 2004;107:86–90.

[10] Laska EM, Sunshine A, Wanderling JA, et al. Quantitative differences in aspirin analgesia in three models of clinical pain. J Clin Pharmacol 1982;22:531–42.

[11] Cooper SA. Single dose analgesic studies: the upside and downside of assay sensitivity. In: Max M, Portenoy R, editors. Advances in pain research and therapy. New York: Raven Press Ltd.; 1991. p. 117–24.

[12] Hyllested M, Jones S, Pedersen JL, et al. Comparative effect of acetaminophen, NSAIDs or their combination in postoperative pain management: a qualitative review. Br J Anaesth 2002; 88:199–214.

[13] Rowlingson JC, Rawal N. Postoperative pain guidelines–targeted to the site of surgery. Reg Anesth Pain Med 2003;28:265–7.

[14] Rosenquist RW, Rosenberg J. Postoperative pain guidelines. Reg Anesth Pain Med 2003; 28:279–88.

[15] Prospect Working Group guidelines. Available at: www.postoppain.org. Accessed November 4, 2004.

[16] Kehlet H. Modification of responses to surgery by neural blockade: clinical implications. In: Cousins MJ, Bridenbaugh PO, editors. Neural blockade in clinical anesthesia and management of pain. Philadelphia: Lippincott-Raven; 1998. p. 129–75.

ELSEVIER
SAUNDERS

Anesthesiology Clin N Am
23 (2005) 211–225

ANESTHESIOLOGY
CLINICS OF
NORTH AMERICA

Organization, Function, and Implementation of Acute Pain Service

Narinder Rawal, MD, PhD

*Department of Anesthesiology and Intensive Care, Örebro University Hospital,
SE-70185, Örebro, Sweden*

Pain relief after surgery continues to be a major medical challenge. Improvement in perioperative analgesia is not only desirable for humanitarian reasons but is also essential for its potential reduction of postoperative morbidity [1–4] and mortality [2]. Unrelieved postoperative pain may delay discharge and recovery and result in an inability to participate in rehabilitation programs, leading to poor outcomes. Recent studies [5] show that undertreatment of pain continues, despite the availability of drugs and techniques for its effective management. It is generally accepted that the solution to the problem of inadequate pain relief lies not so much in the development of new analgesic drugs or technologies but in the development of an appropriate organization to utilize existing expertise.

Although several authors in the late 1970s advocated the introduction of a pain management team to supervise and administer analgesics and to assume the responsibility for teaching and training in postoperative pain management, almost a decade passed before specialized in-hospital postoperative pain services emerged. Recently, various medical and health care organizations have recommended the widespread introduction of an Acute Pain Service (APS) [6–12]. The provision of an APS is presently a prerequisite for accreditation for training by the Royal College of Anaesthetists in the United Kingdom and by the Australian and New Zealand College of Anaesthetists [13].

E-mail address: n.rawal@orebroll.se

Prevalence of acute pain service

Table 1 shows the prevalence of the APS in Europe, North America, Australia, and New Zealand [14–27]. There appears to be an increase in the worldwide number of hospitals with an APS. However, the prevalence of an APS does not mean much in the absence of established standards with respect to the structure and function of an APS [24]. The prevalence does not provide any indication about the nature of service provided, the staffing and facilities, the training and competence of the personnel, or the effectiveness of an APS. Many hospitals consider their services adequate for their needs, although they have only some but not all components of an APS [20]. For example, a recent Canadian survey showed that the percentage of academic hospitals with an APS had increased from 53% in 1993 to 92% in 2004 [26]. However, an APS with anesthesiologists as the sole providers had decreased from 36% to 22% because of growing clinical demands and a reduced number of anesthesiologists. Only 44% of centers had a designated group of APS physicians,

Table 1
National surveys of the prevalence of acute pain services

Study	Region/country	Survey year	Prevalence[a] $\langle n(\%)\rangle$
Zimmerman [14]	Canada	1991	24/47 (53)[b]
Goucke [15]	Australia, New Zealand	1992/1993	37/111 (33)
Rawal [16]	Europe	1993	37/105 (34)
Davies [17]	United Kingdom	1994	77/221 (35)[b]
Windsor [18]	United Kingdom	1994[c]	151/354 (43)
		1990	10/358 (3)
Merry [19]	New Zealand	1994	12/62 (19)
		1996	17/22[d]
Harmer [20]	United Kingdom	1995[e]	97/221 (44)[b]
Ready [21][f]	United States	1995	236/324 (73)
Warfield [22]	United States	1995	126/300 (42)
Neugebauer [23]	Germany	1997	390/1000 (39)
Stamer [24]	Germany	1999	161/446 (36)
O'Higgins [25]	United Kingdom	2000[e]	$\geq$49%[g]
Goldstein [26]	Canada	2004	50/62 (93)[b]
Powell [27]	United Kingdom	2004	270/325 (83)

[a] Formal Acute Pain Service, provision of staff and funding.

[b] Only university affiliated.

[c] Survey was conducted in 1994 and contained a retrospective analysis of 1990 data.

[d] This part of the survey included only 22 publicly funded Crown Health Enterprises with $\geq$150 beds.

[e] Year of survey not stated.

[f] Letter

[g] A total of 118 of 240 Anaesthetic College tutors confirmed the presence of an acute pain team to review epidural analgesia on the wards.

Adapted from Werner MU, Søholm L, Rotbøll-Nielsen P, et al. Does an acute pain service improve postoperative outcome? Anesth Analg 2002;95:1361–72.

although nursing representation was only 55%. Additionally, only 29% of centers reported having an ongoing prospective data collection system. The authors commented that no information was obtained about the management of acute pain in patients who were not followed by the APS, which represented the majority of postoperative patients [26]. Furthermore, recent evidence indicates that some APS face financial problems and may provide only a token service. Although there is a consensus that one of the major functions of an APS is to ensure the safe and effective delivery of postoperative analgesia, many hospitals without an APS may also claim that they provide these services [27,28]. However, it is important to differentiate between the advantages of the analgesic techniques themselves and those conferred by the increased supervision of specialists and the education provided by a dedicated staff of an APS. This suggests a need to develop APS standards with well-defined criteria for evaluating performance and comparing with national benchmarks [27].

Structure and functions of acute pain service

The original organizational model for managing postoperative pain was largely catalyzed by an APS developed in the United States [21] and gradually introduced in the United Kingdom during the 1990s after the landmark report "Pain After Surgery" [7]. Yet the implementation of the APS since 1990 has been piecemeal and haphazard, with successive reports up to the late 1990s providing evidence of significant variation within and among hospitals in the structure and function of an APS [27].

Most major institutions in the United States have an anesthesiology-based APS. The comprehensive pain management teams usually consist of staff and resident anesthesiologists, specially trained nurses, pharmacists, and physical therapists. Sometimes biomedical and infusion pump specialty personnel are also included. Secretarial and billing personnel are also a part of a United States-style APS. Patients under the care of an APS are visited and assessed regularly by members of the team. The anesthesiologist-based APS organization model usually provides "high tech" pain management service to patients receiving epidural analgesia or intravenous patient-controlled analgesia (IV-PCA). However, the costs of the United States-style APS are high and are being questioned increasingly by health care payers. In many institutions, IV-PCA management has now been taken over by surgeons. A downsizing of many APS is taking place in the United States, with further reductions predicted.

There is a clear need for new APS models that provide effective pain relief for all surgical patients. As discussed later, the nurse-based, anesthesiologist-supervised APS model may be an alternative to the conventional physician-based APS model. The United Kingdom Joint Colleges of Surgery and Anesthesia Working Party report [7] recommended that a multidisciplinary team including specialist-nursing staff should run the APS. They further recommended that the services should assume day-to-day responsibility for the management of postoperative pain, in-service training for nursing and medical staff, and research and auditing. Similar recommendations have been made by national expert committees from Australia [6], the United States [8,10], Germany [9], Sweden [11], and again in an updated form by the American Society of Anesthesiologists Task Force [12]. In the United Kingdom, two national surveys [14,15] were conducted to determine the extent to which the recommendations of the Working Party report had been implemented. Unfortunately, there appeared to be a large degree of variation in what was thought to constitute an APS, and some hospitals had only some of the elements recommended by the Working Party report [18,20].

An ideal APS organization should provide optimal pain management for every patient who undergoes surgery, including children and those under-going outpatient surgical procedures. The Joint Commission for Accreditation of Healthcare Organizations, an independent not-for-profit organization that sets health care standards in the United States, recognizes this and now requires that hospitals assess, treat, and document patients' pain, guarantee the competence of their staff in pain assessment and management, and educate patients and their families about effective pain management. Hospitals must also consider the needs of ambulatory surgery patients for information and provide guidelines for their pain management after they are discharged from the hospital [29].

One of the most important activities of an APS is to provide an ongoing review of institutional policies and practices regarding pain control and mechanisms to deal with problems as they arise. The members of the program should meet regularly to provide feedback and discuss opportunities for further improvement. Such meetings are important to provide a forum for assessing the efficiency of the APS, to highlight practical problems, and to find solutions to lesser functioning aspects of the APS [30].

Although each institution may have different requirements for its APS, and modifications of published models may be necessary to accommodate local conditions, the main components of an APS should include the following: (1) designated personnel who are responsible for providing 24-hour APS (in small hospitals 1 or 2 individuals may be adequate); (2) regular pain as-sessment (with appropriate scales for children and patients with cognitive impairment) at rest and movement, the maintenance of pain scores below a predetermined threshold, and regular documentation of pain scores ("make pain visible"); (3) active cooperation with surgeons and ward nurses for the development of protocols and critical pathways to achieve preset goals for postoperative mobilization and rehabilitation; (4) ongoing teaching programs for ward nurses for the provision of safe and cost-effective analgesic techniques; (5) patient education about pain monitoring and treatment options, goals, bene-fits, and adverse effects; and (6) a regular audit of the cost-effectiveness of analgesic techniques and in- and outpatient service satisfaction [29].

Does an acute pain service improve outcome?

It is believed that the introduction of an APS has led to an increase in the appropriate use of specialized analgesic techniques, such as IV-PCA opioid and epidural and perineural analgesia. The implementation of these techniques may represent a true advance in improving analgesia and patient well-being and in reducing postoperative morbidity [12,13]. In addition, an APS may reduce "analgesic gaps" that can occur during the transition from IV-PCA or epidural analgesia to oral analgesic therapy. Although evaluating the safety of analgesic techniques is an important objective of an APS, its role in preventing and reducing adverse events has not been well established. Wheatley et al [31] reported a decrease in the incidence of lower respiratory tract infection from 1.3% to 0.4% after the introduction of an APS. Tsui et al [33] investigated the benefits of an APS program in patients undergoing esophagectomy. The patients were managed either by an APS (n = 299) or received conventional analgesic therapy in a non-APS setting (n = 279). In the APS group, patients received postoperative epidural or systemic opioid infusion, and the non-APS group received intermittent intramuscular injections of morphine. A significantly lower incidence of pulmonary and cardiac complications and shorter hospital stay were reported in patients in the APS group [32]. However, other studies [13,33,34] have not found any reduction of hospital stay in patients managed by an APS.

In a recent literature review, Werner et al [13] evaluated the effects of an APS on postoperative outcome in 44 audits and 4 clinical trials, which included 84,097 postoperative patients. The authors found that the implementation of an APS was associated with a significant decrease in pain intensity. In addition, the introduction of an APS might have been associated with less postoperative nausea and vomiting and urinary retention. However, the authors could not draw clear conclusions about the side effects of analgesic modalities, patient satisfaction, or postoperative morbidity because of a large variability in the studies regarding an APS function and the services provided [13]. McDonnell et al [35] found that the implementation of an APS was associated with initiatives that are hallmarks of good postoperative pain management; however, they did not explore the impact of an APS on postoperative outcomes. Hospital administrators may be more likely to invest in an APS if they are persuaded that implementation results in measurable improvements in patient outcomes, at an affordable cost.

Is acute pain service cost effective?

Cost-benefit analyses are necessary to justify the need for an APS, but no such studies have been conducted. Cost analyses of acute pain management are impeded by the lack of a well-defined baseline and outcome assessment. There is no valid method of assigning financial costs to differing levels of analgesia, and the effect of various analgesic techniques on economic outcomes has not been adequately examined [13]. Cost-effectiveness analyses of postoperative pain management must consider not only the direct costs associated with analgesic drugs, devices, nursing and physician time, and duration of stay in the post-anesthesia care unit, intensive care unit, or surgical ward, as well as postoperative morbidity, but also the indirect costs of improved analgesia and patient satisfaction [13].

Brodner et al [36] have shown that the introduction of a multimodal program with improved pain relief, stress reduction, and early tracheal extubation decreased the number of patients who required a stay in an intensive care unit in the immediate postoperative period after major surgery. Because of faster discharge from the high-dependency areas, cost savings were achieved [36]. In an effort to reduce APS-related costs, several authors have advocated a low-cost nurse-based, anesthesiologist-supervised model [5,37–39] as an alternative to the more expensive physician-based multidisciplinary APS [39–42]. Currently, there is no evidence that a physician-based multidisciplinary APS is superior to a specialist nurse-based, anesthesiologist-supervised APS. Although cost-benefit studies are difficult to perform there is a great need for such studies.

How to implement an acute pain service

It is becoming increasingly clear that simple and less expensive APS models must be developed to improve the quality of postoperative analgesia for every surgical patient (including day surgery patients) in a cost-effective way. At Örebro University Hospital, Örebro, Sweden, a pain specialist nurse-based, anesthesiologist-supervised model has been successfully implemented [5]. The first step to initiating a pain management program is to organize an inter-disciplinary team of interested and motivated individuals who represent diverse professional skills and approaches to patient care.

The section anesthesiologist has the overall responsibility for anesthetic care as well as for postoperative pain management. The anesthesiologist selects the appropriate analgesic modality based on the departmental policy of using the "acute pain analgesic ladder" (Fig. 1). In a recent American Society of Anes-thesiologists practice guidelines publication [12], similar therapies are recom-mended. The guidelines suggest that, unless they are contraindicated, all patients should receive an around-the-clock regimen of nonsteroidal anti-inflammatory drugs, coxibs, or acetaminophen. In addition, a regional blockade with local anesthetics should be considered. The choice of medication, dose, route, and duration of therapy should be individualized [12]. During regular working hours, the section anesthesiologist is available for consultation or any emergency; later on, the anesthesiologist on-call assumes the same function.

A specialist acute pain nurse (APN) plays an important role in the APS. The duties of an APN are described in Table 2. An APN makes daily rounds of all surgical wards. The postoperative pain therapy of individual patients is based on standard orders and protocols developed jointly by the section anesthesiologist,

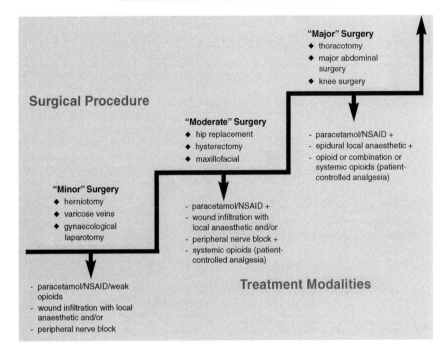

Fig. 1. Acute pain analgesic ladder. EuroPain-European minimum standards for management of postoperative pain. (*Adapted from* Rawal N. Postoperative pain and its management. In: Rawal N, editor. Management of acute and chronic pain. London: BMJ Books; 1998. p. 51–88; with permission.)

surgeon, and ward nurse. The APN facilitate collaboration among anesthesiologists, surgeons, and nurses on surgical wards. The clinical nurse specialists or APN educate ward nurses give necessary support and help initiate and supervise analgesia. This gives the ward nurses the flexibility to administer the analgesics when necessary.

Upgrading the role of ward nurses

The author's model is based on the concept that postoperative pain relief can be greatly improved by providing in-service training for surgical nursing staff about the optimal use of IV-PCA opioids and regional analgesia techniques [5]. Nurses on surgical wards have the responsibility for assessing the patient's pain intensity, administering prescribed analgesic treatments, monitoring their efficacy and adverse effects, and monitoring the extent of regional blockade. At the author's institution, ward nurses have been allowed to administer IV opioids, set up IV-PCA devices, manage epidural analgesia, and change IV-PCA and epidural analgesia drug administration parameters (within prescribed limits). Of note, the nurses were not allowed to do this at the time of implementation of an APS in 1991. Regular teaching and daily visits by the APN have resulted in effective and safe pain relief, which is confirmed by the annual audit data.

Table 2
Organization of acute pain services at Örebro University Hospital, Örebro, Sweden

Healthcare member pain "representatives"	Responsibilities
Director Acute Pain Service	Responsible for coordinating hospital-wide acute pain service and education
Section anesthesiologists	Responsible for pre-, intra-, and postoperative care (including postoperative pain) for their surgical section
Pain "representative" ward surgeons	Responsible for pain management for their surgical ward; helps integration of analgesia techniques into clinical pathways for individual surgical procedures
Pain "representative" day/night nurses	Responsible for implementation of pain management guidelines and monitoring on the ward[a]
Acute pain nurse (specialist pain nurse)	Daily rounds of all surgical wards Data collection for audits Trouble shoots technical problems Refers problem patients to section anesthesiologist (link between surgical ward and anesthesiologist) Bedside teaching of ward nurses

[a] Patients are treated on the basis of standard orders and protocols developed jointly by chiefs of anesthesiology, surgery, and nursing. Pain representatives meet every 3 months to discuss and implement necessary improvements.

The pain "representatives" from each surgical ward meet regularly with the anesthesiologist and the APN to discuss improvements based on annual audit data.

The nursing role must be upgraded if postoperative pain management is to improve on surgical wards. In many countries and institutions, ward nurses are not allowed to administer IV or epidural opioids; they are required to call an APS physician for IV-PCA and epidural analgesia dose adjustments. This is time consuming, cost ineffective, and unnecessary. These restrictions for ward nurses are surprising in view of the increasing trends toward self-treatment by patients. Outside hospitals, diabetic children are allowed to self-administer insulin, and cancer patients are allowed to self-administer epidural and intrathecal analgesics. The use of home ventilators, home dialysis, home-PCA devices, and opioids in noncancer pain is increasingly accepted. Notably, in many hospitals, midwives are allowed to manage epidural analgesia for labor pain, but ward nurses are not allowed to do the same for postoperative pain. There is convincing evidence from many countries and institutions that with appropriate teaching and training ward nurses can monitor and manage analgesic modalities such as IV-PCA and epidural analgesia. Nurse education is widely recognized as an important priority in pain management [5,20,29,30,40]. Recent studies [5,20,40,41] have demonstrated the importance of the ward nurses in improving the efficacy of analgesic regimens. Surgeon and ward nurse participation is crucial in this model.

Defining maximum acceptable pain scores and "making pain visible"

One of the responsibilities of the ward nurse is to routinely document each patient's pain intensity using the visual analog scale (VAS) every 3 hours, and the documentation of treatment efficacy on a vital sign chart is the cornerstone of this model. This assessment includes pain at rest and during movement and also before and after an intervention. In the absence of a formal, documented pain assessment, many of the medical and nursing staff continue to believe that patients who do not report pain do not feel pain. Patients should be informed that their pain will be maintained at or below a predefined threshold level (generally 3 on a 10-point VAS) and that pain scores in excess of the threshold will trigger interventions to reduce pain [29]. It is therefore essential that a maximum acceptable pain score is defined and pain intensity is routinely documented before and after analgesic treatment. A VAS above 3 is promptly treated. Documentation also provides data for the audit and facilitates review and improvement of care. Quality assurance measures can no longer be ignored.

Role of the surgeon

Although all guidelines emphasize the importance of a multidisciplinary APS as a tool to improve postoperative pain relief, in the literature no distinction has been made among the roles of individual members of the multidisciplinary team. The role of the surgeon is far more important than, say, that of the pharmacist; indeed, it would be no exaggeration to state that an APS without the surgeon's cooperation is doomed to fail. The surgeon's participation is important for the development of (1) protocols for all analgesic techniques, keeping in mind that a majority of surgical patients may not need epidural analgesia or IV-PCA techniques for effective analgesia; (2) clinical pathways to achieve preset goals for postoperative mobilization and rehabilitation, which can be expected to reduce hospital stay; (3) strategies for pain management after outpatient surgery (up to 70% and increasing surgical population); and (4) improved ward nurse compliance for the implementation of APS goals, including frequent pain assessment and documentation [29].

Education

One of the most basic yet essential activities of an APS is to develop and implement educational programs for patients and health care providers. For patients, the educational process should begin at the time of the preoperative evaluation. Traditionally, patients have assumed that pain after surgery is inevitable. They are unlikely to be aware of the standard of care they can expect to receive and the potential benefits of effective pain relief. Content should include explaining the importance of adequate pain control, the commitment of hospital staff to providing effective pain control, the various options available to manage postoperative pain, practical information about how to report pain intensity (eg, the VAS or a numerical scale), and how to participate in the pain management plan [5,29,30].

Specialist pain nurse-based APS: does it work?

In the model described above, the only additional cost is that of two APNs. At the author's hospital, approximately 16,000 surgical procedures are performed each year. The low-cost model is designed to benefit all patients (approximately € 3 per patient excluding drug and equipment costs). Regular audits have confirmed that the aims of the author's APS are achieved in over 90% of patients. The number of times anesthesiologists are consulted or called has decreased over the years; currently it is in the range of one to two consultations per week. However, the latest audit showed the need for a more detailed comparison of nighttime and daytime pain relief.

The general principles for this organization model have been accepted and recommended for Swedish hospitals by the Swedish Medical Association [11]. Based on the author's model, Bardiau et al [40] have described the implementation of an APS in a Belgian general hospital of 1005 beds, of which 240 are surgical beds. The process was divided into eight stages over a 3-year period. This program anticipated an improvement in postoperative pain relief for all surgical inpatients and the maintenance of this service over time. First, a pain management committee was formed, including anesthesiologists, surgeons, pharmacists, and nurses. The next month, a survey of nurses' attitudes and knowledge of postoperative care was conducted using an anonymous 35-item questionnaire. The following month, a 10-cm VAS device was introduced for the routine assessment of pain intensity. Then, for a 6-month period, a baseline survey (survey I) was designed to analyze the current practices of pain treatment. Following that, a specialist nurse-based, anesthesiologist-supervised APS model was implemented. Standardized treatment protocols included regular assessments of pain intensity using the VAS every 4 hours and documentation of treatment efficacy by the APN, as well as the use of analgesic regimens developed by the pain management committee. Three months later, a second survey (survey II) of 671 patients was conducted to assess the effect of an APS implementation. Finally, a third confirmation survey (survey III) of 2383 patients was conducted to investigate whether the initial improvements were maintained.

The survey of nurses identified that they lacked knowledge and skills in assessing and managing pain effectively because of the absence of nursing guidelines and pain treatment protocols. Pain relief improved significantly after the implementation of the APS. In addition, acetaminophen consumption increased significantly, whereas the use of nonsteroidal anti-inflammatory drugs increased from 20% in survey I to 64% and 99% in surveys II and III, respectively. At the same time, opioid consumption decreased. The authors concluded that the standardization of analgesic therapies, nursing practice, and regular feedback on performance are essential factors to improving pain management. Organizing teams of anesthesiologists, surgeons, and nurses is necessary for this improvement. Cost-benefit analyses are now needed to further substantiate these results [40].

Audits and continuous quality improvement of acute pain service

An audit is a monitoring and evaluation process that should help to recognize those situations on which attention should be focused, and the analysis of specific aspects of clinical practice leads to the setting of standards against which future practice can be measured and evaluated. Regular audits will show whether the goals of an APS are achieved [29]. Audits of the APS are necessary to assess quality of pain management and to evaluate the adverse events of analgesic techniques such as IV-PCA opioid, epidural analgesia, and peripheral blocks. Such audits would show any problems with these techniques and the need for change in practice. An audit was performed in the northern and Yorkshire regions in the United Kingdom to assess postoperative pain management outcomes [41]. All patients undergoing surgical procedures over a 2-week period in 16 hospitals, ranging from large teaching hospitals with 5500 beds to smaller district general hospitals with fewer than 400 beds, were included in the study. Pain scores at rest and during movement were obtained in the recovery room and at 24 hours and 7 days postoperatively. Data were also collected on the modalities of pain management. The results showed that a large percentage of patients reported unacceptable levels of pain despite changes in practice and the development of an APS. Sites with pain management teams (ie, an APS) did not provide better pain management than those without an APS [41]. Stamer et al [24] reviewed the literature on APS and concluded that despite the guidelines, most APS worldwide did not meet basic quality criteria, which were defined as: regular assessment and documentation of pain scores at least once per day, written protocols for pain management, personnel assignment for an APS, and policies for postoperative pain management during nights and weekends. These studies emphasize the need for regular audits to address the problems of an APS and to justify the cost of the service. Unfortunately, the literature on APS audits is limited.

Future perspectives

The aims of the APS have expanded to embrace not merely a reduction of pain intensity but also the promotion of postoperative comfort and rehabilitation. The widening of objectives, together with the insidious elevation of standards and expectations, have placed a burden on an old order that is often ill equipped to serve the new ambitions [42]. Evidence that the standards are improving can be found in the way that pain is assessed. As pain control has improved, its evaluation has become more demanding. Although the goal of pain management remains a reduction in pain intensity, it is no longer sufficient to measure efficacy at rest but also on mobilization and on coughing for abdominal and thoracic surgery. Expanding the multidisciplinary approach could extend the role of an APS through the entire postoperative course, including patient rehabilitation. Such widening of the role might improve not only overall patient care, but it might convince hospital managers that the APS is worthy of support [42].

Central to concerns about out-of-hours care is the debate over whether the key role of an APS is to provide hands-on direct patient care or to provide a resource for education and training and the promotion of good clinical practice. Powell et al [27] argue that if an APS is well resourced and able to institute the widespread organizational and attitudinal changes required to overcome barriers to pain management, even a daytime APS would promote and maintain good clinical practice over the 24-hour period [27]. However, because many patients perceive nighttime pain as more severe [44], the current "office hours" model of an APS that covers only approximately 50 hours of the 168 hours in a week would seem destined to leave many patients in pain [27].

In the United Kingdom there has been debate about the future direction of the APS. Suggested developments include integrating the APS with other pain services (ie, chronic and palliative care), aligning the APS with critical care outreach teams, and developing comprehensive postoperative rehabilitation programs that would include an APS [43]. The integration of an APS with other pain services (eg, chronic pain and palliative care) may not be appropriate because the practical issues related to the management of postoperative pain are entirely different from chronic pain. The APS anesthesiologist is involved with the pre-, intra-, and postoperative phases, including performing, teaching, and training of regional anesthesia. However, not all chronic pain services include anesthesiologists. Even if the chronic pain physicians are anesthesiologists, they are rarely involved with the delivery of anesthesia per se and may not be familiar with the day-to-day practical issues of postoperative pain management on surgical wards. Therefore, it is unclear whether the problems of postoperative pain can be solved by the development of a more comprehensive service [27]. In the author's institution, the organization of an APS is separate from that of chronic pain. There is good cooperation between the two teams for chronic pain patients who undergo surgery, patients with drug problems, and patients with postoperative complications in which long-term pain relief may be necessary. For organizational purposes, after postoperative day 7, the chronic pain team takes over the management of the patient from the APS.

The APS plays a unique educational role, which might be further expanded as other health care providers are incorporated into the team. In the author's opinion, the key role of the APS may not be to provide hands-on, direct patient care but to provide a resource for education and training as well as to promote good practice based on algorithms and protocols developed jointly by anesthesiologists, surgeons, and nurses. These protocols must be integrated into predefined clinical pathways for each surgical procedure. Furthermore, the integration of newly developed Internet- and evidence-based procedure-specific guidelines into an APS protocol should further optimize postoperative analgesia and outcome [45–48]. These guidelines allow practitioners to modify analgesic therapies based on local circumstances (eg, regulatory issues and the availability of drugs and their costs) (see article by Kehlet elsewhere in this issue).

Summary

Freedom from postoperative pain is a central concern of surgical patients, and the alleviation of pain may contribute to improved clinical outcomes. However, despite long-standing recognition, undertreatment of postoperative pain continues to be a major problem internationally. It is clear that the introduction of an APS has increased the awareness that adequate postoperative pain management contributes to patients' well being. It has become increasingly evident that an organized multidisciplinary team of dedicated physicians and nurses seems to be a fundamental prerequisite for a well-functioning APS program. Although controlled trials are not available, observational studies suggest the effectiveness of an APS in reducing postoperative pain and analgesic adverse effects. In addition, the integration of the newer Internet-based surgical procedure-specific initiatives that provide evidence-based recommendations and allow the clinician to select appropriate analgesic techniques may further improve the efficacy of an APS.

The number of hospitals with an APS is increasing, but there is no consensus regarding the optimal structure and function of an APS. The selection of an appropriate organizational structure may be as important to the success of the APS as the choice of analgesic modalities. In addition, there is an obvious need for developing well-defined criteria on the basis of which the performance of an APS at an individual hospital can be evaluated and compared with national standards. It is important to recognize that quality improvement initiatives must be specifically tailored to the local environment, because there is no single approach that is guaranteed to be successful in all settings. The APS will also need to document their value and demonstrate the justification of allotted resources and expertise. Finally, the integration of effective analgesia into surgical care is mandatory to improve outcome and will depend on close cooperation between the surgeons and anesthesiologists.

Acknowledgments

The author thanks Marianne Welamsson for excellent secretarial assistance.

References

[1] Ballantyne JC, Carr DB, deFerranti S, et al. The comparative effects of postoperative analgesic therapies on pulmonary outcome: cumulative meta-analyses of randomized, controlled trials. Anesth Analg 1998;86:598–612.

[2] Rodgers A, Walker N, Schug S, et al. Reduction of postoperative mortality and morbidity with epidural or spinal anaesthesia: results from overview of randomised trials. BMJ 2000;321: 1493–7.

[3] Kehlet H, Holte K. Effect of postoperative analgesia reduces on surgical outcome. Br J Anaesth 2001;87:62–72.

[4] Beattie WS, Badner NH, Choi P. Epidural analgesia reduces postoperative myocardial infarction: a meta-analysis. Anesth Analg 2001;93:853–8.

[5] Rawal N, Berggren L. Organization of acute pain services – a low cost model. Pain 1994;57: 117–23.

[6] National Health and Medical Research Council of Australia. Acute pain management scientific evidence. Canberra, Australia: Ausinfo; 1999.

[7] Royal College of Surgeons and College of Anaesthetists Working Party on Pain after Surgery. Pain after surgery. London: Royal College of Surgeons; 1990.

[8] Agency for Health Care Policy and Research. Acute pain management: operative and medical procedures and trauma. US Department of Health and Human Services, Publication # 92–0032. Rockville (MD): AHCPR Publications; 1992.

[9] Wulf H, Neugebauer E, Maier C. Die behandlung akuter perioperativer und posttraumatischer schmerzen: empfehlungen einer interdisziplinaeren expertenkommission. New York: G. Thieme; 1997 [in German].

[10] Joint Commission on Accreditation of Healthcare Organizations. 1992 Hospital accreditation standards. Oakbrook Terrace (IL): JCAHO; 2001.

[11] Behandling av postoperativ smärta, riktlinjer och kvalitetsindikatorer [Treatment of postoperative pain, guidelines, and quality indicators]. Svenska Läkaresällskapet [Swedish Medical Association] Förlagshuset Gothia AB, Stockholm. Available at: www.gothia.nu. 2001.

[12] Practice guidelines for acute pain management in the perioperative setting: an updated report by American Society of Anesthesiologists, task force on acute pain management. Anesthesiology 2004;100:1573–81.

[13] Werner MU, Søholm L, Rotbøll-Nielsen P, et al. Does an acute pain service improve postoperative outcome? Anesth Analg 2002;95:1361–72.

[14] Zimmerman DL, Stewart J. Postoperative pain management and acute pain service activity in Canada. Can J Anaesth 1993;40:568–75.

[15] Goucke CR, Owe H. Acute pain management in Australia and New Zealand. Anaesth Intensive Care 1995;23:715–7.

[16] Rawal N, Allvin R, for The EuroPain Acute Pain Working Party. Acute pain services in Europe: a 17-nation survey of 105 hospitals. Eur J Anaesthesiol 1998;15:354–63.

[17] Davies K. Findings of a national survey of acute pain services. Nurs Times 1996;92:31–4.

[18] Windsor AM, Glynn CJ, Mason DG. National provision of acute pain services. Anaesthesia 1996;51:228–31.

[19] Merry A, Jugde MA, Ready B. Acute pain services in New Zealand hospitals: a survey. N Z Med J 1997;110:233–5.

[20] Harmer M, Davies KA. The effect of education, assessment and a standardized prescription on postoperative pain management: the value of clinical audit in the establishment of acute pain services. Anaesthesia 1998;53:424.

[21] Ready LB. How many acute pain services are there in the United States, and who is managing patient-controlled analgesia (letter)? Anesthesiology 1995;82:322.

[22] Warfield CA, Kahn CH. Acute pain management: programs in US hospitals and experiences and attitudes among US adults. Anesthesiology 1995;83:1090–4.

[23] Neugebauer E, Hempel K, Sauerland S, et al. The status of perioperative pain therapy in Germany: results of a representative, anonymous survey of 1,000 surgical clinics – Pain Study Group. Chirurg 1998;69:461–6.

[24] Stamer UM, Mpasios N, Stuber F, et al. A survey of acute pain services in Germany and a discussion of international survey data. Reg Anesth Pain Med 2002;27:125–31.

[25] O'Higgins F, Tuckey JP. Thoracic epidural anaesthesia and analgesia: United Kingdom practice. Acta Anaesthesiol Scand 2000;44:1087–92.

[26] Goldstein DH, Van Den Kerkhof EG, Blaine WC. Acute pain management services have progressed albeit insufficiently in Canadian academic hospitals. Can J Anesth 2004;51:231 – 5.

[27] Powell AE, Davies HTO, Bannister J, et al. Rhetoric and reality on acute pain services in the UK: a national postal questionnaire survey. Br J Anaesth 2004;92:689 – 93.

[28] Harmer M. When is a standard, not a standard: when is it a recommendation? [Editorial]. Anaesthesia 2001;56:611 – 2.

[29] Rawal N. Acute Pain Services revisited – good from far, far from good? [Editorial]. Reg Anesth Pain Med 2002;27:117 – 21.

[30] Blau WS, Dalton AB, Lindley C. Organization of hospital-based acute pain management programs. South Med J 1999;92:465 – 71.

[31] Wheatley RG, Madej TH, Jackson IJ, et al. The first year's experience of an acute pain service. Br J Anaesth 1991;67:353 – 9.

[32] Tsui SL, Law S, Fok M, et al. Postoperative analgesia reduces mortality and morbidity after esophagectomy. Am J Surg 1997;173:472 – 8.

[33] Lempa M, Gerards P, Koch G, et al. Efficacy of an acute pain service – a controlled comparative study of hospitals. Langenbecks Arch Chir Suppl Kongressbd 1998;115:673 – 6.

[34] Rose DK, Cohen MM, Yee DA. Changing the practice of pain management. Anesth Analg 1997;84:764 – 72.

[35] McDonnell A, Nicholl J, Read S. Acute Pain Teams in England: current provision and their role in postoperative pain management. J Clin Nurs 2003;12:387 – 93.

[36] Brodner G, Mertes N, Buerkle H, et al. Acute pain management: analysis, implications and consequences after prospective experience with 6349 surgical patients. Eur J Anaesthesiol 2000;17:566 – 75.

[37] Coleman SA, Booker-Milburn J. Audit of postoperative pain control: influence of a dedicated acute pain nurse. Anaesthesia 1996;51:1093 – 6.

[38] Mackintosh C, Bowles S. Evaluation of a nurse-led acute pain service: can clinical nurse specialists make a difference? J Adv Nurse 1997;25:30 – 7.

[39] Bardiau FM, Braeckman MM, Seidel L, et al. Effectiveness of an acute pain service inception in a general hospital. J Clin Anesth 1999;11:583 – 9.

[40] Bardiau FM, Taviaux NF, Albert A, et al. An intervention study to enhance postoperative pain management. Anest Analg 2003;96:179 – 85.

[41] Taverner T. A regional pain management audit. Nurs Times 2003;99:34 – 7.

[42] Bonnet F. Postoperative pain management: a continuing struggle. European Society of Anaesthesiologists Newsletter 2004;17:8 – 9.

[43] Counsell DJ. The acute pain service: a model for outreach critical care. Anaesthesia 2001; 56:925 – 6.

[44] Closs S, Briggs M, Everitt VE. Implementation of research findings to reduce postoperative pain at night. Int J Nurs Stud 1999;36:21 – 31.

[45] Rosenquist RW, Rosenberg J. Postoperative pain guidelines. Reg Anesth Pain Med 2003; 28:279 – 88.

[46] Rowlingson JC, Rawal N. Postoperative pain guidelines – targeted to the site of surgery. Reg Anesth Pain Med 2003;28:265 – 7.

[47] Rawal N, McCloy RF, for the PROSPECT working group. Incisional and intraperitoneal local anaesthetics in laparoscopic cholecystectomy and abdominal hysterectomy: a systematic review. Reg Anesth Pain Med 2004;29:A307.

[48] Fischer B, Camu F, for the PROSPECT working group. Comparative benefits of epidural analgesia following hysterectomy and colonic resection. Reg Anesth Pain Med 2004;29:A309.

ELSEVIER
SAUNDERS

Anesthesiology Clin N Am
23 (2005) 227–233

ANESTHESIOLOGY
CLINICS OF
NORTH AMERICA

Index

Note: Page numbers of article titles are in **boldface** type.

A

Acetaminophen, as adjuvants to intravenous patient-controlled analgesia, 113
for postoperative pain in children, 165–166
in multimodal approach to postoperative pain management, 188–189
nitric oxide-releasing derivatives of, 191

Acute pain nurses, 216–221

Acute pain service, **211–225**
audits and continuous quality improvement of, 221
cost-effectiveness of, 215–216
impact on outcome, 215
implementation of, 216–221
education, 219–220
role of surgeon in, 219
specialist pain nurse-based, 220–221
upgrading role of ward nurses in, 217–218
prevalence of, 212–213
structure and function of, 213–214

Adjuncts, analgesic, for postoperative pain management, **85–107**
alpha-2 agonists, 90–93
dexmedetomidine, 91, 94
neuraxial clonidine, 91
peripheral nerve blocks with clonidine, 91
systemic clonidine, 90–91
anticonvulsants, 94–95
corticosteroids, 98
epidural administration of, 131
in children, 178–180
alpha-2-agonists, 179
epinephrine, 178
ketamine, 179–180
neostigmine, 180
neuraxial opioids, 179

sodium bicarbonate, 179
tramadol, 180
N-methyl-D-aspartate (NMDA) antagonists, 85–90
amantadine, 90
dextromethorphan, 88–89
ketamine, 86–88
magnesium, 89
neostigmine, 96–98
opioid antagonists, 95–96

Alpha-2 agonists, as adjunct for postoperative pain in children, 179
as analgesic adjunct in postoperative pain management, 90–93
in multimodal approach, 192–193

Amantadine, as analgesic adjunct in postoperative pain management, 90

Anesthetics, local. See *Local anesthetics.*

Anticonvulsants, as analgesic adjuncts in postoperative pain management, 94–95

Antiemetics, as adjuvants to intravenous patient-controlled analgesia, 113–114

Axillary brachial plexus block, for postoperative pain, 145–146

B

Behavioral consequences, of inadequate postoperative pain relief, 23–24

Bone healing, effects of cyclooxygenase-2 inhibitors for postoperative pain management, 61–62

Brachial plexus blocks, for postoperative pain, 141–146
axillary, 145–146
infraclavicular, 144–145
interscalene, 141–143
supraclavicular, 143–144

Bupivacaine, for postoperative pain in children, 176–177

C

Cardiorenal effects, of cyclooxygenase-2 inhibitors for postoperative pain management, 61–62

Catheter techniques, for delivery of local anesthetics for postoperative pain management, 76–77

Caudal analgesia, in children, 170–175
  continuous, 173–174
  high blocks, 172–173
  single-shot, 171–172

Celecoxib, efficacy in postoperative pain management, 53–54

Children, postoperative pain management in, **163–184**
  epidural/caudal blocks, 170–175
  intravenous patient/parent/nurse-controlled analgesia, 168–170
  local anesthetics/adjuncts, 176–180
  nonopioid analgesics, 165–168
  potent opioid analgesics, 168

Cholecystectomy, laparoscopic, procedure-specific postoperative pain management guidelines for, 207–209

Chronic opioid-consuming patients. See *Opioids.*

Chronic pain, postoperative. See *Pain, postoperative, persistent.*

Clonidine, as analgesic adjunct in postoperative pain management, 90–93
  neuraxial, 91
  peripheral nerve blocks with, 91
  systemic, 90–91

Convalescence, postoperative, multimodal analgesia to shorten, 196

Corticosteroids, as analgesic adjuncts in postoperative pain management, 98

Cyclooxygenase-2 (COX-2) inhibitors, in postoperative pain management, contraindications, 63–64
  drug interactions, 63
  efficacy, 51–57
    celecoxib, 53–54
    parecoxib, 56–57
    valdecoxib, 55–56
  expression and function, 50–51
  in children, 167
    in multimodal approach, 189–191
  safety and tolerability, 57–63
    cardiorenal effects, 57–61
    effects on bone and wound healing, 62–63
    gastrointestinal toxicity, 57
    hematologic effects, 57–58
    hepatic effects, 61–62

D

Delivery techniques, novel, for local anesthetics in postoperative pain management, 75–77
  catheter techniques, 76–77
  encapsulated drugs, 75–76

Dexmedetomidine, as analgesic adjunct in postoperative pain management, 91, 94

Dextromethorphan, as analgesic adjunct in postoperative pain management, 88–89
  for postoperative pain in children, 167

E

Education, patient, in acute pain service, 219–220
  on intravenous patient-controlled analgesia, 116–117

Elderly patients, intravenous patient-controlled analgesia in, 118–119

Encapsulated drugs, for delivery of local anesthetics in postoperative pain management, 75–76

Epidural analgesia, for postoperative pain, **125–140**
  benefits and patient outcomes, 126–128
  continuous infusion *versus* patient-controlled, 132
  duration of, 131–132
  factors affecting efficacy of, 129–132
  in children, 170–175
    continuous, 173–175
    patient-controlled, 175–176
  in chronic opioid-consuming patients, 39
  risks of, 132–134
  in multimodal approach to postoperative pain management, 187

Epidural hematoma, risk of, with epidural analgesia, 132–133

Epinephrine, as adjunct for postoperative pain in children, 178

F

Femoral nerve block, for postoperative pain, 148–150

Fentanyl challenge, preoperative, in chronic opioid-consuming patients, 41

G

Gabapentin, as analgesic adjunct in postoperative pain management, 92–93, 94–95
  in multimodal approach, 193

Gastrointestinal toxicity, of cyclooxygenase-2 inhibitors for postoperative pain management, 57

Glucocorticoids, in multimodal approach to postoperative pain management, 193

Guidelines, procedure-specific, for postoperative pain management, **203–210**
  example of, for laparoscopic cholecystectomy, 207–209

H

Hematologic effects, of cyclooxygenase-2 inhibitors for postoperative pain management, 57–58

Hematoma, epidural, risk of, with epidural analgesia, 132–133

Hepatic effects, of cyclooxygenase-2 inhibitors for postoperative pain management, 61–62

Hyperalgesia, sensitization and, 2

I

Incisional pain, mechanisms of, **1–20**
  clinical models of, 2–4
  experimental *versus* clinical models of, 4
  laparotomy models for, 4–5
  plantar incision model for, 5–15
  prevention strategies, 15–16
  schematic for, 16–17

Infection, risk of, with epidural analgesia, 133

Infraclavicular brachial plexus block, for postoperative pain, 144–145

Interscalene brachial plexus block, for postoperative pain, 141–143

Intravenous patient-controlled analgesia. See *Patient-controlled analgesia.*

K

Ketamine, as adjunct for postoperative pain in children, 179–180
  as adjuvant to intravenous patient-controlled analgesia, 113
  as analgesic adjunct in postoperative pain management, 86–88
    role as adjunct to opioids, 86–88
    as continuous bolus infusion, 87
    as single intravenous bolus, 87–88
    epidural, 88
    in patient-controlled analgesia, 86–87
  role in preventive analgesia, 86

L

Laparoscopic cholecystectomy, procedure-specific postoperative pain management guidelines for, 207–209

Laparotomy models, for postoperative pain, 4–5

Levobupivacaine, for postoperative pain in children, 177–178

Liposomal drug delivery, for postoperative pain management, 75–76

Local anesthetics, in postoperative pain management, **73–84**
  beneficial actions, 79–81
  epidural, 130
    combined with opioids, 130–131
  in children, 176–178
    bupivacaine, 176–177
    newer agents, 177–178
  long-lasting, 77–78
  novel delivery techniques, 75–77
    catheter techniques, 76–77
    encapsulated drugs, 75–76
  shift to outpatient surgery and, 74–75
  toxicity issues, 78–79
  unexpected toxicity, 73–74

Lumbar epidural analgesia, continuous, in children, 174

Lumbar plexus block, for postoperative pain, 146–148

M

Magnesium, as analgesic adjunct in postoperative pain management, 89

Models, for postoperative pain, 2–15
    clinical, 2–4
    experimental *versus* clinical, 4
    laparotomy, 4–5
    plantar incision, 5–20

Morbidly obese patients, intravenous
    patient-controlled analgesia in, 118

Multimodal analgesia, for postoperative pain
    management, postoperative and
    rehabilitation, **185–202**
        analgesic options for, 186–193
        as part of preemptive analgesia
            techniques, 195–196
        optimal techniques for, 193–195
        to shorten convalescence, 196

N

N-methyl-D-aspartate (NMDA) antagonists, as
    adjunct in postoperative pain
    management, 85–90
        amantadine, 90
        dextromethorphan, 88–89
        in multimodal approach, 192
        ketamine, 86–88
        magnesium, 89

Neostigmine, as adjunct for postoperative pain
    in children, 180
    as analgesic adjunct in postoperative pain
        management, 96–98
        added to intravenous regional
            anesthesia, 98
        epidural, 97
        intra-articular, 97
        intrathecal, 96–97
        with local anesthetic for brachial
            plexus block, 97–98

Nerve blocks, paravertebral.
    See *Paravertebral nerve blocks*
    peripheral. See *Peripheral nerve blocks*

Neuraxial opioids, as adjunct for postoperative
    pain in children, 179

Nitric oxide, in derivatives of acetaminophen
    and NSAIDs, 191

Nonsteroidal anti-inflammatory drugs
    (NSAIDs), as adjuvants to intravenous
    patient-controlled analgesia, 112–113
    for postoperative pain in children,
        166–167
    in multimodal approach to postoperative
        pain management, 188–189
        nitric oxide-releasing derivatives
            of, 191

Nurses, role in acute pain service, specialist
    pain nurses, 220–221
        upgrading role of ward nurses in,
            217–218

O

Obesity, morbid, intravenous patient-controlled
    analgesia in patients with, 118

Obstructive sleep apnea, intravenous patient-
    controlled analgesia in patients with,
    117–118

Opioid antagonists, as analgesic adjuncts in
    postoperative pain management, 95–96

Opioids, efficacy of epidural analgesia with,
    129–130
    for postoperative pain in children,
        168–176
        epidural/caudal blocks, 170–176
            patient-controlled, 175–176
        intravenous patient/parent/nurse-
            controlled analgesia with,
            168–170
    in multimodal approach to postoperative
        pain management, 186–187
    in postoperative care of chronic opioid-
        consuming patients, **37–48**
        defining threshold for respiratory
            depression, 41–42
        intravenous patient-controlled
            analgesia with an opioid,
            40–41, 117
            practical considerations for,
                44–45
            predicting settings for, 42–43
            transition to oral opioids, 46
        preoperative fentanyl challenge, 41
        preoperative plan for, 38–39
        regional analgesia techniques and
            nonopioid analgesics, 39–40
            epidural analgesia and
                peripheral nerve
                blocks, 39
            nonopioid analgesics, 39–40
        tolerance, 38
    neuraxial, as adjunct for postoperative
        pain in children, 179

Outpatient surgery, shift to, and role of local
    anesthetics, 74–75

P

Pain management, postoperative, 1–225
    acute pain service for, **211–225**
        audits and continuous quality
            improvement of, 221

cost-effectiveness of, 215–216
impact on outcome, 215
implementation of, 216–221
prevalence of, 212–213
structure and function of, 213–214
analgesic adjuncts in, **85–107**
alpha-2 agonists, 90–93
dexmedetomidine, 91, 94
neuraxial clonidine, 91
peripheral nerve blocks with
clonidine, 91
systemic clonidine, 90–91
anticonvulsants, 94–95
corticosteroids, 98
N-methyl-D-aspartate (NMDA)
antagonists, 85–90
amantadine, 90
dextromethorphan, 88–89
ketamine, 86–88
magnesium, 89
neostigmine, 96–98
opioid antagonists, 95–96
cyclooxygenase-2 inhibitors in, **49–72**
contraindications, 63–64
drug interactions, 63
efficacy, 51–57
celecoxib, 53–54
parecoxib, 56–57
valdecoxib, 55–56
expression and function, 50–51
safety and tolerability, 57–63
cardiorenal effects, 57–61
effects on bone and wound
healing, 62–63
gastrointestinal toxicity, 57
hematologic effects, 57–58
hepatic effects, 61–62
epidural analgesia for, **125–140**
benefits and patient outcomes,
126–128
factors affecting efficacy of,
129–132
risks of, 132–134
in children, **163–184**
epidural/caudal blocks, 170–175
intravenous patient/parent/nurse-
controlled analgesia,
168–170
local anesthetics/adjuncts,
176–180
nonopioid analgesics, 165–168
potent opioid analgesics, 168
in chronic opioid-consuming patients,
37–48
defining threshold for respiratory
depression, 41–42
intravenous patient-controlled
analgesia with opioid, 40–41
practical considerations for,
44–45

predicting settings for, 42–43
transition to oral opioids, 46
opioid tolerance, 38
preoperative fentanyl challenge, 41
preoperative plan for, 38–39
regional analgesia techniques and
nonopioid analgesics, 39–40
epidural analgesia and
peripheral nerve
blocks, 39
nonopioid analgesics, 39–40
inadequate, consequences of, **21–36**
for recovery and health care use,
24–25
persistent postoperative pain,
25–31
definition, 25
incidence, 25–26
mechanisms involved in,
28–29
predictors of, 26–28
prevention of, 29–31
physiologic, 21–23
psychologic and behavioral, 23–24
incisional pain, mechanisms of, **1–20**
clinical models of, 2–4
experimental *versus* clinical models
of, 4
laparotomy models for, 4–5
plantar incision model for, 5–15
intravenous patient-controlled analgesia,
109–123
local anesthetics, clinical pharmacology
of, **73–84**
beneficial actions, 79–81
long-lasting, 77–78
novel delivery techniques, 75–77
catheter techniques, 76–77
encapsulated drugs, 75–76
shift to outpatient surgery and,
74–75
toxicity issues, 78–79
unexpected toxicity, 73–74
multimodal analgesia techniques and
rehabilitation, **185–202**
analgesic options for, 186–193
as part of preemptive analgesia
techniques, 195–196
optimal techniques for, 193–195
to shorten convalescence, 196
peripheral nerve blocks and continuous
catheter techniques, **141–162**
brachial plexus blocks, 141–146
axillary, 145–146
infraclavicular, 144–145
interscalene, 141–143
supraclavicular, 143–144
femoral plexus block, 148–150

lumbar plexus block, 146–148
paravertebral nerve block,
   153–154
popliteal fossa sciatic nerve block,
   151–153
sciatic nerve block, 150–151
procedure-specific, **203–210**
   example of, for laparoscopic
      cholecystectomy, 207–209
   initiatives to provide guidelines for,
      205–209
   reasons for, 204–205

Pain scales, for children, 164

Pain scores, defining maximum acceptable in
acute pain service, 219

Pain, postoperative, incisional, mechanisms of,
1–20
   clinical models of, 2–4
   experimental *versus* clinical models
      of, 4
   laparotomy models for, 4–5
   plantar incision model for, 5–15
   prevention strategies, 15–16
   schematic for, 16–17
persistent, as consequence of inadequate
pain relief, 25–31
   definition, 25
   incidence, 25–26
   mechanisms involved in, 28–29
   predictors of, 26–28
   prevention of, 29–31

Paravertebral nerve blocks, for postoperative
pain management, 153–154
   in multimodal approach to,
      187–188

Parecoxib, efficacy in postoperative pain
management, 56–57

Patient-controlled analgesia, intravenous,
109–123
   adjuvant drugs and, 112–114
      added to the IV-PCA solution,
         113–114
      administered separately, 112–113
   choices of opioids for, 111–112
   efficacy of, 109–111
   epidural, in children, 175–176
   in children, 168–170
      epidural, 175–176
   in specific patient populations, 117–119
      elderly patients, 118–119
      morbidly obese patients, 117–118
      opioid-tolerant patients, 117
      sleep apnea patients, 117–118
   opioid-related side effects, 112
   patient factors, 116–117
      patient education, 116–117
      psychological characteristics, 116

program parameters for, 114–116
   bolus dose, 114–115
   concurrent background
      (continuous) infusions,
      115–116
   dose limits, 116
   lockout interval, 115
with opioids, in chronic opioid-
consuming patients, 40–46
   defining threshold for respiratory
      depression, 41–42
   practical considerations for, 44–45
   predicting settings for, 42–44
   preoperative fentanyl challenge, 41
   transition to oral opioids, 46

Pediatrics, postoperative pain management in
children, **163–184**
   epidural/caudal blocks, 170–175
   intravenous patient/parent/nurse-
      controlled analgesia,
      168–170
   local anesthetics/adjuncts,
      176–180
   nonopioid analgesics, 165–168
   potent opioid analgesics, 168

Peripheral nerve blocks, for postoperative pain,
141–162
   brachial plexus blocks, 141–146
      axillary, 145–146
      infraclavicular, 144–145
      interscalene, 141–143
      supraclavicular, 143–144
   femoral plexus block, 148–150
   in chronic opioid-consuming
      patients, 39
   lumbar plexus block, 146–148
   paravertebral nerve block,
      153–154
   popliteal fossa sciatic nerve block,
      151–153
   sciatic nerve block, 150–151
   in multimodal approach to postoperative
      pain management, 187–188

Persistent postoperative pain.
   See *Pain, postoperative, persistent.*

Pharmacology, of pain behaviors after plantar
incision, 8–9
   spinal and parenteral, of incisional pain,
      12–15

Physiologic consequences, of inadequate
postoperative pain relief, 21–23

Plantar incision model, for postoperative pain,
5–15
   dorsal horn neuron sensitization, 12
   nonevoked pain, 5–7
   primary afferent fiber sensitization,
      10–12

primary mechanical hyperalgesia, 7, 10
spinal and parenteral pharmacology of, 12–15

Popliteal fossa sciatic nerve block, for postoperative pain, 151–153

Postoperative pain, models of, clinical, 2–4
experimental *versus* clinical, 4
laparotomy, 4–5
plantar incision, 5–15
persistent, as consequence of inadequate pain relief, 25–31
definition, 25
incidence, 25–26
mechanisms involved in, 28–29
predictors of, 26–28
prevention of, 29–31

Postoperative pain management. See *Pain management.*

Preemptive analgesia, multimodal analgesia as part of, 195–196

Pregabalin, in multimodal approach to postoperative pain management, 193

Procedure-specific postoperative pain management, **203–210**
example of, for laparoscopic cholecystectomy, 207–209
initiatives to provide guidelines for, 205–209
reasons for, 204–205

Psychologic consequences, of inadequate postoperative pain relief, 23–24

R

Regional analgesia, for postoperative pain in chronic opioid-consuming patients, 39

Rehabilitation, postoperative, multimodal analgesia to shorten, 196

Respiratory depression, predicting threshold for, with postoperative opioids in chronic opioid-consuming patients, 41–42

Ropivacaine, for postoperative pain in children, 177–178

S

Sciatic nerve block, for postoperative pain, 150–151

Sensitization, dorsal horn neuron, 12
hyperalgesia and, 2
primary afferent fiber, 10–12

Sleep apnea, obstructive, intravenous patient-controlled analgesia in patients with, 117–118

Sodium bicarbonate, as adjunct for postoperative pain in children, 179

Supraclavicular brachial plexus block, for postoperative pain, 143–144

Surgeons, role in acute pain service, 219

T

Thoracic epidural analgesia, continuous, in children, 174–175

Tolerance, opioid, 38, 117

Toxicity, of local anesthetics in postoperative pain management, 78–79

Tramadol, as adjunct for postoperative pain in children, 180
for postoperative pain in children, 167–168

V

Valdecoxib, efficacy in postoperative pain management, 55–56

W

Wound healing, effects of cyclooxygenase-2 inhibitors for postoperative pain management, 61–62

Changing Your Address?

Make sure your subscription changes too! When you notify us of your new address, you can help make our job easier by including an exact copy of your Clinics label number with your old address (see illustration below.) This number identifies you to our computer system and will speed the processing of your address change. Please be sure this label number accompanies your old address and your corrected address—you can send an old Clinics label with your number on it or just copy it exactly and send it to the address listed below.

We appreciate your help in our attempt to give you continuous coverage. Thank you.

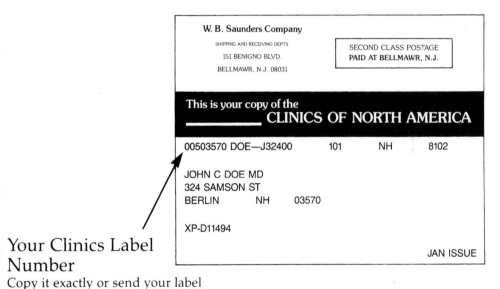

W. B. Saunders Company

SHIPPING AND RECEIVING DEPTS.

151 BENIGNO BLVD.

BELLMAWR, N.J. 08031

SECOND CLASS POSTAGE
PAID AT BELLMAWR, N.J.

This is your copy of the
CLINICS OF NORTH AMERICA

00503570 DOE—J32400   101   NH   8102

JOHN C DOE MD
324 SAMSON ST
BERLIN   NH   03570

XP-D11494

JAN ISSUE

Your Clinics Label Number
Copy it exactly or send your label
along with your address to:
W.B. Saunders Company, Customer Service
Orlando, FL 32887-4800
Call Toll Free 1-800-654-2452

Please allow four to six weeks for delivery of new subscriptions and for processing address changes.